The JF.
Assassination Dissected

The JFK Assassination Dissected

An Analysis by Forensic Pathologist Cyril Wecht

CYRIL H. WECHT, M.D., J.D., *and*
DAWNA KAUFMANN

Foreword by Oliver Stone

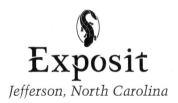

Exposit

Jefferson, North Carolina

ISBN (print) 978–1–4766–8511–3
ISBN (ebook) 978–1–4766–4544–5

Library of Congress and British Library
cataloguing data are available

Library of Congress Control Number 2021049914

On the cover *left to right*: Cyril Wecht (courtesy Andrew Kreig, Esq.);
JFK (National Archives); scalpel YJPTO/Shutterstock

Printed in the United States of America

Exposit is an imprint of McFarland & Company, Inc., Publishers

Exposit
*Box 611, Jefferson, North Carolina 28640
www.expositbooks.com*

Table of Contents

Foreword by Oliver Stone

The term "on the case" means that someone is aware of a particular problem and is trying to solve it. The assassination of President John F. Kennedy is a huge problem for American society in manifold ways. And perhaps no one alive has been on that case as long as Dr. Cyril Wecht has.

Cyril is both an attorney and a forensic pathologist. Therefore, he has an effective skill set for peering into the dark corners of what became the official story of Kennedy's assassination. From his first exposure to the news, in the offices of his friend and colleague Dr. Thomas Noguchi in Los Angeles, Cyril's curiosity sprang up as certain witnesses—like Abraham Zapruder, and Bill and Gayle Newman—seemed to contradict what was the developing, official story. That story said all the shots came from above and behind the president. Yet these witnesses said the shots came from *behind* them, and they were all standing in front of the limousine and to Kennedy's right.

Then the Warren Commission Report was published, with its accompanying volumes of testimony and exhibits. The doctor now began to examine another serious problem with the official story. A significant number of doctors who treated Kennedy in Dallas said they saw a large hole in the rear of Kennedy's skull. One of these witnesses was Kemp Clark. Dr. Clark was chief of neurosurgery at Parkland Memorial Hospital. He was in Trauma Room One with Kennedy. How could he be wrong?

Why was Earl Rose, the medical examiner in Dallas, essentially run over by the Secret Service in its haste to get Kennedy's corpse back to Washington? Dr. Rose was a forensic pathologist, and his office was at Parkland Hospital, directly across from Trauma Room One. For whatever reason, Kennedy's body was flown to the National Naval Medical Center in Bethesda, Maryland. Physicians James J. Humes and J. Thornton Boswell—the man leading the autopsy and his chief assistant—were not board-certified in forensic pathology. As Cyril notes in this book, there isn't any evidence that either man had ever done a gunshot wound autopsy. This while—as Cyril has told me—the leading forensic pathologist in America, Dr. Milton Helpern, was packing his bags and waiting for his phone to ring.

Cyril's reaction to the autopsy report was that it was much too skimpy—only six pages. When he read it, he thought he would not want his name on this document. The Armed Forces Institute of Pathology manual for an autopsy was itself 79 pages long. Perhaps Dr. Helpern could have explained, among many other things, how a single bullet did so much damage to both the president and Governor John Connally, yet was essentially pristine when recovered, as the government claimed. Would Dr. Helpern have made reference in his autopsy to a civilian witness he never talked to as a guide for the direction of the shots? But further, why did the Warren Commission condone this kind of practice?

Cyril made himself familiar with all these issues and all the 26 volumes of evidence. He studied them for a year. He was then asked by a professional colleague to make an address on the Kennedy case at the annual conference of the American Academy of Forensic Sciences (AAFS) in February of 1966. One of the Kennedy pathologists was in attendance. Dr. Pierre Finck was the most qualified of the original prosectors, but he had arrived to the autopsy after it was already underway. After Cyril's speech, Dr. Finck approached Cyril. He told Cyril: "You cannot believe what it was like. It was horrible, horrible. I only wish I could tell you about it."

That AAFS address now made the forensic pathologist the medical man to see for the critics of the Warren Commission Report. The president of the AAFS now began to get calls and meetings with people like Mark Lane and Sylvia Meagher and Josiah Thompson. Through Thompson—who was working on an article for *Life* magazine—Cyril was able to view the Zapruder film at Time-Life in New York. That experience now turned his suspicions about what the Warren Commission had done into a certainty. After watching the differing reactions of Kennedy and Governor John Connally, he now understood that the single bullet theory was not to be taken seriously. It had now, in his description, been reduced to a fantasy.

This work is really two books. It tells the story of Cyril Wecht, as it relates the history of the Kennedy assassination. So readers will not just meet the notable critics named above but also participants in this ongoing drama. Because Cyril was a distinguished professional, he met and debated Arlen Specter, who had served as an assistant counsel for the Warren Commission. (The elevator ride after that encounter is worth reading the book.) Readers will also meet New Orleans D.A. Jim Garrison. The D.A. wanted Cyril to be his expert witness on the autopsy at the trial of Clay Shaw. They went to court to secure Cyril's access to the autopsy materials so he could testify. The judge agreed, but the government lawyers appealed the case. During the investigation of the House Select Committee on Assassinations, Cyril was around for both the first chief counsel, Richard Sprague, and the second, Robert Blakey. The doctor takes pains to note the differences in the two approaches. If readers have not read, listened to, or watched his dissenting opinion before the committee, I strongly advise them to do so. It gives life to the old adage: One man with the truth constitutes a majority.

During that testimony, Cyril noted that, in 1972, he was the first non-governmental forensic pathologist allowed entry into the National Archives in order to inspect the autopsy exhibits. It was his visit that made a disturbing fact public knowledge about President Kennedy's brain. I won't spoil the reveal, but this appalling disclosure explains why no medical investigation can now legally certify the findings of the original autopsy. Add to that the admission during the Clay Shaw trial, Dr. Finck admitted that Kennedy's back wound was not dissected either. So here was a murder-by-gunshot case where neither wound was tracked through the body to determine trajectory. This would not be acceptable in a big-city homicide case. It should be unthinkable for the murder of the President of the United States.

As I said, Cyril and his excellent coauthor, Dawna Kaufmann, have actually written two books. One is about the journey of a young forensic pathologist. Through his eyes, we watch the history of a tragic mystery unfold. Not just the one about who really killed President Kennedy but also why our media and institutions have been unable to solve a crime that so damaged the national psyche.

By his refusal to give in to those formidable forces, Cyril Wecht embodies the eternal flame at Arlington.

Oliver Stone is a director, writer, and producer whose movies about American and world politics have won multiple Oscars, BAFTAs, and Golden Globe Awards. His 1991 film JFK *ignited interest of a new generation to learn about the assassination of President Kennedy and led to the passing of the JFK Records Act, which declassified thousands of government documents on the case. His new two-hour documentary,* JFK Revisited: Through the Looking Glass, *is available worldwide.*

Preface

Over my 50-plus years as a forensic pathologist, I've personally performed more than 21,000 autopsies, and reviewed, consulted on, and signed off on another 41,000 death cases. I've testified for both prosecutors and defense attorneys across the United States and in several foreign countries. I'm also an attorney of long-standing, so the medico-legal world is my bailiwick. Generally, I complete my tasks and go on to the next case. But there is one homicide I think of every day and lament the fact that the victim never received justice.

Our 35th U.S. president, John Fitzgerald Kennedy, was fatally gunned down in Dallas, Texas, on November 22, 1963. He was 46 years old, with a wife and two young children, and he was three years into his first term. The good-looking and affable Democrat from Massachusetts was preparing to run for a second term, and few people would have bet against him winning. However, bullets from at least two assassins cut short his life and left our country in deep mourning from which many of us have never recovered. We're angry that a two-pronged conspiracy was in play—one that planned the murder and pulled it off, and another that covered the tracks of the planners and killers. Even today, there is still a cone of silence over many of the facts of the case that protect those responsible—abetted by craven politicians and journalistic malpractice among the top news outlets in this country that seek to protect the secrets of the assassination squad and reward those people who continue to ignore or mischaracterize the case evidence.

One bright spot is that the majority of Americans believe that our president was *not* struck down by one insignificant weasel with a shady background, who decided to achieve fame that day, then was shot to death himself two days later by someone who didn't want this criminal defendant's case to go to trial. There are citizens who strongly believe rogue elements within our own government are to blame for the president's demise. Go outside our country's borders and the number of people who believe our government has blood on its hands is even higher.

The term "conspiracy theorist" is tossed around by those who resent that we don't buy the official story. They sneer that we can't prove what we claim—while slamming the door on declassifying government files that might help us do that very thing. They want to make us seem like paranoid time-wasters for pursuing this case for all these years. They'd like us to shut up and find a new hobby, one that won't cast aspersions on their past actions and continual cover-up.

But we who are true believers in the idea of governmental malfeasance are not oppressed at being termed conspiracy theorists. We're fine with those two simple words because they cast doubt on the party line. We wear those words proudly, as our badge of honor.

We may all be on the same side against the government fiction, but there is wide diversity in what we believe happened, as well as who might have been involved, and/or why. So we have frequent communication, hold conferences and seminars, and express our views in the media. We debate and reflect, building our arguments with new evidence and witnesses. While giving a wide berth to credible authors and researchers who make valuable additions to the true and tested knowledge base, we sometimes have to stamp out distractions from troublemakers with implausible offerings. One thing is for certain: Until we have all the proof needed behind our contrasting theories, we will adamantly and noisily keep pushing for answers.

Hours after JFK was killed, he was scheduled to attend a Democratic fundraiser in Austin, Texas. He never got the chance to deliver the speech that would have ended with this important message:

> Neither the fanatics nor the faint-hearted are needed. And our duty as a Party is not to our Party alone, but to the nation, and, indeed, to all mankind. Our duty is not merely the preservation of political power but the preservation of peace and freedom. So, let us not be petty when our cause is so great. Let us not quarrel amongst ourselves when our nation's future is at stake.

In my long career, there have been many monumental examples of great difficulty, unpleasantness, and controversy. But, from time to time, any forensic pathologist who aggressively and courageously pursues his or her cases whenever necessary beyond the performance of an autopsy will undoubtedly encounter difficult and unpleasant situations. Every professional person involved in the field of legal medicine is well aware of how these conflicts arise and the manner in which they are sometimes regrettably pursued in an insulting, unsportsmanlike manner.

So, you can sit on the bank of the river and dip your toes in the water, moving gently with the flow—or you can jump in and swim from one place to another, often against the current or tide. If you never attempt to make an impression upon anyone for legitimate reasons, you are unlikely to ever have any "impressionable" moments in your life. When it comes to dipping into the JFK murder, I say, come on in, the water's fine!

I hope this book inspires readers to carry the baton of justice with dedication and enthusiasm and pass it safely to the next generation. There's much more work to do.

The World's Greatest
Murder Mystery

Over the past decades, hundreds of letters and telephone calls have come into my various offices in Pittsburgh, Pennsylvania, from people claiming to have information on the assassination of President John F. Kennedy. Many of them have been helpful, even educational. Others related stories that would be more at home on an irresponsible "fake news" blog.

One elderly gentleman called to say he had reviewed the famed Zapruder home movie of the incident and said it was clear as crystal: Vice President Lyndon Johnson, sitting in a limousine that followed President Kennedy in the motorcade in Dallas, jumped out of his car, ran up alongside the president's limo, pulled a gun from his coat, and started shooting, then darted back to his own car—all completely undetected by those at the scene and by the millions who have reviewed that same film in the years since the shooting.

Another favorite was the woman who purported to have "top-secret" details about JFK's slaying. "The assassin was Marilyn Monroe dressed up as a Secret Service agent," she explained. When I replied that that was impossible since the iconic actress had died the year before, the woman logically answered that the killer was actually the ghost of Monroe.

Others have blamed William Greer, the Secret Service agent who was driving the presidential limousine, or a fellow agent in the follow-up car who fumbled his gun and accidentally shot the leader of the free world. Other fanciful candidates include First Lady Jacqueline Kennedy, who was furious about her husband's well-reported skirt-chasing, and Texas Governor John Connally, who was jealous of all the attention the president was getting on "Big John's" home turf. No tips have come in yet blaming Annie Oakley, Bonnie and Clyde, or zombies from Mars, but give it time....

I can't count the number of times I've been interviewed, written papers, or lectured about the assassination. It's a weekly occurrence. Very few people have spent as much time reviewing the physical evidence in this case as I have. Simply put, it is the world's greatest murder mystery, and the interest in it will not go away—not by the public, and not by me.

Much of my extracurricular time in legal medicine has been spent researching what happened in those brief, horrible seconds in Dallas. There are few events in my life—other than my wedding day or the births of my children—when I can look back 10, 25, or 50-plus years and tell you exactly where I was and what I was doing on that fateful day. For me, as for many Americans, the assassination of President Kennedy is one of those indelible memories.

"The President's Been Shot!"

O n November 22, 1963, I was in Los Angeles visiting a new friend and professional colleague, then–deputy coroner Thomas Noguchi. At the time I was 32 and just getting my career in legal medicine off the ground in my hometown of Pittsburgh. I attained a medical degree from the University of Pittsburgh School of Medicine in 1956 and law degrees from UPitt in 1962 as well as the University of Maryland that same year. I was licensed to practice law in Pennsylvania and was a member of the state bar there, as well as the American Bar Association. I was also a partner at one of the city's leading law firms.

I was a fellow of the American Academy of Forensic Sciences, an organization for which I would serve as president in a few years; the president of the American College of Legal Medicine; a fellow at the Law-Science Academy of America and its vice chancellor; and the director and president of the Pittsburgh Institute of Legal Medicine. I was also an adjunct professor in legal medicine at Pittsburgh's Duquesne University School of Law. (Much later, I would be honored when Duquesne established the Cyril H. Wecht Institute of Forensic Science and Law, for which I am chairman of its advisory board.) In addition, I was a diplomate of the National Board of Medicine and was licensed to practice medicine in Pennsylvania, California, and Maryland.

I had a recent honorable discharge from the U.S. Air Force, where I had been an associate pathologist at Maxwell Air Force Base in Montgomery, Alabama, and served as a captain in the USAF's Medical Corps. Following my military service, I finished a research fellowship in forensic pathology at the Baltimore Medical Examiner's office, then returned to Pittsburgh and was working as a pathologist and acting chief of laboratory services at the Leech Farm Veterans Administration hospital.

Tom Noguchi was not yet the chief medical examiner at the Los Angeles County Coroner's office. But he was definitely an up-and-coming forensic pathologist in that office, with a great intellect and curiosity about death investigations. I still consider him a cherished associate. Tom would later become known for performing autopsies on a number of notable personalities, such as Marilyn Monroe, Natalie Wood, Sharon Tate, Janis Joplin, William Holden, John Belushi, and Senator Robert "Bobby" F. Kennedy. Noguchi was also the model for the coroner character for the TV drama *Quincy, M.E.,* that ran on NBC-TV from 1976 to 1983.

As is typical for physicians in our profession, Tom and I were comparing and contrasting the cases we've had and speaking of changes we'd like to implement to better serve our communities. It was late morning, California time, and we were standing in the middle of an autopsy room, corpses of all kinds around us. Just then, Tom's secretary, appearing distraught, came rushing into the room and whispered into his ear. Stunned, Tom turned to me and exclaimed, "The president's been shot!"

Information was sketchy at that point. We learned that President Kennedy and his wife, Jacqueline, had been campaigning in Dallas, Texas, and were part of a motorcade through the city's streets. The Kennedys shared a limousine with the state's governor, John Connally, and his wife, Nellie. The president, the governor, and possibly others in different vehicles in the motorcade were shot, but it wasn't clear how badly they were injured. The motorcade was en route to the nearest trauma center, Parkland Memorial Hospital. In the split second following Noguchi's shocking revelation, we shared dozens of thoughts and questions: Why would someone do this? Has the person been caught? How bad are the injuries? Is the president dead? What we didn't have were answers.

Back in 1963, cell phones, computers, electronic tablets, and the Internet were years from being invented. Few offices had television sets, and for those that had one, the picture was in black-and-white, with a rabbit ear–style antenna to stabilize the image. Not only did Tom's office not have a TV set, but even radio transmission was fuzzy there. We quickly left to go to a local restaurant that had a television and spent the next two hours absorbing every word that was broadcast about the shooting.

As we walked in and sat down, the image of CBS News anchor Walter Cronkite was live on the air, doing an audio-only bulletin from a tiny voice-over studio. *As the World Turns*, the soap opera that had been airing on the network, was interrupted and replaced with a card that announced the news bulletin. It was 12:40 p.m. in Dallas.

In those early days of television, the broadcasters didn't just point a camera at the talent and go live on the air. It took about 20 minutes for the vacuum tubes to warm up and for the camera operator and the technician in the booth to tinker with the settings to get a usable picture and sound. During that time, Cronkite kept hearing conflicting stories about Kennedy's and Connally's condition and, as managing editor of the CBS Evening News, he wanted to wait for official notice. By 1:00 p.m., Cronkite had moved to the newsroom and was live on nationwide television. He seemed disheveled, in his white shirt sleeves, with no jacket. He sat at his desk, with papers piled high and three black telephones that were his lifelines to the field reporters and his producers in the broadcast booth.

Cronkite introduced footage from the Dallas affiliate, KRLD-TV, showing a group of JFK's supporters who had been awaiting his arrival at the city's Trade Mart, where Kennedy was scheduled to deliver a speech. A voice-over of newsman Eddie Barker said that he heard that the president was dead, but the information was unconfirmed. Also unconfirmed was that Governor Connally was in the operating room. Barker, who was also the station's news director, said that the president had been whisked to Parkland. The president, he added, was undoubtedly in the emergency room on the first floor of that hospital. He reported that "the attempted assassins—we now hear that it was a man and a woman—who fired the shots were on the ledge of a building near the Houston Street underpass."

With the footage showing devastated-looking people milling around the Mart, Cronkite's own voice interrupted to report that blood transfusions had been given to the president. Tom and I took a measured breath of relief, hoping that indicated the president was still alive and could survive whatever happened. Cronkite filled the screen again, as he strained to listen to an off-camera voice. It was Barker declaring that the president was dead. "Totally unconfirmed," Cronkite snapped, looking miffed at the less-than-solid information. But Barker repeated that Kennedy had been fatally shot "by an assassin at the intersection of Elm and Houston Streets, just as he was going into the underpass."

I knew that intersection. It was the main thoroughfare to the Stemmons Freeway, which goes in and out of Dallas. The triple underpass where Elm, Main, and Commerce Streets merge is the one the reporter mentioned. It's a very open, public area. With the undoubted presence of so many Secret Service agents, I wondered how in the world an assassin could shoot at least two people, wounding one of them very seriously. Did someone with a pistol rush the car? If so, why weren't we hearing about him or her being shot in return, or pulled to the ground and arrested?

Somebody in the restaurant said he had heard on the radio that Kennedy's head "exploded" from the gunshot. Tom and I exchanged worried glances. If that was true, the prognosis didn't bode well for JFK. We spoke of the excellent medical examiner in Dallas, Dr. Earl Rose, and felt the president's autopsy, if needed, would be done by an experienced professional.

Cronkite, who was nervously putting on and taking off his thick, black-framed glasses, then announced that a Catholic priest had administered Last Rites to the president. While falling short of making a pronouncement of JFK's death, he added that sheriff's deputies had taken a young man into custody at the scene, "a man 25 years old." Tom and I couldn't resist speculating about a future trial. Assuming there would be an arrest, the trial of the killer would be in Dallas where there were not only tough prosecutors, but also aggressive defense attorneys. Such a trial would bring out the A-team for both sides, we agreed. Even if the defendant had no money and would be assigned a public defender, there would likely be many famed attorneys willing to step in and represent him pro bono, for the notoriety and publicity. There would be no shame in that as even the worst criminal deserves a good defense.

CBS' other reporter on the scene, Dan Rather, also told Cronkite the president was dead, but the veteran anchor again insisted there was no official confirmation. Vice President Lyndon Johnson, Cronkite stated, had been "slightly wounded in the arm"—information that proved to be untrue. Mostly he stuck to facts, such as how our U.S. Ambassador to the United Nations, Adlai Stevenson, had been assaulted in Dallas just the month before as he left a dinner meeting.

Meanwhile, sources from ABC, UPI, and the Associated Press were also working sources to uncover the story. As we flipped the channels back and forth, ABC's Dallas affiliate WFAA-TV was broadcasting a homemaking series that was abruptly interrupted live by the station's out-of-breath program director, Jay Watson, with news of the double shooting. ABC Radio anchor Don Gardiner would make the first official announcement of JFK's death, followed by ABC-TV showing a photo of the president with the caption: John F. Kennedy, 1917–1963.

Back on CBS, Cronkite's voice trembled as he reacted to a news bulletin… "From Dallas, Texas, this flash, apparently official: President Kennedy died at one p.m., Central Standard Time. Two o'clock, Eastern Standard time, some 38 minutes ago. … Vice President Johnson has left the hospital in Dallas, but we do not know to where he has proceeded. Presumably, he will be taking the oath of office shortly and become the 36th president of the United States."

I changed the channel on the television to NBC, then to ABC News again, in the off-chance one of them would have different, better news. Within 10 minutes of the assassination, a married couple—Bill and Gayle Newman—and their two small sons, who can be all seen in footage of the grassy knoll, were whisked to the WFAA-TV studio for a live interview with Watson. The interview was also taped, and that version, which ran nationally, was what Tom and I saw. It's distinctive as a vivid account from two of the people closest to the president's car when he received his shot to the head. With their children on their laps, the distraught Newmans, both 22 years old, explained how they had been standing on the curb on the north side of Elm Street as the motorcade approached. Yards behind them was a curved white structure known as a "pergola," which was next to a wooden fence.

Bill, an electrician, said he heard a gunshot and saw the president jump up in his seat. Within seconds, as the car was directly next to his family, Newman said another shot "apparently from behind us hit the president in the temple." Since he and his wife were facing the street, "behind us" would have referred to the pergola and fence area. He further explained the location as "up on top of the hill, the little mound near the garden."

Gayle, a housewife, added that the president was shot on the right side of his head and that Governor Connally, who was turned to the side, grabbed his stomach. Both Newmans said they first thought the gunshots were firecrackers until they saw the blood on the president. That's when they went into protective mode and laid atop their little boys.

A short time later, Watson apologized for an earlier comment that erroneously stated that "six to eight" people had been shot. Bill Newman was interviewed again and repeated his earlier observation. Watson, who had also been at the site, said he heard three gunshots, whereas Newman only recalled hearing two but admitted he was busy taking care of his wife and kids. In Gayle's second interview, she repeated her original story, adding: "President Kennedy grabbed his—looked like he grabbed his ear and blood kept gushing out." She pointed to her right ear as she described the point of impact. The family had initially gone to the airport to see the first family, but couldn't get a good look, so they drove to Dealey Plaza. They wanted their older son to have a memory to stay with him, not realizing that that would be quite the understatement.

Despite the confused initial reports, with details that would later prove to be false, there was no escaping the reality: President Kennedy was dead from an assassin's bullet. The world as we knew it had changed, and we were only beginning to see the ramifications of what that would mean.

Within minutes after the shots were fired, Dallas sheriff's deputies in Dealey Plaza scattered to look for the shooter. Officers went into the Texas School Book Depository, the closest building to the plaza. Two deputies went to the sixth floor, where they saw boxes of books piled high. As one walked to the window in the southeast corner where he believed the shooter could have been, the other found a rifle on the other side of the room, stuck in a crevice, its barrel upright. The news accounts indicated that the "sniper's nest" had been found. Tom Noguchi and I discussed the procedural process. Investigators would soon learn if the rifle were registered and, if so, to whom. And they would be able to match the bullets to those that hit Kennedy and Connally. Further, paraffin tests would be conducted on the rifle to find any fingerprints.

We wondered who might have had access to that window. Was the shooter an employee, whose presence there would not be questioned? Or could the shooter have killed other people on the way to the sniper window? There were no mentions of anyone injured in the building, but the news was quickly breaking in many directions. Who knew what could happen next? Many of the TV bulletins added to the confusion, which is what often happens with live broadcasts. One televised interview from the scene indicated there might have been a second gunman firing from in front of the president's car as it passed through Dealey Plaza. Dallas County District Attorney Henry Wade even stated: "Preliminary reports indicate more than one person was involved."

All I could do was take a deep breath while the news unfolded. As a forensic pathologist, I had dealt with death on a daily basis, but here was a president, very much in the prime of life, killed on a sunny day, in a public place, with scores of people and Secret Service agents around. I had the sudden realization that no one is ever really completely safe, and no one is immortal. How dare an assassin—or assassins—rob this country of its leader? Was it someone who hated his policies? A political critic? A foreign fiend? I wanted answers about the killer's motivation and hoped for swift justice. And as we sat and watched the news that awful day, I never imagined how closely involved I would later become in the investigation into the shooting of President Kennedy.

Who Was
John Fitzgerald Kennedy?

Jack Kennedy was born on May 29, 1917, in Brookline, Massachusetts, the second of nine children in an Irish, Roman Catholic family. His father, Joseph P. Kennedy, Sr., was a businessman who would become America's ambassador to Great Britain. Rose Fitzgerald, Jack's mother, was the daughter of Boston mayor John F. Fitzgerald, who served three terms in Congress. Jack attended boarding schools and later attained a bachelor of science degree from Harvard College. He joined the U.S. Navy in 1941 and the next year served as a lieutenant on a patrol torpedo (PT) boat. In the South Pacific, his boat was rammed by a Japanese destroyer, and he saved the life of one badly burned crewman by swimming to shore with the man's life jacket strap in his mouth. Before his honorable discharge, Kennedy received a Purple Heart and numerous other medals for bravery.

JFK's older brother, Joe Jr., was the family's designee for an eventual political career, but he died at age 29 when his U.S. Navy plane exploded over England in 1944. Jack became his brother's proxy. His first election won him a congressional seat that lasted six years, then, in 1952, he defeated Republican incumbent Henry Cabot Lodge, Jr., for the U.S. Senate. By the end of the decade, Joe had his eye on the presidency for his son. With his father's influence and his own natural charisma, John Kennedy easily picked off the challengers—Minnesota Senator Hubert Humphrey, Jr., and Texas Senator Lyndon B. Johnson—to win the 1960 Democratic primary election. Kennedy's speech at the national convention promised a "New Frontier" to tackle the nation's problems, and he assuaged concerns about his Catholicism, saying that no one asked about his religion when he was on that PT boat. Still, understanding how he needed to secure votes in the conservative southern states, he signed up Lyndon Johnson as his vice-presidential running mate. Johnson had a good record on civil rights, which Kennedy had not yet come around to embrace.

Kennedy's opponent on the Republican ticket was Richard M. Nixon, then Eisenhower's vice president, and a former U.S. senator from California. That fall, the two candidates faced off on the first televised presidential debate in U.S. history. Americans who only heard the debates on the radio assumed Nixon won, but TV viewers had a different experience. They saw Kennedy, whose boyish good looks

were enhanced by a television makeup artist, and a Nixon who had refused the powder and looked sweaty and in need of a shave. Nixon also seemed ill-at-ease and
jumpy, whereas Kennedy's easy smile was in evidence. On Election Day—November
8, 1960—a record of 68.8 million Americans cast their ballots, with Kennedy winning
by a razor-thin margin of 120,000 votes, despite rumors of voter fraud in Illinois and
Texas. Nixon's advisers told him to contest the election, but the former vice president
refused and offered a gracious congratulation to Kennedy.

Besides his father, JFK had another secret weapon in his political endeav-
ors—his wife. Jacqueline Lee Bouvier was born on July 28, 1929, in Southampton,
New York, to stockbroker John Bouvier III. He and Jacqueline's mother, Janet Lee,
divorced in 1940. Two years later, Janet wed Hugh Auchincloss, the heir to Standard Oil. Jackie, as she was known, had a younger sister, Caroline Lee (later known
as Lee Radziwill), from her parents' first marriage, and two younger step-siblings.
Raised Roman Catholic, she attended boarding schools and made her society debut
in 1947. She spent two years at Vassar College before moving to France for advanced
studies. In 1951, she graduated from George Washington University with a bachelor of arts degree in French literature. The *Washington Times-Herald* newspaper
hired Jackie to be its roving reporter, taking photos of people on the street and adding snappy captions. She spoke fluent French and Spanish, and passable Italian and
Polish.

In 1952, Jackie and Rep. Jack Kennedy met at a party. After he won his U.S. Senate
seat, the two began dating and became engaged. They married at St. Mary's Church,
at Newport, Rhode Island, on September 12, 1953, and settled into life in McLean,
Virginia.

Health woes plagued Jack, beginning with an emergency appendectomy when
he was 13. At 17, he spent time at the Mayo Clinic in Rochester, Minnesota, where
he was diagnosed with colitis, an inflammation of the colon that would give him
persistent abdominal cramping. When still a teen, he hurt his back while playing sports, then later re-injured himself in the PT boat incident. His chronic spinal pain was debilitating, requiring two surgeries. He wore a back brace for the
rest of his life. He also had been diagnosed with Addison's disease, a rare disorder
of the adrenal gland. And he had hypothyroidism, an underperforming thyroid
gland that does not produce enough hormones and can evoke physical and emotional symptoms. JFK managed his ailments by taking a variety of prescription
medications.

Jack and Jackie had two children who grew up in the public eye, but there were
actually five pregnancies. The first, in 1955, ended in an early miscarriage. On August
23, 1956, daughter Arabella Kennedy, was delivered stillborn. November 27, 1957,
brought the birth of Caroline Bouvier Kennedy. Today, Caroline is an author and
attorney. Since 1986, she's been married to art designer Edwin Schlossberg. Caroline
and their three children are the only living direct descendants of Jack and Jackie Kennedy. John Fitzgerald Kennedy, Jr., nicknamed John-John, came along on November

25, 1960. He became a lawyer, author, and editor-in-chief of his own magazine, *George*, but died in 1999, at the age of 38, while piloting his private plane. The crash also killed his wife, Carolyn Bessette, and her sister, Lauren. Patrick Bouvier Kennedy was born on August 7, 1963, surviving two days before perishing from hyaline membrane disease, a lung dysfunction common in premature infants.

Kennedy as President

The murder of John F. Kennedy and the way it was investigated have been a source of constant intrigue throughout most of my adult life. As a young forensic pathologist, I was not yet immersed in the world of politics, although, as a fellow Democrat, I had voted for and supported the senator from Massachusetts in the 1960 election. During Kennedy's campaign stop in Pittsburgh, I was a face in the crowd listening to one of his many dynamic speeches. He talked of a need for reassessing our values. "The time has come for Americans to look inward, to discover the greatness, the charity in each of us," Kennedy told us that day. "Sure, we should strive to prosper. But we should also lend a helping hand to those who have tried but failed, to those who have not had the same opportunities and successes as we have found."

After defeating Richard Nixon in the presidential election, Kennedy became America's 35th president and the first Roman Catholic to hold that office. At 43, he was the youngest man elected to the job. JFK's swearing-in ceremony was the first to be broadcast in color, and I certainly felt a great sense of satisfaction as I watched the event with my wife, Sigrid, on our Admiral 10-inch black-and-white TV. His speech was inspiring as he proclaimed, "to friend and foe alike that the torch has been passed to a new generation of Americans born in this century, tempered by war, disciplined by a hard and bitter peace, proud of our ancient heritage, and unwilling to witness or permit the slow undoing of those human rights to which this nation has always been committed and to which we are committed today at home and around the world." Toward the end of his address, he asked Americans to lend a hand for our joint success, uttering the famous words: "Ask not what your country can do for you. Ask what you can do for your country."

Kennedy's enthusiasm wasn't just earth-bound. He saw the value of extending the fledgling U.S. space program and beefed up its funding. By 1961, America was already in second place to Russia's cosmonaut program for single astronaut flight around the Earth. Kennedy raised the stakes by promising to send U.S. astronauts to the moon by the end of the decade. He would accomplish that goal, even though he would not live to see it.

As JFK assumed the presidency, he inherited the Eisenhower administration's distaste for Fidel Castro, Cuba's prime minister, whose ties to the communist Soviet Union were deep. Eisenhower had allocated millions of dollars in a Central

Intelligence Agency plot to overthrow Castro, abetted by Cuban exiles and Mafia muscle from Miami, who were eager to reestablish gambling casinos that Castro had shut down. JFK signed off on the proposed invasion on the island's southern coast. On April 13, 1961, American forces—including five infantry battalions, one paratrooper battalion, and 16 B-26 bombers—attacked at the Bay of Pigs and were bested by Castro's better-prepared forces. The spectacular defeat was embarrassing for Kennedy, who took his lumps but shared blame with the CIA. He obtained resignations from CIA Director Allen Dulles, Deputy Director Charles Cabell, and Deputy Director for Plans Richard Bissell, and vowed he would "splinter the CIA in a thousand pieces and scatter it to the winds."

Castro continued to be a thorn in the side of the Kennedy administration, and a series of half-baked, almost comical assassination schemes ensued, including using an exploding cigar, a toxic wetsuit, a ballpoint hypodermic needle, heavy metal poisons to make Castro's beard fall out, and more. If some of these murderous ideas make Cuba seem like America's comedy relief, other encounters were deadly serious. The Cuban Missile Crisis in October 1962 brought the world to the brink of nuclear war. President Kennedy was pitted against Soviet Premier Nikita Khrushchev in a tense political and military standoff over the presence of Russian nuclear-armed missiles on the Cuban coast, 90 miles from Florida. For 13 days, Kennedy, guided by his brother, U.S. Attorney General Robert Kennedy, played bully games with the Russians until, thankfully, the two countries agreed to terms: the Soviets would remove their missiles from Cuba, whereas the United States promised not to invade Cuba and would also remove its missiles from Turkey. Despite Kennedy's legitimate beef with communism, he sought a better relationship with Khrushchev and told U.S. diplomats to keep channels open with their Soviet counterparts.

Kennedy's stance on civil rights, which seemed perfectly reasonable to me, was revolutionary at the time and condemned in some circles. When Alabama Governor George Wallace stood in the doorway at the University of Alabama, refusing to allow two African American students to enter, JFK dispatched the National Guard until the segregationist politician backed down. In a speech on June 11, 1963, Kennedy explained his actions, calling it a "moral issue," one "as old as the Scriptures and as clear as the American Constitution." The president pledged that the very next week, he would ask the U.S. Congress to enact legislation so that black citizens would no longer be deprived the rights enjoyed by every other American in schools, restaurants, movie theaters, voting booths, housing, and employment.

On June 12, Medgar Evers was slain by a gunshot in the driveway of his Jackson, Mississippi, home. The black, 37-year-old civil rights activist had helped overturn segregation at the University of Mississippi after his law school application was rejected due to his race. Evers had survived previous assassination attempts in the days before his death, including a Molotov cocktail hurled at him, and nearly being run down by a car. The bullet that tore through his back and entered his heart was probably not survivable, but it didn't help that the hospital where he was brought delayed accepting him as a patient because of his color. A white supremacist, Byron De La Beckwith, was arrested for the murder, but in two trials, both all-white, all-male juries deadlocked without convicting him. In 1994, Evers' body was exhumed by Dr. Michael Baden, and modern forensic testing finally nailed De La Beckwith, who died in prison in 2001. Evers was buried at Arlington National Cemetery with full military honors.

It must be inconceivable to younger generations today that racial separation existed so vociferously in our recent past, but Kennedy's proposals became part of the Civil Rights Act of 1964—another achievement he would not be alive to witness. Of course, there's still not racial parity in this country, and every so often riots erupt to remind us that we must try harder.

In the early 1960s, fear of communism was pervasive in the Western world. Americans remembered too well the murderous Nazi regime and Stalinist leaders of World War II. In 1954, President Eisenhower had warned about the "domino theory," whereby all of Asia—China, Korea, Vietnam, Laos, Cambodia, Thailand, Malaysia, Indonesia, Burma, and India—could fall like communist dominoes. The same threat was later perceived in countries of South America where so-called "people's movements" were taking place, from Chile, Nicaragua, Grenada, El Salvador, and Guatemala. Europe was also the scene of much concern, with our forces watching intently as the Soviet government tried to protect East Germans from the lure of Western decadence. Plans were made for the Russians to build a 12-foor high concrete wall, 96 miles in length, to surround West Berlin and make it impossible for East Berliners to defect to a freer society. Construction of the wall began in June 1961. The vivid symbol of the Cold War was the site of one of JFK's most rousing speeches. On June 26, 1963, he stood at the wall and exclaimed solidarity with the West Germans. "Today, in the world of freedom, the proudest boast is 'Ich bin ein Berliner,'" he announced. On that day, like all free men around the world, he was, indeed, a Berliner. A throng of 1.1 million, 58 percent of the city's residents, cheered him on.

Americans' exuberance for the Kennedy administration was offset by national paranoia. News broadcasts monitored above-ground nuclear tests that the United States, Russia, and other countries conducted, and rumors proved true that the Soviet Union had created a 50-megaton bomb, the most potent nuke on the planet. Many U.S. citizens built bomb shelters in their basements, stocking them with provisions in case of a communist attack. Elementary school children of the era practiced regular "duck and cover" drills as a countermeasure against nuclear attack. Civil defense sirens would sound, and teachers would order the students to hide under their desks. It wasn't until later that most sensible people realized that the underside of a wooden desk wouldn't really offer sufficient protection if our air and water supplies were contaminated.

Another trouble spot handed down from the Eisenhower administration was Southeast Asia. The U.S. government had been gradually supporting the South Vietnamese army to stand against communist forces from the North. Kennedy agreed that Vietnam was a fitting location to prove our anti-communist resolve. He boosted the number of U.S. military advisers in Vietnam from 700 to 16,000, and increased special operations forces and helicopters, while the civil war continued to get bloodier.

Matters deteriorated when Ngo Dinh Diem, the Catholic president of South Vietnam, fell out of favor with the U.S. government. A coup d'etat was approved by Henry Cabot Lodge, Jr., the American ambassador to South Vietnam. On November 2, 1963, Diem and his brother, Ngo Dinh Nhu, were both assassinated by a leader of the CIA-backed South Vietnamese army. But rather than stabilizing the southern government, the dual assassinations only energized the northern forces led by Ho Chi Minh.

Since President Diem's assassination came only 20 days before Kennedy's, it is difficult to speculate how JFK would have handled the Vietnam War if he had lived and won reelection. Historians will debate this point, as well as whether the fear of communism was so contrived that we wrongfully interceded in a conflict we had little business being involved in and couldn't possibly win. Under President Johnson, the war raged on, with most citizens eventually showing contempt for his leadership. The American people grew tired of seeing the lives of military personnel being risked for reasons that were becoming more untenable by the day.

In the spring of 1962, Kennedy had instructed Secretary of Defense Robert McNamara to draft a withdrawal plan that would have all U.S. personnel back on American soil by the end of 1965. On October 11, 1963, Kennedy signed National Security Action Memo 263, initiating a withdrawal of 1,000 Americans stationed in Vietnam. While Diem's death and the turmoil that followed altered that timeline, Kennedy was still resolved to reduce America's commitment.

President Kennedy faced a lot of challenges in his short administration. He served only 1,036 days in office—two years, ten months and three days. The immense crises he faced were indicative of how our citizens viewed each other and the world. Our hopes for the future were acutely delineated. The majority of Americans really liked this president and almost certainly would have given him a second term to follow through on the tasks he started. But JFK also had made a lot of formidable enemies. When you consider the individuals who wanted him dead, you only have to look at the triumphs and tragedies of his time in office to begin making a list of suspects.

November 22, 1963

President Kennedy, the First Lady, and their retinue began their Texas trip in San Antonio on Thursday, November 21. Jacqueline didn't normally travel with JFK on domestic trips, but he prevailed upon her the importance of winning over Texans, and she agreed to go. On their first day in the Lone Star State, they also visited Houston and Fort Worth, where they spent the night at the Hotel Texas. The pair would travel to Dallas the next day, then fly with Vice President Lyndon B. Johnson and his spouse, Lady Bird, to unwind at their ranch in Stonewall, Texas, on the northern bank of the Pedernales River, about 250 miles southwest of Dallas.

On the morning of the 22nd, JFK woke at 7:30 a.m. and went down to greet a few thousand people who were waiting for him in the rain outside the hotel. When someone shouted to ask where Jackie was, the president pointed to their 8th floor suite and said with a wink: "Mrs. Kennedy is organizing herself. It takes her a little longer—but, of course, she looks better than we do when she does it."

The Kennedys then went to a Chamber of Commerce breakfast, where Kennedy gave a well-received speech. In attendance were the Johnsons and Texas Governor John Connally and his wife, Nellie. In the audience were hundreds of governmental, municipal, civic, business, academic, and community leaders. Kennedy's speech addressed topics like Fort Worth's pivotal role in aviation, military history, and national defense, and expressed his hope for peace in the world and progress in the nation's space program. JFK joked that he didn't understand why his vice president was getting a better reaction from the crowd than they had given to him—he knew the answer. Johnson was on his home turf, having been born and raised in Texas, and his political career had begun there, first as a U.S. congressman and then as a U.S. senator, before Kennedy chose him as second in command.

The president also poked fun at his attractive wife, saying she regretted that the short stint they had in Fort Worth meant she wouldn't be able to go shopping at Neiman Marcus. Jackie, typically stylish, wore a pink, wool boucle double-breasted suit with navy blue trim, a blue blouse, a pink pillbox hat by Halston, blue pumps, and short white gloves, and carried a blue handbag. A coordinating coat in a darker shade of pink stayed on the plane. Although the suit was widely thought to be a Chanel design, it was actually a knockoff made by a Manhattan fashion label. She had worn the outfit on two previous public occasions, and Jack Kennedy suggested _ar it for the Dallas trip to show off her casual elegance amid the fur-wearing, diamond-dripping Republicans they would be encountering. The president wore a dark gray suit, a white shirt with muted vertical stripes, and a dark blue patterned tie.

After the breakfast, the Kennedys and their entourage flew in Air Force One from Fort Worth's Amon Carter Field, northwest of Love Field airport in Dallas. The Johnsons, Connallys, and others flew in Air Force Two. Although it was only a trip of about 40 minutes by car, the decision to fly was made "for security reasons." The Kennedys, Johnsons, and Connallys met up at Love Field at 11:40 a.m. The Kennedys walked across the tarmac, holding hands until someone handed her a giant bouquet of long-stemmed red roses. She smiled at the surprising color, commenting that she thought Texans would give her yellow roses. The First Lady carried the blooms on her lap when she got into her limousine. Someone gave a bouquet of yellow roses to Nellie Connally, who held them on her lap inside the vehicle. Lady Bird Johnson was also given yellow roses, which she took to her car. Ten minutes later, the group left Love Field in their designated vehicles.

There were 23 cars and 15 motorcycles in the motorcade. A white Ford sedan was the police pilot car, staying a quarter mile ahead to clear the way. Another white Ford sedan, the lead car, was immediately in front of the presidential limousine.

The presidential limousine was a royal blue 1961 Lincoln Continental four-door convertible, with dark blue leather interior. It was 21 feet, eight inches long, and weighed about 7,500 pounds. Its Secret Service code name was X-100. The limousine was transported from Washington, D.C., to Texas—or any other location on the agenda—courtesy of a military C-130 transport aircraft. A non-bulletproof steel and plastic roof panel had been removed that day to allow for the amiable JFK to enjoy close contact with supporters in the crowd.

Kennedy's car was driven by Secret Service agent William Greer, whose supervisor, Roy Kellerman, was in the front passenger seat. The Connallys were seated on folded-down jump seats, with Nellie behind Greer and John behind Kellerman. Behind the Connallys were the Kennedys, with Jackie on Nellie's side and the president behind the governor. Connally had been wearing an off-white Stetson hat that he took off in the car and held on his lap. The rear seat could be hydraulically controlled to elevate the president and anyone sitting next to him by 10½ inches. The controls were solely operated by the president.

Two radio telephones were in the car and, if needed, flashing red lights and a siren. Four retractable steps were on the vehicle's exterior for Secret Service agents, with another two steps on the rear bumper for additional agents. Two permanent grab handles were affixed to the trunk lid. Two flagstaffs were on the exterior, curved front panel, with the American flag always displayed on the passenger side. On the driver's side was the flag of whatever state or country the limousine was visiting.

A black 1956 Cadillac convertible was the follow-up car, driven by Secret Serviceman Samuel A. Kinney, and carrying seven other agents, including four who stood on running boards outside the vehicle. The agents scanned the crowds, windows, and

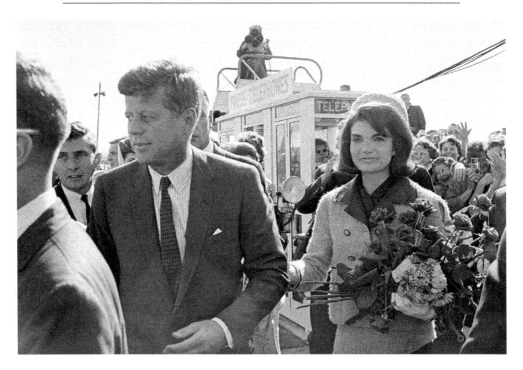

After deplaning from Air Force One at Dallas' Love Field Airport, Jack and Jackie Kennedy had just over an hour of happiness left (AP Photo/File).

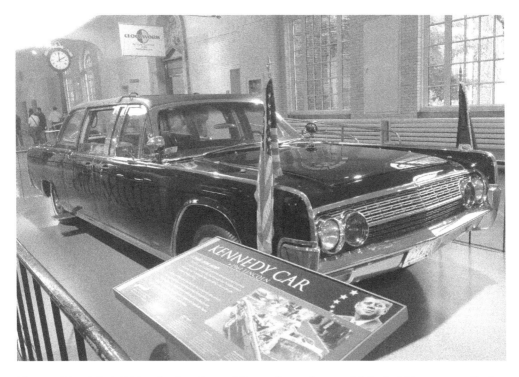

The presidential 1961 Lincoln Continental limousine—shown with its bubble top—on display at the Henry Ford Museum in Dearborn, Michigan (courtesy Randy O. Sacia).

rooftops, looking for potential troublemakers. By mandate, the Secret Service car was never to be more than a five-foot distance from the president's car. On the floor of the agents' car was a Thompson submachine gun, ready to fire, if necessary. Other cars in the motorcade were driven by Texas state highway patrolmen. Their passengers were the Johnsons; U.S. Senator Ralph W. Yarborough; staffers of the president and Mrs. Kennedy; local politicians; members of the media; law enforcement; and the president's personal doctor, USN Rear Admiral George G. Burkley.

The procession was to curl through the streets of Dallas, then hit the freeway for the brief trip to the city's Trade Mart, where the president was to give a luncheon speech to business leaders. That evening, a Democratic fundraiser requiring the president's attendance was planned in Austin. As JFK's limousine passed through the suburbs of the "Big D," the Kennedys were genuinely pleased by the smiling, waving crowds they saw. Old and young, rich and poor, white, black, and brown—and everyone red, white, and blue. There was one short and unexpected stop. JFK spotted a family with a banner that read: "Please Mr. President, get out and shake our hands. Our neighbors said you wouldn't." So, with a big chuckle, Kennedy took a moment to do that.

The motorcade drove on, now in the thick of the downtown district. People were piled on the sidewalks, on both sides of the street. The president and governor waved at the folks to their right, while the first ladies waved at those to their left. And it was noisy. Between people in the crowd whooping to get the president's attention and the revving of the motorcycles, any conversation within the limousine had to be very loud. As they were just about to veer left onto Elm Street, Nellie Connally turned to Kennedy and shouted: "Mr. President, you can't say that Dallas doesn't love you." His reply was a wide smile.

"Nut Country"

Not everyone in Dallas was happy to see the president. Handbills had been circulated showing his face full front and in profile, as if it were a mug shot. In bold black lettering, the words "Wanted for Treason" were at the top. Under that was an unhinged rant, suggesting that Kennedy was dedicated to turning "the U.S. over to the communist controlled United Nations."

The author was Robert A. Surrey, a 38-year-old former printer in Dallas who paid $60 to have the handbills printed. They were widely distributed on the streets of Dallas for two days before Kennedy's arrival. Surrey also had a business with Major General Edwin A. Walker, an ultra-conservative Texan who despised Kennedy.

The president had far wealthier and more committed enemies within Dallas. Haroldson Lafayette Hunt—known by his initials, H.L.—was an oil billionaire who supported rabidly anti-communist groups such as the John Birch Society and William F. Buckley Jr.'s Young Americans for Freedom. Hunt's fortune helped finance the political campaigns of Senator Joseph McCarthy, the Republican firebrand from Wisconsin. Hunt also funded tax-exempt "news" organizations, like *Facts Forum* and *Lifeline*, which filled the airwaves with paranoia-inducing programs about communists infiltrating our government and the United Nations' plan to take away America's freedoms. Hunt was married three times and had 15 children. His proclivity for playing dirty in business deals made him the inspiration for the fictional character J.R. Ewing on the long-running CBS series *Dallas*.

On November 4, 1963, Hunt's security chief, an ex–FBI agent named Paul Rothermel, wrote his boss a memo regarding "unconfirmed reports of possible violence" during Kennedy's upcoming motorcade through Dallas. Rothermel had solid sources in the local FBI and Dallas police department, and with individuals close to General Walker. After the assassination, H.L. Hunt was whisked out of Texas and put into hiding at Washington, D.C.'s Mayflower Hotel for several weeks, courtesy of the Bureau. From his elegant foxhole, Hunt issued this statement: "Every American, whatever the faith of his views or his political affiliations, suffers a personal loss when a president dies. … Freedom is in fearful danger when a president dies by violence." Allan Maley, the secretary-treasurer of the Dallas AFL-CIO, made his own declaration: "There is no use beating around the bush. Dallas is a sick city. There are powerful leaders who have encouraged or condoned, or at best remained silent, while the preachment of hate helped condition a citizenry to support the most reactionary sort of political philosophy."

Kennedy wasn't much loved at the city's leading newspaper either. The *Dallas Morning News* had once been owned by businessman George Bannerman Dealey. Under his progressive leadership, the paper took an editorial stand against the Ku Klux Klan and refused to publish questionable advertising. But when Dealey died in 1946, his son E.M. "Ted" Dealey inherited the paper, and things changed.

Ted Dealey was a zealous right-winger and, by the 1960s, his hatred of Kennedy was almost irrational. In 1961, when Dealey attended a White House function with other Texas publishers, he surprised everyone in the room by whipping out a 500-word prepared statement and reading it to President Kennedy. Part of the lecture included: "We can annihilate Russia and should make that clear to the Soviet government. ... The general opinion of the grassroots thinking in this country is that you and your administration are weak sisters. We need a man on horseback to lead this nation, and many people in Texas and the Southwest think you are riding on [your daughter] Caroline's tricycle." Kennedy turned red with anger, looked Dealey in the eye, and snapped: "The difference between you and me, Mr. Dealey, is that I was elected president of this country and you were not. I have the responsibility for the lives of 180 million Americans, which you have not, and I didn't get elected by arriving at soft judgments. Wars are easier to talk about than they are to fight. I'm just as tough as you are, Mr. Dealey."

On the day of Kennedy's visit to Dallas, Dealey accepted an advertisement his father would have rejected. It was a full-page, black-bordered screed that appeared in Section 1, page 14. "Welcome, Mr. Kennedy to Dallas," it began, followed by itemized accusations that criticized JFK's "philosophy and politics," as well as his handling of matters in Cuba, Latin America, Southeast Asia, and Europe. It also claimed the president curried favor with Russia and the Communist Party, all contentions a reasonable person would view as paranoid blather. At the bottom of the ad was a notice that it was paid for by the "American Fact-Finding Committee" and its chairman, Bernard Weissman of Dallas.

According to information developed later during the Warren Commission investigation of Kennedy's assassination, the ad was the creation of four oil industry workers and former U.S. army members with ties to the local Young Americans for Freedom chapter. The American Fact-Finding Committee was not a real organization, but a title the foursome chose to sound authentic. Bernard Weissman's name was used because he was Jewish, and the others felt a Semitic name would lead away from their Christian roots. The men said they intended no personal harm to the president and only took out the ad as a dignified protest to Kennedy's policies. The advertisement cost about $1,500 and was paid for by H.L. Hunt's son, Nelson Bunker Hunt, and some of his business associates. Investigators could find no link between the people behind the ad and anyone involved in the murder of the president. Kennedy had read the ad that morning while still in Fort Worth and handed the newspaper to his wife, saying, "We're heading into nut country today."

Dealey Plaza
and the "Grassy Knoll"

To guarantee that citizens who wanted to see their president would know where to view the motorcade, both local newspapers—the *Dallas Morning News* and the *Dallas Times-Herald*—published the 10-mile route on Tuesday, November 19. The presidential parade would travel southeast from Love Field Airport to Mockingbird Lane, turning onto Lemmon Avenue, then onto Turtle Creek Boulevard, turning south onto Cedar Springs Road. They'd pass through downtown until North Harwood Street and then go west onto Main Street to Houston Street, the site of Dealey Plaza.

Dealey Plaza is a city park of about 15 acres. Established in 1940, it was named for newspaper publisher George Dealey. The motorcade would make a wide left turn onto Elm Street—a one-way thoroughfare—go under a railroad bridge known as the "Triple Underpass" to the Stemmons Freeway, then continue on to the Trade Mart. (The Triple Underpass is still there today, consisting of three access routes: Commerce Street on the left, the Thornton Freeway in the middle, and the Stemmons Freeway North on the right.)

As the underpass was in sight, Jacqueline Kennedy thought to herself that the tunnel would be cooler than the oppressive heat from the sun that was beating down on them and blinding everyone in the car. It's been fiercely debated whether there had been an original plan to have the motorcade just come straight down Main Street and get directly on the freeway, avoiding the turn onto Elm that would take them past the sniper. On November 16, a reporter for the *Dallas Morning News* wrote that the route would go straight down Main Street, and on the 22nd, a crudely drawn map that ran in a small box on that paper's front page was too imprecise to discern. Years later, Gerald Behn, the Secret Service agent-in-charge of the president's detail, along with two other agents, told author Vincent Palamara that the route had, indeed, been changed.

The motorcade's journey down Houston Street was only one block long but showed off the city's finest buildings. The Old Red Courthouse, a castle-like structure, was on the southeast corner of Main and Houston. On the west side of Houston, separated by Main Street, were matching reflecting pools, with a continuous row of white columns and a spread of lawn. By the south pool was a statue, and by the north

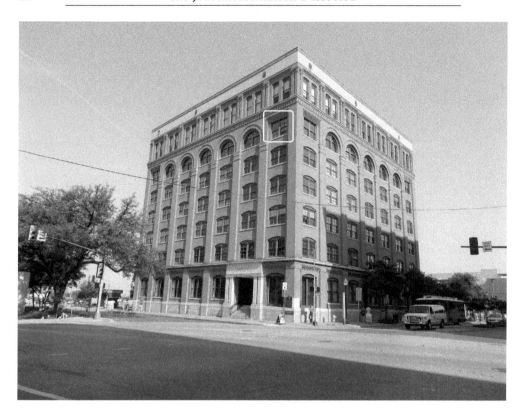

The Texas School Book Depository's sixth-floor window is highlighted to show where authorities claim Lee Harvey Oswald was positioned when he shot President Kennedy (courtesy Randy O. Sacia).

pool was an obelisk. On the east side of Houston were the buildings for the County Records and County Criminal Courts.

On the northeast corner of Houston and Elm was the Dal-Tex building, the epicenter for textiles, where a man named Abraham Zapruder kept offices on the fourth and fifth floors for his dressmaking business. On the northwest corner of Houston and Elm was the Texas School Book Depository building, a seven-story orange brick building at 411 Elm Street. It was constructed in 1898 as a five-story building and, five years later, almost burned to the ground when lightning hit it. In 1903, it was constructed in its present form. In 1963, the edifice was used as a warehouse for textbooks for the school district. In November of that year, a former U.S. Marine named Lee Harvey Oswald worked there as a temporary employee. On the depository's rooftop was a prominent Hertz Rent-a-Car billboard with a digital clock and temperature display. The structure, currently the Dallas County Administration Building, is a Recorded Texas Historic Landmark. It houses the Sixth Floor Museum, which was established in 1989 and is dedicated to assassinated-related exhibits.

Running along the north side of Elm Street, the fan-shaped lawn covers the ground from the depository to the underpass. A curved, white pergola is set back on the lawn and elevated by three steps. Made of concrete, it is an open, airy pavilion with five columns that give the appearance of creating small rooms. On either side is a larger room without a door. There are no windows and no foliage growing on the structure. The design is symmetrical and artistic but somewhat impractical. Because there are no benches, it is not a place suitable for bringing a lunch or even sitting and reading. The area remains now as it was in 1963, except that the trees that are behind and beside the pergola are much taller and fuller than they were then. Beyond the west side of the pergola is a white retaining wall of about four feet tall. A few yards behind it is a five-foot-tall wooden picket fence with a car parking area behind it and trees on either side. Concrete steps with a metal handrail at the top run just east of the fence down to the sidewalk. This is the location known as the "grassy knoll," a term United Press International bureau chief Patrick Conway made up on-the-fly to describe the landscape.

Abraham Zapruder

On either side of the Dealey Plaza pergola is a concrete pedestal approximately four feet tall. The pedestal on the west side is where Abraham Zapruder stood when he shot the world's most famous home movie. Zapruder, 58, was born in the Ukrainian city of Kovel but immigrated to Brooklyn, New York, as a teenager. He later began working in the garment industry and in 1940 relocated to Dallas with his wife, Lillian, and their two children, Henry and Myrna. He opened a dressmaking company called Jennifer Juniors that had its offices in the Dal-Tex building near Dealey Plaza.

On November 22, 1963, Zapruder had planned to film the motorcade with his new camera. But when it rained early that morning, he left the camera at home. Later, after the clouds lifted, Zapruder's assistant, Lillian Rogers, persuaded him to run home and get the camera, which he did. "Mr. Z," as his employees called him, and his receptionist, Marilyn Sitzman, walked to the pergola area to look for the best vantage point for him to shoot his footage, and he jumped onto the nearby concrete pedestal. Marilyn stood behind him, holding his leg so he would keep his balance.

Zapruder was a Democrat who liked President Kennedy and was enthusiastic about the prospect of being able to capture him on film. It would be his first time using the camera—a Bell & Howell Zoomatic Director Series Model 414 PD—which was state-of-the art for that era. Zapruder used Kodachrome II 8 millimeter safety film and a Varamat 9–27 millimeter f1.8 telephoto lens set for full close-ups.

As the motorcade rounded the corner from Houston Street to Elm Street, Zapruder held his camera to his eye and started filming. He followed the presidential limousine as it moved at a pace of around 12–15 miles per hour down Elm Street, right past him, and continued toward the Stemmons Freeway entrance. The footage captured Secret Service agent William Greer behind the wheel of the vehicle with his supervisor Roy Kellerman in the front passenger seat. Governor John Connally and his wife Nellie sat behind them and, on the rear bench seat, were President and Mrs. Kennedy.

Most witnesses would later say they heard three shots, within about six seconds. In quick succession: Kennedy reacted to a gunshot to his throat; Connally appeared to be shot as well. Finally, there was a spray of blood and brain matter when another bullet blasted open the right side of the president's head, and he fell against his wife.

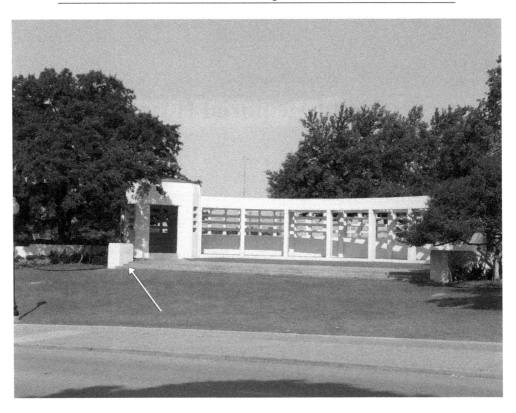

The arrow marks the pedestal where local businessman Abraham Zapruder stood with his new camera to film what would become history's most tragic home movie (courtesy Randy O. Sacia).

Then, Jacqueline Kennedy crawled onto the trunk of the limousine to grab something, as her designated Secret Service agent, later identified as Clint Hill, jumped onto the rear of the car and pushed her back inside. He signaled his colleagues in the follow-up car with a thumb's down before covering both Kennedys' bodies with his own. The limousine then sped forward toward the underpass and disappeared from sight.

Zapruder's footage was only 26.6 seconds long and had no sound. It consisted of 486 frames, meaning the film ran through the camera at 18.3 frames per second. Sometimes it was out of focus or out of frame, and because it was hand-held and not on a tripod, the images were shaky. Still, I can think of no other footage more realistic and dramatic. The Zapruder film is probably the most historically valuable footage ever shot. It has provided endless education for investigators, media, and students of the assassination, and will continue to do so far into the future.

Zapruder's film was not broadcast nationally until March 1975. But I had the opportunity to view the footage much earlier, which I will discuss in a subsequent chapter.

Parkland Memorial Hospital

Parkland Memorial Hospital is located at 4900 Harry Hines Boulevard in Dallas. It was, and is, the chief teaching medical facility in the area and is affiliated with the University of Texas Southwestern Medical School. A new 17-story facility was built across the street and opened in 2015.

In 1963, Parkland's emergency room would treat some 99,280 patients. That's 272 per day or about one every five minutes. The two trauma rooms on the main floor are where a patient would, with luck, be stabilized before he or she was brought upstairs for surgery, sent to a department for specialized tests, moved into a recovery room, or discharged. The area outside the trauma rooms was colloquially called "the pit." Parkland was the medical epicenter for the Kennedy assassination, as its emergency personnel treated the president and Governor Connally. Two days later, the alleged assassin, Lee Harvey Oswald, who suffered a gunshot wound, would be pronounced dead there. And four years later, nightclub owner Jack Ruby, who shot Oswald, died there of a pulmonary embolism and lung cancer.

On November 22, Kennedy and Connally were brought into the emergency rooms at 12:38 p.m. and logged as Patient 24740 and 24743, respectively. Two other people came in at the same time, which explains the gap in the numbering. By the time the president's body left the hospital at 2:19 p.m., seven other emergency patients were admitted. Among the 23 other patients undergoing treatment in the trauma area that day were a boy who was bleeding from a fall; a man who had chest pains; a woman who complained of nervousness; and individuals who had automobile crash injuries, dog bites, and infections. There were other deaths at Parkland that day and 18 births. With the shooting of President Kennedy and Governor Connally, Parkland Hospital had become the temporary seats of the governments of the United States and the state of Texas.

From a telephone in the presidential motorcade, Parkland personnel were notified that the president and possibly others had been shot and that the wounded would be arriving within minutes. Head emergency room nurse Doris Nelson, who took the call, alerted personnel to prepare Trauma Room One for the president. She called upon operating room supervisor Audrey Bell to begin making arrangements in Trauma Room Two across the hall. Both gray-tiled rooms were very small but stocked with all the modern equipment of the day. Other surgical arenas could be opened, if needed. Nurse Janie Wester also received a phone call, advising her that the president would be arriving soon and that she should be ready for two possible procedures. One was a craniotomy, or a surgical exploration of the head, and the other was a thoracotomy, or the exploration of the heart, lungs, and esophagus. She assigned personnel to set up two rooms for these tests, but they were never needed.

It was a wild four-mile ride on the Stemmons Freeway at speeds of up to 80 miles per hour, with sirens blaring. The presidential limousine passed the Trade Mart, where Kennedy was scheduled to give his speech, and exited the freeway at Wycliff Avenue. The car turned right at Industrial Boulevard and travelled a couple of blocks north to the hospital. As the limousine pulled into the ambulance parking area at the back of the hospital, gurneys were waiting. A photograph published in the *Fort Worth Star Telegram* showed the car's interior after everyone went inside. Pools of blood, chunks of brain tissue, and Nellie's crushed roses were chilling reminders of what had happened there. The other motorcade vehicles, which had been following the president's car, parked where they could find spaces. Dr. Bill Midgett, a second-year obstetrics-gynecology resident, greeted the limo, assisted by Nurse Pat Hutton from his unit. Secret Service agents first took Governor Connally out of the vehicle. It was evident that he had a gunshot wound to the back of his right shoulder blade. But he was alert and didn't seem to be in mortal danger. He was placed on a stretcher, and Mrs. Connally followed him out of the car.

Agent Clint Hill popped up from his position covering both Kennedys, but Jackie remained hunched over her husband, cradling him and whispering in his ear. Hill helped her out of the car as she muttered: "They murdered my husband." Jackie's pink suit was stained with so much blood, there was a fear that she had also been shot. Her white gloves were almost completely red, and brain tissue clung to her purse. She grabbed the red roses and took them with her. Hill then turned to the president who was facedown on the back seat. As several of the agents lifted JFK out of the car and onto a stretcher, Hill removed his coat and put it over the president's face and shoulders to stymie any photographers who might try to snap a gruesome picture. Jackie Kennedy laid her roses and her pink hat on top of her husband's supine body.

Merriman Smith, with United Press International, managed to corner Hill and ask him how badly the president was hit. Hill's glum response was, "He's dead." Smith became the first newsman to carry the unconfirmed news to the American public. Cell phone technology was decades from being implemented in 1963, so there was always a mad dash to find a telephone if a reporter needed to call in his or her story. Mr. Smith had better luck than most in finding ones at Parkland.

As President Kennedy and Governor Connally were rolled into their respective trauma rooms, Jackie Kennedy and Nellie Connally followed their husbands inside. They were soon joined by Secret Service and FBI agents, Dallas police officers, sheriff deputies, Vice President and Lady Bird Johnson, other politicians, Kennedy staffers, JFK's personal physician George Burkley, and news gatherers who flooded the scene. Resident doctors James Carrico and Richard B. Dulany helped guide the stretchers through the pit and into their proper trauma rooms. Carrico then went into Kennedy's room, while Dulany went with Connally.

Lyndon Johnson, who had recently been treated for a coronary condition, held his chest. His face was ashen. He was brought to a small cubicle near the nurses' station where an agent would keep him separated from everyone except his wife, Lady Bird, and select associates. Curtains were drawn on the glass walls for his protection. At some point, Mrs. Johnson, accompanied by two Secret Servicemen, made a brief departure from the room to lend comfort to Jackie Kennedy and Nellie Connally.

Agent Kellerman excused himself to find a phone to call the White House Detail in Washington, D.C. He apprised his supervisor, Secret Service Special Agent-in-Charge Gerald A. Behn, that the president and governor had been hit by bullets and were in surgery at Parkland. There was commotion in the pit and hallways, with people barking orders. An FBI agent ran down the corridor, only to be stopped by a Secret Serviceman who was carrying a Thompson submachine gun. With a loud "thud," the Secret Serviceman smashed the FBI agent in the face with the weapon, causing the agent to crumble to the floor, unconscious and with a broken jaw. Nurse Wester helped keep unnecessary traffic out of the Trauma Room One and the hallway before she went to Trauma Room Two and assisted the doctors working on Governor Connally.

A Secret Service agent ordered that some of the Texas state highway patrolmen who had been driving other vehicles in the motorcade stand guard over the president's limousine. They put the bubble top on the limousine, told the press the car was off-limits, and blocked off the area with police tape. Supposedly at Lyndon Johnson's order, the exterior of the vehicle was washed down. When you consider that this was a murder and that the limousine was the crime scene, it's unimaginable that someone—even the U.S. vice-president—would have the lack of intelligence to command such an act. It's a crime to tamper with evidence, but there would be even greater forensic affronts ahead. Some medical students watched as agents tidied up the car. When a student commented to a friend that there was a bullet hole in the windshield, a Secret Serviceman who heard the remark jumped in the car and drove it away.

Inside Trauma Room One, the emergency crew wheeled in President Kennedy and transferred him to an operating table, face up. His legs were elevated, which is standard procedure for a patient in shock. As the president was rolled past her, Mrs. Kennedy grabbed her pink hat from his gurney and put it back on her head. Under the bright light of the operating arena, the surgical team surrounded the president. His famous eyes were wide open, and his pupils were fixed and dilated. His mouth was slack. Such a familiar face, yet so strangely lifeless. "Moribund" was the word one of the doctors used. There was no obtainable pulse or blood pressure and only a faint suggestion of a heartbeat. Kennedy's chest was making jerky contractions, as he struggled to breathe.

The president's coat, tie, and shirt were removed and set aside. He was not wearing an undershirt. A white sheet was draped over the lower portion of his body, and a stainless steel bucket on wheels—known as a "kick bucket"—was placed to collect the blood that was dripping from him. The surgeons recognized that Kennedy's condition as "four-plus," meaning the worst-case scenario. Yet these doctors and nurses did not want President Kennedy to die on their watch. No matter what their individual political feelings were—whether they were JFK's fan or foe, Democrat or Republican—they were all Americans in that moment. Together, as they fought back tears, they would undertake every possible measure to save this man. I can make no criticism of the medical and surgical treatment administered by everyone on the Parkland Hospital staff on November 22, 1963.

Dr. Malcolm O. Perry, Parkland's attending surgeon and vascular consultant, and senior surgical resident Carrico led the procedure. They were assisted by Drs. Ronald Jones, chief surgical resident; William "Kemp" Clark, neurological surgery chairman; Paul Peters, assistant professor of urology; Charles Baxter and Robert Nelson McClelland, assistant professors of surgery; Fouad Bashour, chief of cardiology; and Donald W. Seldin, chief of medicine. Dr. Tom Shires, the chair of the hospital's department of surgery, was at a conference in Galveston that afternoon.

Other surgical residents and/or interns included Drs. Bill Midgett, Don Teel Curtis, Charles A. Crenshaw, Kenneth E. Salyer, Martin G. White, Lito Porto, Richard Brooks Dulany, Joe D. Goldstrich, Phillip Earle Williams, Jr., and William Zedelitz. Anesthesiologists present were Dr. Marion T. "Pepper" Jenkins, the chief of the

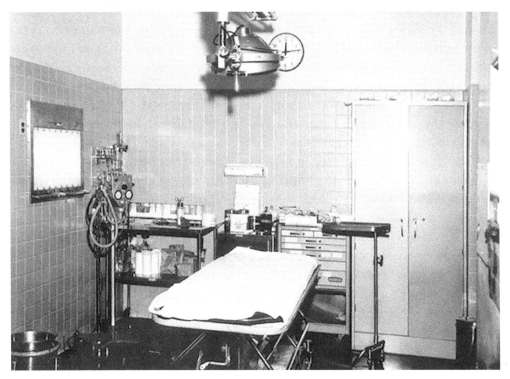

Some 30 dedicated doctors and nurses tried in vain to save JFK's life in Parkland Hospital's tiny Trauma Room One (courtesy Parkland Health & Hospital System, 1963).

department; and his associates, Drs. Jackie Hansen Hunt, Adolph H. Giesecke, and Gene C. Akin. Among the nurses who worked on the president were Doris M. Nelson, the supervising emergency room nurse; assistant supervisor Jane C. Wester; head nurses Ruth J. Standridge and Audrey Bell; and Pat Hutton, Diane Bowron, and Margaret M. Henchcliffe.

Some of the doctors and nurses were only in the Trauma Room One long enough to perform a particular task or until they learned their expertise wasn't needed. Then, they either left to go into Trauma Room Two or somewhere else in the hospital. It's possible that some of the medical personnel in Kennedy's room were not logged onto any official list. But the important thing to know is that many hands worked together that day to try to achieve a miracle.

Drs. Jim Carrico and Ronald Jones were the first to begin work. They knew the ABCs of lifesaving: Airway, Breathing, Circulation. One of the nurses started an IV bag of Ringer's lactate, the sterile solution that contains sodium lactate and three types of chloride, to provide fluid resuscitation after traumatic blood loss. The Parkland team could see that President Kennedy's face was extremely swollen and blue. His thick reddish-brown hair almost disguised his massive head injury, but when Carrico and Jones pulled back the flap and saw the extensive defect that had blasted away so much brain and skull tissue, they knew that any life-sustaining attempts would be a mere formality. The entire right hemisphere of Kennedy's brain was missing, beginning at his hairline and extending to behind his right ear. Pieces of skull that hadn't been blown off were clinging to blood-matted hair. And part of his cerebellum—the rear portion of the brain that helps with balance and coordination—was shredded and dangling from the back of his head like a blood-soaked sponge. But the doctors couldn't explore that damage; they had to keep the patient breathing.

The president had sustained another wound—there was a small, round opening about the diameter of a pencil, in Kennedy's front throat, but there would be no tracking to determine that bullet's trajectory. Since all the attention was paid to Kennedy's front side as they worked to keep him alive, no one turned him over to look for wounds on his back. It had no bearing on their task at hand. Dr. Carrico injected the president with a steroid called Solu-Cortef, the trade name for sodium hydrocortisone succinate, which is used to treat adrenal deficiency—but that ailment was the least of Kennedy's problems in the trauma room.

Carrico placed an endotracheal tube into the president's mouth and down his throat to keep his airway open. Anesthesiology fellow Hunt had brought in a respiration machine for artificial ventilation, before she went to Governor Connally's trauma room—so, Dr. Don Curtis, a dentist and resident in oral surgery, attached the endotracheal tube to the breathing machine. Soon, a 100-percent oxygen infusion was going into the president. More doctors and nurses entered the Trauma Room One. Someone asked what Kennedy's blood type was, and neither his wife nor his physician knew. But Roy Kellerman, the president's Secret Service agent, knew and shouted that JFK's type was O Rh positive. That blood was obtained from the blood bank and put in his IV bag. (The Secret Service now carries pints of the U.S. president's own blood type, in case of an emergency. The pints are kept chilled in the trunk of the presidential limousine and/or on Air Force One.)

Dr. Charles Baxter looked at Jackie and said, "Mrs. Kennedy, I think you should step outside." Nurse Doris Nelson walked over to the First Lady and suggested she'd be more comfortable waiting in the hallway. A chair was moved outside the door, and Jackie sat there for a few minutes. Then someone came out of the trauma room and remarked that the president was still breathing. Jackie stood and plaintively asked, "Do you mean he may live?" When no one would answer her, she went back into the operating room and stood or sat in the corner with Dr. Burkley. A nurse asked if the First Lady would like a wet towel to clean off her hands or clothing, but she refused. She was steely and eerily calm.

Dr. Charles Crenshaw, a third-year resident, and first-year resident Salyer got the IV going and hung a bag of blood. Crenshaw noticed that Secret Service agent Clint Hill was in a frenzied, disoriented state and waving his .38 caliber handgun. Crenshaw motioned to Baxter, as if to ask what should be done about Agent Hill, but before Baxter could respond, Nurse Nelson interceded. She boldly went to Hill and said, "Whoever shot the president is not in this room." Hill just stared at her. Pointing at each doctor, she continued, "He's okay, he's okay, he's okay," until she indicated every man in the room. "Now, put your gun away, so we can get to work." Hill said nothing but left the emergency room. In the hallway, he took a phone call from Attorney General Robert Kennedy and gave him the horrific news. Hill would later go to work for the new president, Lyndon Johnson, and stay with the Secret Service until his retirement in 1975. But he never quite got over what he experienced that day in November 1963 and battled depression and alcoholism for many years.

Crenshaw recounted the Parkland showdown and more in his superb book, *JFK: Conspiracy of Silence* (coauthored with Jens Hansen and J. Gary Shaw, Signet/Penguin Books 1992). It was republished under the title, *JFK Has Been Shot: A Parkland Hospital Surgeon Speaks Out* (Pinnacle True Crime Books, 2013), with a fresh "Personal Reflections" chapter by me.

There was still a question as to whether Kennedy had an adequate pulse, so Drs. Jones and Paul Peters pulled the president's pants down to his knees to get to his femoral artery at the junction of the leg and the trunk. When they touched the area, they got a very weak rhythm. The physicians noticed JFK was wearing a cream-colored back brace. Similar to a corset, it fully encircled his midsection, and was about eight- to 11-inches tall and about an ⅛-inch thick. Kennedy was also wearing an Ace bandage wrapped around his pelvis in a figure-8 fashion, encompassing both of his thighs and his lower trunk. Peters would later remark that he was surprised that the president was wearing a $3 bandage but that he likely needed the pelvis support for his chronic back pain. They removed the bandage and pushed aside the brace to palpate the area. Assisted by Nurses Bowron and Henchcliffe, Dr. Crenshaw removed the president's slacks the rest of the way, as well as his right sock and shoes. Crenshaw saw that one of the shoes had a ¾-inch lift in it, indicating that one of JFK's legs was shorter than the other. He decided to preserve what dignity was possible by leaving on Kennedy's undershorts.

The doctors embarked on three simultaneous "cutdowns" to supply President Kennedy's body with fluids. Drs. Crenshaw and Salyer did the procedure to the right leg, while Dr. Curtis worked on the left one. Dr. Jones did a cutdown on the left arm. First nurses sterilized each area and draped a sterile sheet with a window hole over it. Then, the doctors made a small incision about two inches above each ankle and below the elbow, and a vein was dissected free at each location. A cannula, or 18-gauge catheter, was placed in each vein in the direction of the heart, and a purse string ligature was tied around the catheter at one end. An IV was plugged into the flange of each catheter, and more Ringer's lactate began flowing. The wound was then closed with sutures. Dr. Curtis, whose expertise was dental surgery, may have tied his knot too closely to the ligature. His cutdown was ineffective and infiltrated into the tissues. Drs. Martin White and William Zedelitz stepped in to start another ankle cutdown, but when the one on the other ankle seemed successful, theirs was canceled.

Dr. Pepper Jenkins, the chief of anesthesiology, was at his usual position, at the patient's head. He began manually squeezing more oxygen into the president's lungs. As the oxygen began circulating, the bullet hole in JFK's throat began bubbling blood, and the clumps of brain dangling from his skull took on a more vibrant color. But Jenkins knew the artificial respiration wasn't going to save the president's life. Every time there was a heart compression, his head wound would seep blood, meaning there was massive vascular damage. When Jenkins spotted two priests come through the door, he turned his duties over to an associate and walked to the clergymen. The Vincentian priests, Fathers Oscar L. Huber and James N. Thompson, were affiliated with the nearby Holy Trinity Catholic Church. Huber had watched the presidential motorcade and returned to the church when Thompson told him about the shooting. They drove to Parkland and were astounded that they could simply talk their way into Trauma Room One. They didn't realize that someone on Mrs. Kennedy's behalf had requested a priest, and when Holy Trinity received the call, a parish official advised that two priests were already en route. Not being Catholic, Jenkins didn't know when the proper time was to administer Last Rites, the church's sacrament for a dying believer. Huber explained that it was usually before the soul leaves the body. But, in cases like this one, the priest said, the ritual could occur after Kennedy was declared dead.

Dr. Perry was only 34 years old but had considerable surgical experience, with as many as 200 gunshot wound cases. He entered the trauma room and decided the best course to help Kennedy breathe would be to bypass his nose and mouth. He spotted the small, circular opening that was slowly bleeding at the front of the president's throat. Perry asked Carrico if that was a hole he had made for a tracheotomy, but Carrico replied that it was a bullet hole. They washed away the blood, and

Perry could see that the edges of the hole were clean and not jagged. Perry feared that the bullet's path might have compromised critical areas, from the carotid artery to the jugular vein and lungs. Therefore, the tracheotomy incision would have to be made as low on the throat as possible. The bullet wound would provide the ideal location for a breathing tube to go directly into Kennedy's trachea, or wind-pipe. Both doctors agreed that the first course of action would be to keep the patient breathing.

Perry expanded the bullet hole with an incision about an inch wide, below the president's Adam's apple and to the right of the midline. Due to the presence of free air and blood around the endotracheal tube, Perry determined that the trachea was somewhat deviated to the left. Dr. Robert McClelland wielded a retractor to keep the tissue open while Perry used his scalpel to sever some of the strap muscles on its other side to reach the trachea. Dr. Baxter helped in the procedure. The endotracheal tube was then removed from JFK's mouth, and Perry inserted a tracheostomy tube into the chest. Drs. Jenkins and Buddy Giesecke then linked the tube to the respiratory machine to better control the circulatory system. Drs. Fouad Bashour and Donald Seldin entered the room. The former saw that there was a cardiac issue for which he could be helpful, but the latter saw there were no kidney issues, so he left the room. Bashour felt Kennedy's extremities and found them to be cold and connected the patient to a machine that measures heartbeats, known as a "torpedo." He got a blip, but it was likely from the artificial ventilation.

There was worry about subcutaneous emphysema, or air bubbles below the skin, so Perry requested that chest tubes be inserted to expand the president's chest cavity, seal the drainage, and protect the lungs. Drs. Peters and Baxter each made a small horizontal incision in the upper anterior chest wall on both sides, by the nipples. McClelland and Jones inserted the chest tube on the left side, and Peters and Baxter did the same for the right side. Trocars, or sharp-pointed instruments, were plunged into each incision, and rubber tubes with air holes were inserted. Then, the trocars were removed. The other ends of the tubes were put into water-sealed drainage bags to form negative pressure and expand the lungs. More pure oxygen began flowing into JFK's organs. All of this happened within about four minutes from Perry's arrival to the emergency room.

Next to enter the trauma room was neurosurgeon Clark. He inspected the head wound and noted that the president's eyes were deviated outward, slightly skewed, and did not react to light. He lifted up Kennedy's head and saw the large, gaping wound to the posterior part, with cerebral and cerebellar tissue damaged and exposed. He also noted the extreme amount of blood on the table, the floor, and the clothes of many of the people present. Dr. Baxter asked him: "Kemp, tell us how bad that head injury is, because we are losing him." Clark glumly replied: "My God, the whole right side of his head is shot off. We've got nothing to work with." Shaking his head at the futility of the situation, Clark felt for a carotid pulse but found none. He began an external cardiac massage with a defibrillator and requested that a more sensitive cardiac monitor be connected. Dr. Bashour was ready and switched over to a cardiotachyscope.

Dr. Perry, who was in a more advantageous position, took over with manual cardiac massage. For a brief moment, there was an elevation in the electrical activity of the heart, but it didn't last. Pepper Jenkins noted that the electrocardiogram reading was flat-lining, and Perry asked whether they should open Kennedy's chest and massage his heart. But Clark and Jenkins said it wouldn't do any good. The brain injury and loss of blood was too severe to sustain life. Just then, what remaining spark there was flickered out as the straight green line transversed the heart scope. There was no neurological or muscular response to the resuscitation attempts. The doctors could do no more. Jenkins shut off the breathing machine. Someone closed Kennedy's eyes, and Dr. Baxter covered him with a sheet.

The doctors who flooded into the trauma room that day had been dressed in their normal suits, white shirts, and ties. As they embarked on their life-saving mission, there was no time to don hospital scrubs. They all put on surgical gloves, and some tossed their jackets into a pile. When their duties were finished, their clothing and shoes were splattered with JFK's red blood and tissues, a grim souvenir of their historic day.

At 1:00 p.m., President John F. Kennedy was pronounced dead by Dr. Perry. Dr. Clark filled out and signed the death certificate, which he gave to Admiral Burkley, the commander-in-chief's physician. Clark walked over to Mrs. Kennedy, who had been watching everything. He advised her that her husband was deceased, and she nodded her head in acknowledgment. She thanked him and his team for doing all they could. As the medical personnel filtered out of the room, some wept. No doubt, every one of them reflected on the sorrowful page of history they had just witnessed. At that moment, they didn't consider their deeds and words would be reviewed in detail for decades to come but knew they had shared a life-altering experience.

The last remaining doctor in Trauma Room One was Pepper Jenkins, the anesthesiologist. The two priests and Mrs. Kennedy were also present. Without saying a word, the shell-shocked new widow approached Jenkins and opened her hand to give him a piece of skull and brain tissue she had been holding. It was a fragment she had grabbed as it flew onto the limousine trunk. Jenkins would later describe it as the worst heartbreak he had ever witnessed. When he was finally alone, he went to his office and made a Dictaphone recording of everything he observed, and even drew a diagram of all the people in the room that day. Jenkins, who died in 1994, testified to the Warren Commission about what he observed in that horrible half-hour. He resisted talking about it publicly and eschewed offers to write a book. But he used his diagram to assist Oliver Stone when the movie director filmed his masterpiece, *JFK*. Jenkins helped obtain vintage surgical equipment and set it up to perfectly replicate Trauma Room One in November 1963. My own experience with that film will be recounted in a subsequent chapter.

Father Huber prepared to administer Last Rites to the fallen leader. The ceremony gives spiritual aid to a dying Roman Catholic, absolving him or her of sin and blessing the person's eyes, ears, nose, mouth, hands, and for a male, loins. Huber's fellow priest, Father Thompson, observed. Several of the doctors returned for the benediction, including Baxter, McClelland, Bashour, and Crenshaw. They stood with Jenkins and some of the nurses with their heads respectfully bowed. The white sheet covered all of the president's body except for his bare right foot. Jackie knelt down and kissed her husband's big toe. Then she reached under the sheet for Jack Kennedy's right hand and pressed it against her cheek as she rose to her feet. At the end of the priest's blessing, Jackie took off her wedding ring and placed it on her husband's little finger, then kissed his cheek.

The Battle Over the Body

Following the brief religious ceremony, the priests departed, and the physicians stepped outside the trauma room, so that the nurses could prepare the president for transport to the medical examiner's office. Mrs. Kennedy sat in the hallway, as she smoked a cigarette. Someone had ordered a casket from the local Oneal Funeral Home. Aubrey Rike, who worked there, brought in the casket on a wheeled table. Outside, an ambulance was standing by to swoop away the president's corpse.

Nurses removed the rest of JFK's clothes. All of his clothing, his Ace bandage, and his back brace were put into two shopping bags and given to Secret Service agent Greer, who would bring them back to Washington, D.C. Nurse Pat Hutton removed the IVs and other tubes from the patient. When she took the tracheostomy tube from the president's throat, the wound that had been surgically expanded closed up on its own, so one would barely know there had been surgery. The bullet hole remained apparent. Supervising Nurse Nelson inspected the president's body as it was lifted into the coffin. She saw that the back of his head was missing. "There was no hair back there," she told investigators. "Some of his head was blown away and his brains were on the stretcher." Nurse Bowron cleaned the large defect in his head and packed it with gauze squares. Hutton told Nelson the bleeding was so bad that even though they had wrapped four white sheets around his head, the blood had seeped through. Nelson told her to find a plastic mattress pad with which to line the casket, and Hutton and Henchcliffe did so. The president's nude body, with the sheets around his head, was then placed in the casket.

Nurse Jeanette Standridge, who had finished her duties in Trauma Room Two, came into Kennedy's room with a mop. The black rubber floor was covered with empty bottles and boxes, tubing, bloody gauze and bandages, Jackie's roses, brain tissue and blood, and other detritus of the herculean task that was attempted there. After she and some orderlies picked up the debris, they swabbed and sterilized the floor, walls, and equipment. Before long, Trauma Room One was readied for its next patient, who might not even know what had occurred within those walls just minutes before.

Texas, like every other state in the nation, adheres to a law mandating that an autopsy be performed by the local jurisdiction in which the death occurred. An autopsy is required when a death is suspicious, unexpected, or outside the care of an attending doctor. The procedure is conducted by a licensed physician whose training and skills are used to determine the manner and cause of the death.

A "manner of death" has five possible classifications: homicide, suicide, accident, natural, or undetermined. A "cause of death" refers to the way in which the person died: gunshot, stabbing, blunt force trauma, asphyxia, drowning, drug overdose, poisoning, etc. The findings of manner and cause of death are then entered into the official record in the form of an autopsy report. John Fitzgerald Kennedy's manner of death was clearly a homicide, and his cause of death was from a gunshot or gunshots. Even though he perished on an operating table, with more than a dozen physicians surrounding him, his death still required an autopsy. Then, his wounds could be inspected, tracked, and evaluated. Information about the bullet or bullets that might be surgically removed would become useful for police in helping to find the suspected shooter and for prosecutors who would be taking that suspect to court and trying him or her for the murder. At least, that's how it was supposed to work.

Earl Forrest Rose, 37, was the board-certified medical examiner for the Dallas Coroner's office. While working in that office, he also obtained a law degree from Southern Methodist University in Dallas. Dr. Rose's office was at Parkland Hospital, across the corridor from Trauma Room One. When he heard that President Kennedy had expired, he went to talk to Secret Service supervisor Roy Kellerman, the Secret Serviceman with the machine gun, and Dr. George Burkley, who were standing near the body that had been placed in the casket. The two agents advised Rose that they would be leaving with the body at once and that the autopsy would be performed at a military facility near Washington, D.C.

Rose politely informed them of the state law that gave him jurisdiction of the procedure and said that there was a need to preserve the "chain of custody." The body was evidence, and there had to be a well-documented trail of who had access and possession of the body from when it was declared dead to when it was buried. In any legal matter that would follow, violating the chain of custody would give a defense attorney a wide berth to point at sloppy or aberrant handling of the chief piece of evidence. Besides, Rose said, this case would be tried in Dallas because, at its essence, it was a homicide that occurred in Dallas County.

Just as politely, Kellerman and Burkley told him that none of that applied to this death. Federal prosecutors might take over this case, since the decedent was the president of the United States. This was uncharted territory, they acknowledged, but the feds were on the scene and would trump local authorities. Governor John Connally was in no condition to mediate. After he was stabilized in Trauma Room Two, he was brought up to the surgical suite on the second floor, where he was presently undergoing an operation. Rose explained that he already had a craniotomy room that Nurse Wester had previously set up and that he could quickly surgically remove the president's skull and inspect the damage to it and his throat. Then everyone would know the ammunition and directionality of the bullet or bullets that penetrated the president. He also needed to maintain possession of any bullet or fragments found in the body, he argued. It was Rose's duty, too, to study the clothing the president wore when he was shot and to visit the crime scene.

Kellerman, the other agent, and Burkley didn't care about any of that. Rose would later tell Dr. Robert McClelland that the agent who didn't have the machine gun—presumably, Kellerman—put his arms under Rose's armpits, lifted him into the air, and set him down gently against a wall. It wasn't an action designed to hurt Dr. Rose but to show him who was boss. The men informed Rose that the nation was currently without a president. Lyndon Johnson was en route to Air Force One where he would be given the oath of office while the plane was on the tarmac. That would officially promote him from second-in-line to commander-in-chief. Then, without delay, Johnson would fly back to Washington, D.C. But the vice president was refusing to be sworn in without Mrs. Kennedy, President Kennedy, and his casket onboard. Rose was the only bump in the road for a smooth transition from one administration to the next. Surely, he had to understand that.

Plus, they stated, Mrs. Kennedy wouldn't even consider leaving Dallas on Air Force One without her husband. The poor woman who suffered so intensely needed to get to the White House to be with her very young children and advise them of their daddy's death before they heard it from someone else. Only an insensitive and cruel person would want to get in the way of that. (Caroline would end up hearing the bad news from the children's nanny, Maud Shaw, at the direction of Jackie's mother, which angered Jackie.) Kellerman and Burkley stated that the widow was stained with her husband's blood and brain matter from stem to stern and desperately needed to return home to change her clothes.

Rose's head was spinning. He felt he needed backup, so he called for Vernon Stembridge, the chief of surgical pathology, and Sidney Stewart, a pathology resident, to help him hold his ground. A police officer was also there. All three doctors explained the state law again and their intent to perform the president's autopsy in Dallas. It could be done in as quickly as 45 minutes, they said—an impossibly short time, in my view. The body could then be shipped to Washington immediately afterward. Rose didn't understand why Johnson couldn't be sworn in as the plane was in the air. He reasoned that Mrs. Kennedy could remain in Dallas until her husband was ready and then join him on a subsequent flight. The Johnsons could take Air Force One, and the Kennedys could take Air Force Two. Rose's staff would do everything to make Mrs. Kennedy comfortable for the extra hour or so that she was in town. Or she could return now on Air Force One and be with her children and in clean clothing sooner, then see the president's body when it arrived in her town.

That was unthinkable, Kellerman said, with Dr. Burkley echoing the comments. Johnson wanted Mrs. Kennedy there to witness his swearing-in. That's all there was to it. Besides, they snarled, it didn't matter what Rose thought. He was just wasting their precious time. Tempers flared, obscenities flew, and shoving ensued between the two sides. More Secret Service and FBI agents showed up to fortify the decision to take JFK's body at once.

Rose blocked the exit of the doorway with his body. His pathology associates stood behind him. Aubrey Rike held onto the casket that his company had supplied, which was being pushed and pulled by the warring factions. Not only were the Dallas pathologists overruled, but the feds also had firearms and could use them if they needed to. First Kellerman showed his gun, then the other Secret Servicemen pushed back their suit coats to show that they, too, were armed. Rose's two colleagues stormed out of the room and called for a local Justice of the Peace, Theron Ward, to arbitrate. But Ward passed the buck and said he would have to consult with Dallas County District Attorney Henry Wade. In a phone call, Wade said he felt that any bullet recovered would have to be turned over to Dallas Police Chief Jesse Curry. In a separate call, Curry confirmed that opinion. But Justice of the Peace Ward ignored the advice of the two local authorities who outranked him and, with a nod of the head, let Kellerman wheel away the casket containing JFK's body. Texas law be damned.

The Stretcher Bullet

Parkland Memorial Hospital in 1963 consisted of five floors: the basement; the ground floor where the emergency entrance, the pit, and the trauma rooms were; the first floor; the second floor where the surgical suites were; and the third floor. A small self-service elevator took passengers up and down. Around 1:00 p.m., the hospital's senior engineer, Darrell C. Tomlinson, was called by his supervisor. Normally, Tomlinson's duties were to maintain the building's heating and air conditioning units, but, on this day, there was a special order. He was assigned to manually operate the elevator, using a key so that the car would only travel between the ground floor and the second floor.

After Governor Connally was brought on a stretcher into the second floor operating room, Tomlinson took the empty stretcher down to the ground floor. He positioned it against the south wall, beside another empty stretcher. I will call the Connally stretcher "A" and the other one "B." Stretcher A had white sheets and a black mattress pad, whereas Stretcher B had a black mattress pad; bloody sheets; surgical instruments; and items such as gauze, a sponge, and paper wrapping that might have been from a hypodermic needle. Tomlinson would later say he didn't know who the patient on Stretcher B had been. A doctor needing to use the men's room moved Stretcher B aside and left it there after he exited the bathroom. Tomlinson walked to that stretcher and gave it a little kick to get it back in line. He heard a rattle and saw that a virtually intact bullet had rolled out from under the mattress pad. He picked it up and put it in his pocket.

Tomlinson would soon turn the bullet over to hospital security director O.P. Wright. Wright attempted to give custody of the bullet to an FBI agent, who refused to take it. Secret Service agent Richard Johnson would later take custody of the bullet and sign a receipt for it, then turned it over to Secret Service Chief James Rowley. That bullet would be ballistically linked to the Mannlicher-Carcano rifle that was purportedly fired by Lee Harvey Oswald. The Warren Commission Report, the official guide to the investigation, would conclude that the bullet fell out of Governor Connally's thigh when he was moved off the stretcher. However, Tomlinson was consistent in his testimony to the Commission, as well as in frequent interviews, that the bullet was found on Stretcher B and not Stretcher A on which Connally was transported. Despite the clarity of his remembrance, the Commission concluded that Tomlinson had been mistaken. I, as well as most serious Kennedy assassination researchers, believe Tomlinson's account. At home that night, Tomlinson was awakened by a phone call just before 1:00 a.m. An FBI agent was calling to tell him to "keep his mouth shut" about the bullet he found.

Much later, Tomlinson, Wright, and Johnson were shown a bullet said to be the one they had handled that day. But because there had been a broken chain of evidence, all three men declined to identify it as the bullet they had previously seen. Neither Wright nor Johnson was questioned by the Warren Commissioners. And even later, O.P. Wright would tell Kennedy researcher Josiah Thompson that the bullet Tomlinson had given him had a nose that was pointed. The bullet that the federal authorities showed him had a rounded nose.

For reasons you will come to understand, this copper-jacketed missile was dubbed the "magic bullet," a nickname I believe Mark Lane created that has stuck through the years. The bullet's first feat of prestidigitation was how it managed to jump from one stretcher to the other and deposit itself under the mattress pad until it was ready for its grand debut. And since I will later explain the implausibility of a bullet falling neatly out of human flesh, consider the alternative: that it was placed on that stretcher by someone intent to have that bullet traced back to a specific weapon. Now, who could have assisted in such a magic trick? While no one observed the bullet being planted, some very solid sources encountered Jack Ruby at the hospital that afternoon.

Veteran reporter Seth Kantor, who had been riding in the motorcade's press car, saw Ruby at Parkland that day. Kantor, 37, had first met Ruby in 1960 while working at the *Dallas Times-Herald*. Ruby owned local strip clubs and would occasionally stop by the newsroom to pitch human interest stories about his dancers. In November 1963, Kantor was writing for the Scripps-Howard chain of newspapers and arrived at Parkland, desperate to confirm that the president had died and learn the condition of the vice president. In the pandemonium, Ruby came up behind him, pulled on his jacket, and addressed him by name. They exchanged comments about what a terrible thing had happened, then Ruby asked him if he should close his clubs for the next three nights. Kantor said that would probably be a good idea.

KXOL Radio newsman Roy Stamps was on a pay phone at Parkland, trying to make a call, when he saw Ruby enter with a TV crew, carrying some of their equipment. They acknowledged each other. Stamps had met Ruby dozens of times before, so he was firm in his identification of him. Housewife Wilma Tice didn't know Ruby and didn't recognize him until she saw photos of him in the press following Oswald's murder. She told the Warren Commission that she was at the hospital, standing just a couple of feet from Ruby and a man who was holding a suitcase. She overheard the man call Ruby "Jack" and mention that Governor Connally might need a new kidney. Jack replied that, if true, he would donate one of his. (Connally would not require a kidney donation.) Tice also testified that she had received a phone call at home, in which a male voice she didn't recognize told her to "keep her mouth shut."

The Warren Commission didn't interview Stamps—and, although they deposed both Kantor and Tice, it was determined that the witnesses were just wrong. The Commissioners chose to go with Jack Ruby's account instead. He insisted he wasn't at Parkland the day that JFK was shot. If Jack Ruby were at Parkland while the president was being treated, why wouldn't he admit it? Maybe because it would tie him to a higher degree of involvement in the case than he—or his handlers—were willing to admit.

The Arrest
of Lee Harvey Oswald

As Tom Noguchi and I settled back to watch more news coverage, we wondered what had happened with the young man we heard had been arrested. And what more did police learn about the so-called sniper's nest? Soon, every TV channel had the updates. When Dallas police officers ran into the Texas School Book Depository building, they navigated through boxes that were stacked on the sixth floor. Near the window of the southeast corner were three expended cartridge cases, laid out on the floor. On the other side of the room was a rifle, sticking out of a crevice. A police affidavit identified it as a 7.65 mm German Mauser. The next day, the rifle's description would be amended to that of an Italian Mannlicher-Carcano. Ballistics reports matched the gun to the bullets.

As depository superintendent Roy Truly escorted police officer M.L. Baker through the building, they encountered Lee Harvey Oswald in the second floor lunchroom. Oswald was nonchalantly drinking a bottle of Coca Cola that he had just bought from a vending machine. This was no more than 90 seconds since the last gunshot was fired. If Oswald had been the rifleman on the alleged sixth-floor sniper's perch, he would have had to run down four flights of stairs to get to the lunchroom. Such an act would have caused his pulse to race. But when Truly and Baker spoke with him, Oswald wasn't out of breath at all.

According to the Warren Commission, Oswald left the depository, walked seven short blocks east on Elm Street, and boarded a westward bus. He was spotted there by Mary Bledsoe, a former landlady who recognized him. When the bus became stuck in traffic, due to the motorcade and assassination, Oswald got off and walked to a taxi a few blocks away. He asked his driver to take him a location a few blocks beyond where Oswald had been living. A restaurant owner named A.C. Johnson and his wife, Gladys, owned a rooming house at 1026 North Beckley Avenue. Its location was in Dallas' Oak Cliff district, about two miles southwest of Dealey Plaza. On October 14, Oswald rented one of the 17 bedrooms there and moved in. When Oswald signed the register for the $8-per-week room, he wrote his name as "O.H. Lee." It would not be until after JFK's murder and Oswald's subsequent arrest—when cops found the Beckley address in his pocket and went to the house—that the Johnsons learned their tenant's actual name. Oswald's room was a former library and, at about 8 by 12', one of

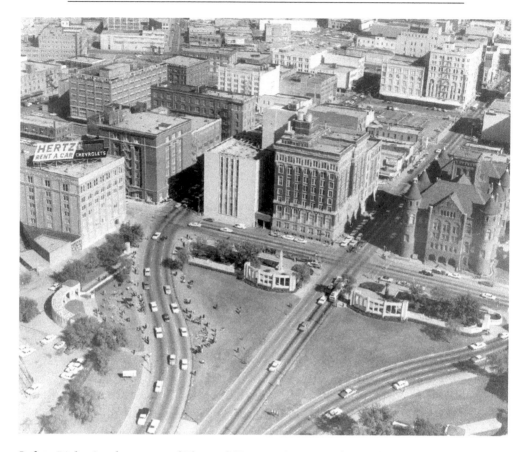

Left to Right: On the corner of Elm and Houston Streets is the Book Depository, under the Hertz sign; behind it is the Dal-Tex Building; across Elm is the Records Building, and the County Jail on Houston and Main Streets. The motorcade could have come straight down Main to get to the freeway, so why did it make the right turn onto Houston, then left onto Elm? A sniper's nest assassin would have had a cleaner shot at an approaching car, rather than one departing—but were gunmen also atop the other buildings or on the grassy knoll in the bushes by the left lower quadrant? (Robert J. Groden Collection).

the smaller rentals in the home, but it had windows on one wall and curtains. He was also allowed to use the living room and refrigerator.

Earlene Roberts was the residence's live-in housekeeper. The man she knew as "Mr. Lee" kept to himself and seldom smiled or talked to anyone there. She and the Johnsons liked him because he kept his room neat and didn't monopolize the bathroom he shared with five other men. Sometimes he would use the pay phone. He could be heard talking to someone in Russian. On most Fridays he would announce that he was going out of town, and he'd return on Monday. Just after 1:00 p.m., Roberts' friend told her that the president had been shot, so Earlene tried to get reception on the living room's television set. There was audio, but the picture kept flickering in and out. As she was adjusting the TV's rabbit ears antenna, Oswald entered in a rush. Roberts remarked, "You sure are in a hurry," but he didn't respond or even look at her as he passed by. During the three or four minutes that Oswald was in his room,

Roberts heard two toots of a horn and looked out the front window. Outside was a Dallas police cruiser, slowly pulling away. She could see two uniformed officers in the car. Oswald exited his room and left the home, walking in a southeast direction. Roberts told investigators that he wore some kind of a shirt when he entered and came out of his room wearing a jacket. She saw him zip it up as he left. She couldn't recall his pants' color and didn't see him holding a gun or having one tucked into his waistband. But investigators believed he took a .38 handgun with him and used it shortly thereafter.

At 1:15 p.m., at the corner of 10th Street and Patton Avenue, less than a mile southeast of the boarding house, Dallas police officer J.D. Tippit was fatally shot outside of his patrol car. Tippit, whose "J.D." were only initials and did not represent actual names, was a 39-year-old former U.S. Army paratrooper. He was awarded a Bronze Star during the last airborne deployment over Germany in World War II. A married father of three, he joined the Dallas police force in 1952 and later earned a medal for bravery for disarming a fugitive. Like many underpaid officers, he supplemented his income by working as a security guard at a restaurant. That afternoon, Tippit, wearing his police uniform, drove his normal beat through the streets of Oak Cliff. While he usually patrolled with a partner, on this round he was alone in his squad car. By 12:54 p.m., he had heard several police radio transmissions to be on the lookout for a male suspected in the death of President Kennedy. The perpetrator was described as a "white male, about 30, 5'8", black hair, slender, wearing a white jacket, white shirt, and dark slacks."

Tippit pulled up alongside a man who fit that description. The man was walking in the same direction as Tippit and stopped beside the police cruiser. The two exchanged words, with the man speaking through the car's passenger vent window. Tippit got out of his car and stood by the driver's door, with his gun removed from his holster. But the other man shot first. In a rapid burst, three shots were fired into the officer's chest, causing him to fall backward, into the street. The gunman then fired one additional shot into Tippit's right temple. Tippit died at the scene, without having fired his gun. Dallas medical examiner Earl Rose, who was barred from performing the president's autopsy, conducted Tippit's postmortem at the Parkland morgue, beginning at 3:15 p.m. that day. The shots blasted through the patrolman's heart, right lung, liver, and brain.

A number of witnesses heard or saw aspects of Tippit's crime scene. Unfortunately, the stories they told were wildly divergent. Most heard two or three shots, whereas others heard five or six. And most missed the actual shooting, only catching its immediate aftermath. One used the cruiser's radio to call in the shooting, another picked up the gun and put it inside the vehicle, and a few would help paramedics load the fallen cop's body into the ambulance. Several witnesses saw the gunman run from the scene, whereas others saw him casually stroll away, reloading his gun as he turned the corner. Domingo Benavides told investigators that he saw the shooter take spent bullet casings from his gun and toss them into the street. Benavides picked up two of the shells and put them in his pack of cigarettes, which he turned over to detectives later. Most described the shooter as having dark hair, a fair complexion, being in his 20s or 30s, 5'10" or under, and of average weight. The gunman's clothing was generally viewed as dark trousers, a dark shirt over a white T-shirt, and wearing a tan-gray jacket. Such a jacket was even found under a vehicle in a nearby used car lot. (No DNA testing existed in those days, so there was no confirmation of who had been wearing the jacket.) Many of the observers were brought to police headquarters and asked to view a four-man lineup that included Lee Harvey Oswald, who had subsequently been taken into custody. Most, but not all, identified Oswald as resembling the man they saw leaving the Tippit murder.

If there were to be a trial of the man who killed J.D. Tippit, these sightings and inconsistencies would come into play to help or hinder either side. But in the world of the Warren Commission, the witnesses who told differing stories were often repeatedly grilled by Dallas police or the FBI until their stories were locked into a scenario that pointed to Oswald as the shooter. At that point, they would be questioned by Commission attorneys, and, only then, their accounts would be made part of the public record.

You could search the Commission's full 26 volumes of evidence and testimony, and you'd never see the narrative of Acquilla Clemons. Her observations were not disclosed until assassination researcher/lawyer Mark Lane interviewed her on film for a 1966 television program. Clemons lived near the murder site and knew Tippit as a regular patrolman for the area. She was sitting on her front porch when she saw him gunned down. But Clemons saw two men involved in the attack. The shooter was short and heavy. The other man was tall and thin, and wore khaki pants and a white shirt. Neither description comports to Oswald's appearance or what he was said to be wearing that day. Clemons added that once Tippit was on the ground, the shooter waved off the other man, and they left the scene in opposite directions. She told Lane she was soon visited by a man who didn't give his name but carried a handgun. He told her that she should not repeat her story to others "or she might get hurt."

The Warren Commission stated that only one female, Helen Markham, was an eyewitness to the shooting. The panel also stated that the FBI did not interview any other female who claimed to have witnessed the shooting, and the Commission had no information about any other female witness. Markham was a local waitress who said she saw the shooting. In fact, she claimed she had been alone with Tippit for 20 minutes as he struggled to talk to her before he died. She described the gunman as being short and small, with bushy hair and a ruddy complexion, and dressed in a white shirt and brown jacket. At first, she said the man wore light-gray trousers, then she said they were dark colored. Markham was so addled, she put the work shoes she had been carrying on the roof of Tippit's squad car and never asked for them back. She also fainted at the scene, was taken to Parkland Hospital, and later released to police custody to view the four-man lineup. At first, she said she didn't recognize any of the men as the shooter, but after seeing a TV news clip of Oswald, she identified him in the lineup. She was interviewed on three occasions by lawyers for the Warren Commission and initially insisted that she never gave an interview to Mark Lane. But Lane had an audio tape of the interview, which he furnished to the Commissioners. When they played it for Markham, she denied it was her voice on the tape. Then she said it was her voice, but instead of acknowledging that Lane was asking the questions, she said it was a Dallas policeman.

And yet, the Warren Commission lawyers preferred to believe Helen Markham over Acquilla Clemons. It was easier for them to manipulate Markham to do their bidding than to investigate the doors that Clemons' account opened. They wanted one killer—Lee Harvey Oswald—and anything that led to him possibly having an associate or being part of a conspiracy was to be denied at all costs. The Commissioners would have an ongoing practice of cherry-picking witness testimony that helped their theory while ignoring that which did not. They were also adept at shaping testimony by pre-interviewing witnesses prior to going on record. All of which seems a very skewed way of conducting business if the goal was to find the truth.

From our table at the restaurant, Tom Noguchi and I had no inkling what the Tippit witnesses would be telling the Commissioners. It would be days before the Warren Commission would even be conceived. At that point, all we knew was that a Dallas police officer had been shot to death near where the president had died, and there were rumblings that the same shooter might be responsible for both crimes. Police cars with their sirens blaring rushed to the Tippit shooting site.

Investigators claimed the man believed to be Oswald turned right onto West Jefferson Boulevard, discarded his jacket, and continued walking west for a few more blocks. He passed a shoe store, whose manager, Johnny Brewer, had just heard about the wanted fugitive on his radio. He saw a man quickly step into his doorway and face him, as a patrol car drove by. Then the man left. Brewer followed at a safe distance and saw the man duck into the Texas Theatre movie house, a couple doors away. Two war movies were on the marquee. Brewer notified cashier Julia Postal that a suspicious man had walked into the theater without buying a ticket, and she phoned the police. The time was 1:40 p.m. Moments later, a floor of police cars arrived at the theater and officers, with their guns drawn, ran inside. The house lights came on. Accompanied by patrolman M.N. McDonald, Brewer looked over the moviegoers until he spotted the man he saw sneak into the theater. As McDonald ordered the suspect to his feet, the man drew a gun from his waistband with one hand and swung a punch at the officer with the other hand. Other policemen—including R.C. Nelson, who was usually Tippit's partner—ran to the rescue. The suspect received a cut over his right eye and a black left eye. Soon he was in handcuffs and under arrest.

Lee Harvey Oswald was the person arrested. I won't argue whether he was the person who shot Officer J.D. Tippit. The timeline and many details seem to fit. But there were many holes in the narrative that might have been patched if Oswald had been allowed to offer a defense. As you will learn, he was not afforded that opportunity. Some assassination researchers believe that Tippit had more involvement in the

Kennedy case than has been revealed. Several believe he might have been sacrificed to incite more public anger toward Oswald as a plausible presidential assassin if he was already a stone-cold cop killer. Other critics feel that Tippit was supposed to kill Oswald, which could explain why he didn't radio in his sighting of a wanted suspect before confronting him. And one writer wondered whether an extra uniform jacket hanging in Tippit's cruiser might have been there to aid Oswald's escape, suggesting that as proof Oswald was not the patrolman's shooter. I wish I knew the answer.

LBJ Becomes President

Aboard Air Force One, as previously noted, Lyndon B. Johnson would not allow the plane to depart Love Field until Jackie Kennedy and the casket carrying her husband were onboard. U.S. District Court Judge Sarah T. Hughes arrived, wearing a polka dot suit because she didn't have time to stop and get her robe. She also didn't bring a Bible, so a Catholic missal found in a drawer in what had been JFK's airborne bedroom would be used instead.

At Parkland, Kennedy's casket was loaded into a hearse. Jackie, her Secret Service agent Clint Hill, and Dr. Burkley rode in the back, while two other Secret Service agents and supervisor Roy Kellerman were in the front. Escorted by police, the hearse sped off and soon arrived on the tarmac of Love Field. The Secret Service agents quickly realized that the plane's doorway was too narrow for the coffin to make it through, so they broke off one of its handles. Staff Sergeant John Hames and other flight stewards had made room at the back of the presidential plane by taking out a bulkhead and four seats, and the coffin was finally loaded and locked into place. Lady Bird Johnson, noting that Mrs. Kennedy was still in her blood-caked clothing, asked if she would like to change her outfit. But Jackie declined, stating: "I want them to see what they have done to Jack."

It was 2:38 p.m. CST when Vice President Johnson began the swearing-in process as the next president of the United States. His wife stood to his right, and Mrs. Kennedy was on his left. Judge Hughes said these words, and Johnson repeated them: "I do solemnly swear that I will faithfully execute the Office of the President of the United States and will, to the best of my ability, preserve, protect, and defend the Constitution of the United States." At the conclusion of Johnson's oath, the roar of Air Force One's engines could be heard. Hughes disembarked, and the rest of those onboard settled into their seats for the journey back to Washington, D.C. By 2:47 p.m., the jet was in the air. It would arrive at Andrews Air Force Base at 5:58 p.m. EST.

After the swearing in of Johnson, Dr. Noguchi and I decided this would be a good opportunity to leave the restaurant and continue our news viewing at his home. Later, he would drive me to my hotel. After being imbued with the dreadful details of the death of this young president in front of his wife, I craved to hear the voice of my spouse, Sigrid. She was in Pittsburgh caring for our sons: David, who was 18 months

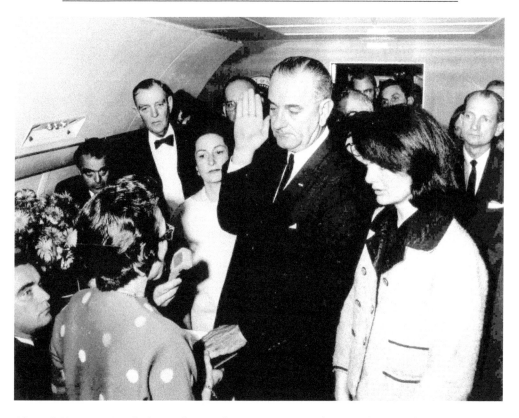

Aboard Air Force One before it departed Texas, Vice President Lyndon B. Johnson was sworn in as our 36th U.S. president. Jacqueline Kennedy is on his left, and his wife Lady Bird is on his right. President Kennedy's body is in a casket nearby (Cecil Stoughton, The White House via Associated Press).

old, and Danny, who had just been born in September. Sigrid had been closely watching the news coverage as well and brought up the two Kennedy children, who would now be without a father. Jacqueline and her children would have to move from the White House, which was their home and not just a national landmark. As much as I would have liked to return home myself, I had other business to attend to in Los Angeles. I told Sigrid I would stick to my itinerary and see her and our boys on Sunday, November 24.

Who Was
Lee Harvey Oswald?

After an unsettling night in a Los Angeles hotel, I awoke on Saturday, November 23, 1963, hoping I had had the world's worst dream. I had an appointment at a law firm to give a day-long deposition. It couldn't be postponed because there was a court date coming up, and these were the days before such activities could be done remotely.

The attorneys I was meeting with had been listening to the radio, so when I arrived, they filled me in on what had happened overnight. I learned about impromptu press conferences with Lee Harvey Oswald where he requested legal assistance. All the lawyers in the room, me included, would have relished the chance to speak with him, not because we were convinced of his innocence—far from it—but because it would have given us unique insight into the thought processes of what well could be a diseased mind. If Oswald were the president's assassin and killer of a Dallas policeman, he must have had some powerful motivation that would be interesting to know. But if he were just a patsy, as he suggested, that would be even *more* fascinating.

Lee Harvey Oswald was born in New Orleans, Louisiana, on October 18, 1939, making him 24 at the time of the assassination. His mother, Marguerite, was a 32-year-old law firm receptionist when Lee was born. She had divorced her first husband, Edward John Pic, Jr., in 1931, when she was three months pregnant with their son, John. The elder Pic supported the child for 18 years but never saw him after the boy's first birthday. Marguerite wed Robert Edward Lee Oswald, a divorced insurance man, in 1933. It was a happy marriage, with son Robert born the next year. But two months before Lee's birth, his father had a fatal heart attack, which sent the family scrambling. All three boys were placed in a children's home as their mother struggled to support the family.

In 1943, she met Edwin A. Ekdahl, whose engineering job would relocate him to Texas. Marguerite joined him there, first with Lee and then with the other boys. Marguerite and Edwin married in 1945, and he was a devoted father figure to the children. While the older boys attended a military boarding school, Marguerite traveled with her husband and Lee, with whom she had an especially close bond. Eventually, the family moved to a large home with an acre of land in the Fort Worth suburb of Benbrook. But the Ekdahl marriage fell apart, due to Edwin's infidelity and Marguerite's claims that he was too controlling with money. In 1946, Marguerite moved back to Covington, Louisiana, with her three sons, and the attending upheaval caused Lee to have to repeat the first grade. The Ekdahls reconciled and moved back to Fort Worth, but their difficulties continued until 1948, when they divorced. Marguerite restored her last name to Oswald.

By 1952, Marguerite and her sons moved to New York City, where Lee attended a Lutheran Church school and displayed chronic truancy. While he amused himself with reading, he wouldn't interact with kids his own age. One psychologist evaluated the 13-year-old as "in the upper range of bright normal intelligence," whereas another diagnosed him as having a schizoid personality with passive-aggressive instincts.

Marguerite's older sister Lillian lived in New Orleans with her husband, ex-boxer Charles "Dutz" Murret, and their five children, and Lee visited frequently over the years. During the Warren Commission investigation, Dutz was described as a steamship clerk. But the House Select Committee on Assassinations later uncovered that Murret was an illegal bookmaker with ties to local organized crime.

The Mafia chief in New Orleans at the time was Carlos Marcello, a wealthy illegal alien from Sicily who was capable of extreme violence. Marcello, who was called "The Little Man," was barely five feet tall and shaped like a fireplug but carried himself with confidence. Marcello was no fan of the Kennedy brothers. In 1959, he appeared before a U.S. Senate panel that was investigating organized crime and labor racketeering in America. Then–Senator John F. Kennedy served on the panel, while his brother, Bobby, was the committee's chief counsel. Marcello took the Fifth Amendment scores of times. While that action was within his rights, it angered the U.S. Justice Department, which began proceedings to deport him—but Marcello's lawyers always kept him protected in his many mansions.

Once John Kennedy was elected president and appointed his brother Bobby as U.S. attorney general, the heat was turned up. In April 1961, RFK had federal agents deport Marcello, putting him on a C-130 transport plane, flying him to Guatemala, and dumping him in the jungle in his silk suit and alligator shoes. He had no cash or provisions and two broken ribs. Within three days, he was able to make a phone call to his wife, who arranged his rescue. Two months later, a furious Marcello was back in the states. Bobby Kennedy demanded that the FBI step up its prosecutions against Marcello and his ilk. But long-time Bureau director J. Edgar Hoover refused to acknowledge that our country had a problem with organized crime. Perhaps it was due to his cozy relationships with the very criminal element that encouraged his racetrack and casino visits, making certain that he won more than his fair share. To Hoover, Marcello was simply a businessman who owned a tomato canning company and lived the American dream.

By 1963, Marcello took the Kennedys' animosity toward him personally and plotted revenge. He told an associate that if Jack were eliminated, all the troubles with Bobby would go away. Marcello had two lieutenants with connections to Dutz Murret, one of whom the committee also linked to Jack Ruby. Murret died in 1964.

Oswald and his mother moved back to New Orleans in 1954. The next year, shortly after starting the 10th grade, Lee quit school and worked as an office clerk. He joined the Civil Air Patrol (CAP), the civilian auxiliary of the USAF. According to other cadets in his program, Lee attended several meetings over a two-month period. Then, as now, members performed search-and-rescue operations, disaster relief, and humanitarian services, training cadets for a career in aerospace or the military. Some CAP members were pilots with private aircraft for their volunteer missions. One such member was David Ferrie, of whom you will read more about in a future chapter. A famous black-and-white photo purports to show Ferrie with a group of cadets, one of which is said to be a teenaged Lee Oswald. You can find the photo on the internet and decide for yourself if it portrays the two men: The "young Oswald" looks like other photos I've seen of Lee as a teen, but the face of the person depicted as Ferrie is obscured by his helmet.

Lee and his mother returned to Fort Worth where he promised her he would finish school. He re-enrolled in the 10th grade, but again dropped out and never received a diploma. In 1956, at 17, Oswald enlisted in the U.S. Marine Corps, perhaps to emulate his brother Robert, who was already in the service. Lee began his three-year tour of duty with boot camp at the Second Training Battalion in San Diego, California. From there, he was posted to the Naval Air Technical Training Center in Jacksonville, Florida, and then Keesler Air Force Base in Biloxi, Mississippi.

In July 1957, he was brought to the Marine Corps Air Station at El Toro, California, where he received combat infantry training, specializing in radar, aviation electronics, and aircraft surveillance. Oswald's spotless record permitted him to handle classified material marked "Confidential," and he was given a security clearance. The next month, he sailed to Japan on the USS *Bexar* and joined the Marine Air Squadron No. 1 at Atsugi. This outpost was a critical one for the U.S. military, which used it to monitor Russian air and sea traffic, and dispatch the CIA's U-2 jets for espionage missions. The U-2 could soar at an altitude of 70,000 feet, allowing it to escape anti-aircraft weaponry. Its camera would take high-resolution photos of Soviet military installations.

Captain Francis Gary Powers was one of the elite U-2 pilots. On May 1, 1960, his plane was shot down over Russian air space. Powers broke two rules that U-2 pilots were trained to adhere to if shot down: He didn't self-destruct the aircraft before he parachuted from it, and he refused to scratch himself with the poisoned coin our government furnished to its spy pilots, so they could die of suicide and keep their secrets intact. The Russian military gleefully recovered the plane's sophisticated equipment. Powers was captured, convicted of espionage, held in a Soviet prison, and used for anti–American propaganda. In 1962, Powers and an American student who was also in Russian custody were bartered for Soviet spy Colonel Rudolf Abel, who had been arrested by the FBI and was being held in an American prison. The dramatic exchange took place on a Berlin bridge.

Oswald's proficiency with a rifle was tested twice while in the Marines. Shortly after enlisting, he scored a 212, two points over the minimum requirement to earn the title of "sharpshooter." His skills dropped for his May 1959 test, when he only scored 191, just one point over the minimum for a "marksman," the lowest level for Marine rifle-firing. A colleague who trained with Oswald, Nelson Delgado, told the Warren Commission that Lee got a lot of "Maggie's drawers," which was Marine-speak for total misses. As JFK researcher Mark Lane would tell me later, Delgado was visited by FBI agents who pressed him to change his remembrance so that it reflected that Oswald was a better shot.

In November 1957, Oswald accidentally shot himself in the elbow with an unauthorized small, short-barreled pistol. He was punished with a court martial, then court martialed again when he got into a scuffle with a sergeant. He was briefly imprisoned in the brig, and he was demoted from private first class to just a private. While on night-time guard duty in the Philippines, he earned more punishment by firing his rifle blindly into the jungle. In 1958, Oswald returned to the El Toro air station. Some of his fellow Marines thought he was college educated because he was so well read. He also liked to play chess and would regale his military buddies with thoughts about socialism. When his buddies saw him studying Russian magazines, they nicknamed him "Oswaldkovitch." The Marines tested Oswald's proficiency in Russian, and he received an average score, but does that imply that the USMC was teaching him the language? And if so, why? Foreign language training was not part of the typical Marine protocol.

In 1963, Victor L. Marchetti, Jr., was a CIA agent specializing in Cold War espionage but would later quit and write books that were critical of the U.S. intelligence community. Marchetti described how the Office of Naval Intelligence established a program where several dozen young American men were assigned to appear disenchanted about the United States and would be sent into Russia or Eastern Europe. Their goal was to be recruited as KGB agents, but they'd actually function as "double agents," since their true loyalties would remain with America. The men were trained in U.S. Naval installations abroad. At the Marine base in Atsugi, one of Oswald's case officers was Gerry Patrick Hemming, who had worked for Fidel Castro as a CIA double agent, then turned virulently anti–Castro once he left Cuba. Was Oswald part of the ONI program Marchetti described, and was Hemming his handler?

In September 1959, Oswald received a hardship discharge from the Marines, after requesting that he be allowed to tend to his ailing mother in Fort Worth. His mother had bruised her nose and missed a day of work, and on that basis he got a hardship discharge? That's hard to fathom. He spent two days with her and then traveled to New Orleans. From Louisiana, he sailed to Le Havre, France, and then to Southampton, England. There he told authorities he planned to stay in the United Kingdom for a week and then go to a school in Switzerland. But on that same day, he flew to Helsinki, Finland, where he received a Soviet visa. He took a train to Moscow and arrived on October 16, two days before his 20th birthday. Upon his arrival, he told representatives of the Moscow Intourist office that he wanted to renounce his U.S. citizenship and become a citizen of what he called the "great Soviet Union."

On October 21, the day his travel visa was set to expire, he was informed that his request was denied. He would have to leave the country that night. When the Intourist guide arrived at Oswald's hotel to escort him from the country, she found him in the bathtub, with his wrist slashed by a razor. Although the cut was minor, there was a lot of blood. Soviet officials had to consider that it was a legitimate suicide attempt, so they admitted him to a hospital for a week of psychiatric observation. During that time, he was debriefed by skeptical bureaucrats about his reasons for wanting to stay in Russia. He showed them his identification, including his Marine Corps discharge papers, and told them he was a radar operator. If he were able to become a Soviet citizen, he hinted, he would be generous with the information he had acquired in the U.S. military.

On October 31, Oswald met with Richard Snyder of the U.S. Embassy and stated that he was adamant about forfeiting his American citizenship. Snyder accepted Oswald's passport, but for all his big talk, Oswald never surrendered his citizenship. Oswald repeated to Snyder what he had told the Soviets about sharing his military secrets, which made news back in the states and resulted in his Marines discharge being changed from "honorable hardship" to "undesirable." Oswald told the Soviets he wanted to attend their Patrice Lumumba University in Moscow, but they dispatched him to Minsk, the capital of the then–Byelorussian Soviet Socialist Republic, 420 miles away. He was given a job as a lathe operator in a factory that manufactured radios, televisions, and military electronics. A local diplomat was assigned to teach Oswald Russian, and he was given a free studio apartment in a nice building. He was under constant surveillance.

By January 1961, Oswald was rethinking his new life. He wrote in his diary that Minsk was boring, and his job was dull. He asked the embassy in Moscow to return his U.S. passport and offered to return to the states if any charges against him would be dropped. Two months later, he attended a local dance and met Marina Nikolayevna Prusakova, a 19-year-old pharmacy worker. She grew up with her mother and stepfather in Severodvinsk in western Russia, until her mother died and her stepfather rejected her. In 1957, she moved to Minsk to live with her uncle, Ilya Prusakov, who worked for the Ministry for Internal Affairs. Oswald and Marina dated for six weeks and then married. Their daughter June Lee Oswald was born the following February.

In May 1962, the Oswalds applied to the U.S. Embassy for documents that would allow Marina to immigrate to America. Days later, the embassy gave Oswald $436 and his repatriation papers. The family arrived in the states and settled in Fort Worth, where Oswald's mother and brother lived. Oswald, Marina, and June lived with both relatives for a short time.

Marguerite Oswald, who was now working as a private duty nurse, had a confrontation with her son. She told him how she had supported him in the press when he defected to the Soviet Union. She told reporters that it was Oswald's right as an American, but that won her few fans and lost her many jobs. For a long time while

Oswald was abroad, she hadn't heard from him and was anxious about his safety. She had even planned to go to Washington, D.C., in 1961 and try to meet with President Kennedy, to see if he could tell her whether her son was living or dead. She canceled her trip after he wrote and sent her gifts, such as teas, embroidered linen napkins, a scarf, and candy for Christmas.

According to her February 10, 1964, Warren Commission testimony, while Marguerite was still fretting about her son's safety, she planned to write a book about what she deemed his "so-called defection." After Oswald returned to Texas, she told that to him, and he hit the roof. "Mother, you are not going to write a book," he scolded. "Lee, don't tell me what to do," she said. "I cannot write the book now because, honey, you are alive and back."

But, as she explained to the Commission counsel J. Lee Rankin, who was questioning her, she didn't like her son quashing her idea. After all, it was *her* story, too. "It has nothing to do with you and Marina. It is my life, because of your defection," she argued. "Mother, I tell you," Oswald said, "you are not to write a book. They could kill her and her family." Left unexplained was who "they" referred to. The KGB? The CIA? Rankin never bothered to ask.

Marguerite Oswald was a talkative woman who appeared to feel that by talking honestly to the Commissioners, she would gain important insight into her son. In the same round of questioning, Marguerite added this morsel: "I said to Lee, 'Lee, I want to know one thing. Why is it you decided to return back to the United States when you had a job in Russia? And, as far as I know, you seemed to be pretty well off, because of the gifts that you have sent me. And you are married to a Russian girl, and she would be better off in her homeland than here. I want to know.' He said, 'Mother, not even Marina knows why I have returned to the United States.' And that is all the information I ever got out of my son."

Compare and contrast Oswald's experience with my own. In the 1970s, after I attended forensic science conferences in Moscow and Leningrad, I was visited in Pittsburgh by two FBI agents who spent more than an hour asking me all sorts of questions, which I was happy to answer. This was long after the end of the Cold War. So, it's inconceivable to me that at the height of the "Spy vs. Spy" mentality of the early 1960s, someone whose travels were so hinky and dramatic as Oswald's were would not have caused alarm bells to go off.

In what universe could someone renounce his citizenship, go to an enemy country, offer military secrets, and then be welcomed back to his homeland and even given money, as if he had done nothing wrong? Why weren't Oswald's acts considered threats to the security of the United States? Why wasn't he tried for treason for participating in a plan to harm his government? The answer is: Lee Harvey Oswald had friends in high places within the U.S. government.

Once Oswald got acclimated in Texas, he merited some official attention by local FBI agents. But instead of being the subject of intense perusal by the feds, he was asked to become an informant. Oswald had announced that he would write a memoir on Soviet life, which put him in touch with anti-communist Russian émigrés in the community, known as the "White Russians." Although he soon lost interest in the book project, his new friends from Minsk latched onto the young Oswald family and did many favors for them. Oswald repaid their kindness by reporting on their activities to his FBI contact. According to the Warren Commission, as of September 1962, Oswald began receiving a $200 monthly stipend as FBI informant number S172. His Bureau handler was Special Agent James P. Hosty, Jr., who would admit to keeping a file on Oswald but denied paying him. Hosty added that his office did not even keep files with that numeric identification.

George de Mohrenschildt

In October 1962, Oswald met George de Mohrenschildt, 51, an elegant petroleum geologist born in Minsk. De Mohrenschildt's father had been a wealthy anti-communist but was arrested during the Bolshevik revolution. The family escaped to Poland, where de Mohrenschildt spent his adolescence. In 1938, he received a doctor of science degree in international commerce from the University of Liège in Belgium. That year, he moved to New York City, where British intelligence told our government he was a German spy.

His older brother, Dimitri, was already living on Long Island and working for the Office of Strategic Services, the forerunner of the CIA, providing wartime espionage support for the U.S. military. Through Dimitri, George got to know Jacqueline Bouvier, the future First Lady along with other members of the Bouvier family. As a child, Jackie would sit on de Mohrenschildt's lap and call him "Uncle George." When George's application to join the OSS was rejected amid rumors that he was a Nazi sympathizer—a claim de Mohrenschildt strongly denied—he moved south and attained a master's degree in petroleum geology from the University of Texas in 1945. In the late 1940s, he moved to Venezuela, where he worked for Pantepec Oil, a firm founded by the father of short-term CIA agent and future conservative writer and television personality William F. Buckley, Jr.

De Mohrenschildt obtained U.S. citizenship in 1949, then launched an oil investment firm that brought him back to Texas and into the circle of the H.L. Hunt, Clint Murchison, and the most important oil barons of the area. He joined the right-wing Texas Crusade for Freedom, which boasted members such as Ted Dealey, the ultra-conservative newspaper publisher, and Earle Cabell, the future mayor of Dallas, whose brother, Charles Cabell, was forced to resign his CIA deputy director post after the Bay of Pigs failure.

De Mohrenschildt's fourth wife, Eugenia "Jeanne" Fomenko, was 47 when her husband met Oswald. She was born in Harbin, China, to Russian-born parents. Her father was a railroad executive who did classified work for the U.S. government before being killed by the communists. Jeanne worked as an architect and professional dancer in China, then moved to Brooklyn, where she worked as a model and fashion designer. By 1956, she had relocated to Dallas, where she met de Mohrenschildt. They would marry three years later.

In 1957, at the request of the U.S. State Department, de Mohrenschildt traveled to Yugoslavia to do a geological field survey. He was accused of drawing sketches of military installations and quickly returned to the United States. Upon his return, he was debriefed by the CIA in Washington, D.C., and Dallas. In 1960, de Mohrenschildt's only son, Sergei, from his third marriage, died of cystic fibrosis. De Mohrenschildt persuaded Jeanne to give up her thriving career for a walking tour that would help him recover from his grief. For 10 months, they—and their toy Manchester terrier, Nero—walked 3,000 miles from Texas through Mexico and Central America to the Panama Canal, and back.

Following their return to America, De Mohrenschildt filed an account of his trip with the State Department. The local man who would debrief George was J. Walton Moore, a Dallas-based CIA agent with the Domestic Contacts Division. Moore told de Mohrenschildt about Oswald, who had spent time in Minsk and had a Russian wife. The de Mohrenschildts held a party for the Minsk

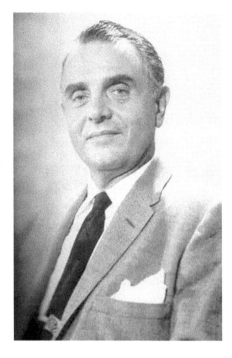

International Man of Mystery George de Mohrenschildt agreed to "babysit" Lee Harvey Oswald for the Central Intelligence Agency in exchange for business favors. It was an arrangement he would come to regret (Robert J. Groden Collection).

contingent, and the Oswalds were invited. Also at the party was a married couple with young children, Michael and Ruth Paine. Michael was a research engineer with a security clearance at the plant of defense contractor Bell Helicopter. Ruth was a housewife and amateur singer. She wanted to improve her Russian-language skills because she worked part-time teaching Russian at a boys' school in Dallas. For that reason, and because she was a Quaker who liked to do good deeds, Ruth took Marina Oswald under her wing.

George de Mohrenschildt was one of the most intriguing individuals in the annals of the Kennedy assassination, and I had an unforgettable encounter with him, which you will read about later.

Oswald in Police Custody

After his arrest, Oswald was brought to the third floor of Dallas' police headquarters where the chief of the homicide and robbery bureau, Captain J. Will Fritz, personally questioned him. Soon, agents from the FBI and Secret Service joined the session. Oswald denied having anything to do with the slayings of either President Kennedy or Officer J.D. Tippit. He denied that he owned a rifle and, later, when shown a photograph of him holding a rifle and handgun, claimed that his face had been superimposed onto someone else's body. He clammed up when asked about why his wallet contained a Selective Service card with his photograph and the name "Alek J. Hidell." Handwriting on the mail order form used to buy the rifle would eventually be linked to Oswald. The revolver Oswald had when arrested was deemed the type used in the Tippit shooting and had been sent to the lab for ballistics testing. Oswald was brought before numerous witnesses for lineups and, at 7:10 p.m., was charged with the patrolman's murder.

Oswald's grilling lasted from Friday afternoon until Sunday morning, with frequent trips from Fritz's office to a holding cell while law enforcement prepared for a new round of questions. Each time Oswald would be marched down the hallway, he'd pass more than 100 print, radio, and television reporters who were awaiting information. Jack Ruby was in the crowd, too.

TV viewers were spellbound by Oswald's answers to the media questions. He admitted working at the book depository but denied shooting either the president or the patrolman. He was "just a patsy," he insisted. And despite repeatedly asking for legal representation, he said the police officers grilling him were not providing a lawyer.

Eventually Oswald was able to place a cold call to New York firebrand attorney John Jacob Abt, who was counsel for the American Communist Party. Abt was away for the weekend and missed the call. Oswald's mother visited him in jail and was startled by his black, swollen eye and the scratches on his face. She asked if the officers were mistreating him, but he said no. In fact, there was no indication that he was harmed once he arrived at police headquarters—until Sunday morning, when he died there.

The President's Autopsy

In the evening of Friday, November 22, 1963, Air Force One bearing the president's body arrived at Andrews Air Force Base in Maryland. The plane was met by Attorney General Robert F. Kennedy, and he stood next to his sister-in-law Jackie as the casket was downloaded by an elevator forklift. Hundreds of reporters were on the tarmac covering the live broadcast. FBI Special Agents James W. Sibert and his supervisor, Francis X. O'Neill, Jr., were assigned to escort President Kennedy's coffin to the morgue. They would also chronicle the autopsy and collect evidence from the procedure.

The casket, Jackie, and Bobby were put in a Navy ambulance and driven to the National Naval Medical Center in Bethesda, Maryland, about 20 miles away. At 7:35 p.m. EST, JFK's body arrived in Bethesda. The casket was opened, and the president was found naked and wrapped in white sheets, including one around his head that was saturated with blood. His clothes were not with his body. The corpse was placed on a gurney and wheeled to the radiology department where full body and head X-rays were taken. Photographs were also taken. At 8:00 p.m., the president's post-mortem examination commenced and would continue for more than three hours. During the procedure, Jackie and Bobby waited on the 17th floor of the medical center, where they were eventually joined by other family members.

United States Navy Commander James J. Humes of the Medical Corps was the lead autopsy doctor for the procedure. Dr. Humes was also the director of laboratories of the Naval Medical School at Bethesda's Naval Medical Center. His duties included supervision of all of the laboratory operations at the medical center for anatomic pathology, composed of examining surgical specimens from postmortem examinations. He was also responsible for clinical pathology, involving the examination of blood and various body fluids. Therefore, it was surprising for me to learn that he was not a board-certified forensic pathologist, whose occupation it is to perform medico-legal autopsies and arrive at a cause and manner of death. Humes' job involved analyzing samples from autopsies that someone else had performed. A lay person might not see that distinction but to anyone in my field, it's a vastly different discipline. This is not to cast aspersions on the quality of Humes' work in his specialty, but it does not translate to experience as a medical examiner. Your dentist might be familiar with mouths and teeth, but if you develop an oral tumor, he or she would wisely send you to someone with specific expertise in tumors. While Humes had training at the Armed Forces Institute of Pathology at Washington's Walter Reed Army Hospital and had seen victims of violent deaths, including those who died from gunshots, he had never performed an autopsy on a gunshot victim before. Still, he was on duty at the facility when he got the call that President Kennedy's body would be shipped there and would need an immediate autopsy.

Humes brought in an associate to assist: USN Commander J. Thornton Boswell, the chief of pathology at the Naval Medical School. Boswell was also not a forensic pathologist, board-certified or otherwise. Like Humes, Boswell had never performed a gunshot wound autopsy in his professional career. After the autopsy was underway, a third doctor joined the proceedings: U.S. Army Lieutenant Colonel Pierre Finck, an expert in the wound ballistics section at AFIP that dealt with casualties caused by military-type weapons, not civilian gunshot wounds as those found in Kennedy. I knew Dr. Finck from my own training at AFIP and, in a future chapter, will describe a most interesting encounter I had with him. (Walter Reed National Military Medical Center is now a tri-service military health-care facility that incorporates the former Bethesda Naval Hospital. It is the headquarters for the Joint Task Force National Capital Region Medical. AFIP was shuttered in 2011, with its work continuing under the aegis of the Joint Pathology Center, in Silver Spring, Maryland.)

In the military chain of command at Bethesda that night, Commander Humes reported to Captain John H. Stover, Jr., the commanding officer of the Naval Medical School. Stover's equal was Captain Robert O. Canada, the commanding officer of the Naval Hospital. Both Stover and Canada reported to Rear Admiral Calvin B. Galloway, the commanding officer of the Medical Center. Galloway's senior was Vice Admiral Edward C. Kenney, the surgeon general of the Navy and chief of the Bureau of Medicine and Science. Kenney's senior was the undersecretary of the Navy and its acting secretary, a civilian named Paul B. Fay, who was a close friend of Jack Kennedy, going back to their PT boat days. Fay worked on Kennedy's political campaigns and was also an usher at Kennedy's wedding. He resigned from his acting secretary post on November 28 but remained as undersecretary until 1965.

The chief of naval operations and highest ranking officer in the Navy was Admiral David L. McDonald, a member of the Joint Chiefs of Staff. Members of the JCS were the senior leaders from all of the military branches who advise the secretary of defense and the president. On the Army side, also sitting with the JCS, was General Earle G. Wheeler, who would the next year become the chairman of the JCS. The surgeon general of the Army was Lieutenant General Leonard D. Heaton who, aside from his administrative duties, performed surgeries on notable Army veterans such as President Eisenhower, Generals Douglas MacArthur and George C. Marshall, and Secretary of State John Foster Dulles. The chairman of the JCS in 1963 was Maxwell D. Taylor, an Army four-star general who Kennedy appointed after the failed Bay of Pigs invasion, which the president blamed largely on the military for not providing adequate intelligence. Kennedy and his brother, Robert, were such fans of Taylor the latter sibling would name one of his sons after him. The secretary of defense was Robert S. McNamara, who used his term in office to escalate the Vietnam War, a move he would vocally regret in his later years.

Although the other military branches—U.S. Air Force, Marine Corps, Coast Guard, and National Guard—had their own medical personnel, the autopsy of President Kennedy mostly seemed to involve top brass members of the Navy and Army. And someone at the highest level of authority made the decision that the president's autopsy would be performed by doctors who were outside their comfort zone and, in my opinion, easily controlled.

Besides Commanders Humes and Boswell, and Colonel Finck, other physicians who attended the president's autopsy were Admirals Kenney and Galloway, and Captains Canada and Stover. The president's physician, Rear Admiral George Burkley, who was attached to the USN Medical Corps., was present, as was Bethesda's chief of surgery, USN Captain David P. Osborne. Other USN medical personnel who were in the morgue that night included, according to a list compiled by FBI agents Jim Sibert and his supervisor, Frank O'Neill: John Thomas Stringer, Jr., medical photographer; Floyd Albert Riebe, medical photographer and Stringer's assistant; Petty Officer Raymond Oswald, medical photographer on call; Paul Kelly O'Connor, laboratory technologist; James Curtis Jenkins, laboratory technologist; Edward F. Reed, X-ray technician; Jerrol F. Custer, X-ray technician; Jan Gail Rudnicki, Dr. Boswell's lab tech assistant; Petty Officer James E. Metzler, hospital corpsman; Commander James H. Ebersole, assistant chief of radiology; Lieutenant Commander Gregory H. Cross, surgical resident; and Chief Petty Officer Chester H. Boyers, in charge of the pathology division, who visited the autopsy room during the final stages to type receipts given by the FBI and Secret Service for items obtained.

Lieutenant Robert Frederick Karnei, Jr., was the senior resident pathologist (but not a forensic pathologist) who usually performed autopsies at the Bethesda facility. If there was anything that required a specialist's expertise, he knew to ask for assistance. On November 22, he was called by Admiral Galloway in the late afternoon and told to be at the morgue to observe, but not conduct, the president's procedure. Karnei became the liaison for various people who were there, assigned Marine Corps guards throughout the building, and was told by Admiral Kenney to make sure no one entered without clearance. Karnei said he was prepared to shoot anyone who disobeyed his orders. He was in and out of the autopsy room to run errands, including ushering people up to the tower's 17th floor where Mrs. Kennedy and Senator Robert Kennedy were waiting. Karnei also helped Humes and Boswell find things, since, in his words, they were "not so familiar with the morgue."

In an interview later, Karnei said he couldn't be sure who was directing the activities but that "at any one time there was a maximum of a dozen people" in the morgue, with others in the anteroom where there was a telephone. Karnei stated that in cases of a head wound like that sustained by the president, it would be usual to bring in a neuropathologist to consult, but that wasn't done. He added that the general procedure would be to bring the brain to the AFIP for sectioning and microscopic study. Two days after the autopsy, Karnei signed a nondisclosure statement that would silence him for 10 years. Just prior to that time elapsing, he signed another agreement extending the period to another 15 years. He told an interviewer he "got the impression" the surgeon general provided the forms at the request of the Kennedy family. Dr. Karnei was not questioned by the Warren Commissioners about what he experienced regarding the assassination.

Additional military personnel who were present: U.S. Air Force Brigadier General Godfrey McHugh, military aide to the president and in charge of Air Force One; U.S. Army Major General Philip C. Wehle, commanding officer of the Military District of Washington, D.C., in charge of making arrangements for the president's funeral and lying in state; Army 2nd Lieutenant Richard A. Lipsey, junior aide to Gen. Wehle; and Army 1st Lieutenant Samuel A. Bird, head of the Old Guard, which escorts the president at ceremonial and memorial events. Non-medical personnel from law-enforcement/security who were in the morgue that night: FBI agents Sibert and O'Neill; and Secret Servicemen William Greer and his supervisor, Roy Kellerman (respectively, the driver and passenger of the presidential limousine in Dallas), and another agent, John J. O'Leary.

At the termination of the autopsy, four representatives from Joseph Gawler's Sons Funeral Home of Washington, D.C., entered the autopsy room to prepare the president's body for viewing and burial, a process that took three to four hours. It's also possible that other individuals, unnamed and unidentified, were present that night. Although the news stated that the autopsy had taken place and mentioned the names of the three doctors who performed it, few details were disclosed beyond that. The world would have to wait for the release of the autopsy report. One could only guess how long that might take.

Governor John Connally's Wounds

John Connally was a Lone Star state native who graduated from the University of Texas School of Law. He married Idenell "Nellie" Brill in 1940, and they had two sons and two daughters. (Their eldest child, Kathleen, died in a shooting accident in 1959.) Connally enlisted in the U.S. Navy and served in the South Pacific during World War II. When he was honorably discharged in 1946, he had attained the rank of lieutenant commander. After his military stint, Connally returned to Austin, Texas, to practice law, specializing in high-end real estate and oil leases. He eventually moved to Fort Worth where he represented wealthy clients with strong ties to Democrat politics. Connally moved his family to Washington, D.C., when long-time friend Lyndon Johnson, then a newly-elected U.S. senator, offered him a job as a chief aide.

At the 1960 Democratic presidential convention, when Kennedy and Johnson were rivals, Connally supported his buddy, LBJ. Connally cautioned certain journalists that if Kennedy were elected, he might not be able to complete his term in office, due to his adrenal deficiency. All was forgiven when Kennedy won the nomination and realized he needed the Southern Democrat voting bloc. Johnson became JFK's vice presidential choice, and the party prevailed at the polls. In 1961, at Johnson's urging, Kennedy named Connally to the post of secretary of the Navy. He held the job for almost a year, then resigned so he could move his family back to Texas and seek the 1962 gubernatorial nomination. The conservative Democrat campaigned hard, becoming a fixture on television and radio, and winning the race. He would stay in office until 1969. During Johnson's term as president, Connally became more hawkish, advising LBJ to take an aggressive stance in Vietnam.

The 1968 presidential race found Connally snubbed by Hubert Humphrey who would not choose him as a vice presidential running mate. While endorsing Humphrey on the surface, Connally formed a bond with the Republican candidate, Richard Nixon. When Nixon won the presidency, Connally was appointed to his cabinet, eventually becoming the U.S. treasury secretary in 1972. The next year, Johnson died in January, and, in May, Connally switched party affiliations from Democrat to Republican. He remained active in GOP politics until his death from lung disease in 1993. Nellie Connally died in 2006.

Connally was 46 years old when he was hit by gunfire in the presidential limousine in Dallas. At Parkland Hospital, he underwent nearly four hours of surgery to repair wounds to his chest, wrist, and thigh. Dr. Robert Shaw presided over Connally's procedures, assisted by Drs. James Boland, James Duke, Charles F. Gregory, William Osborn, Charles Baxter, Robert McClelland, Jackie Hunt, Buddy Giesecke, David Stewart, Charles Crenshaw, David Mebane, Don Patman, and George T. "Tom" Shires (Parkland's chief of surgery).

The high-velocity bullet that hit the governor was a full-metal jacketed missile, designed not to fragment or expand. It entered his back under the right armpit. Then it went through his body, tore through four inches of rib, ruptured his lung, and exited his chest, about two inches below and to the left of his right nipple. The bullet continued through the back side of his right wrist and finally landed in his left thigh. No bullet fragments were recovered from his chest. Connally's thoracic injuries consisted of a comminuted fracture of the fifth rib, lacerations of the middle lobe, and hematoma of the lower lobe of the right lung. Dr. Shaw told the Warren Commission that the patient had a "sucking wound of the chest" that would not have allowed him to breathe or talk in a normal manner. This calls into question exactly how and when Connally was able to shout out, "Oh my God, they're going to kill us all," as one eyewitness stated.

The governor, who went to his grave supporting the Warren Commission's findings, nevertheless maintained that he was hit by the second of three bullets. The first one, according to his testimony, passed through JFK's neck, causing Connally to look around. He was not wounded then, he stated. But the second one hit him and took his breath away, bathing him in blood. He had only a moment to realize how much pain he felt when he heard the third shot, which blew apart Kennedy's head. His testimony is inconsistent with the single-bullet theory that would have had him hit by the missile that went through Kennedy's neck.

Once Connally's chest trauma was repaired, doctors operated on his wrist and thigh. The wrist defect was a through-and-through injury, meaning the bullet passed completely through and exited. It traveled through his jacket cuff, into his shirt's doubled French cuff, and shattered the distal radius (wrist bone) at its thickest point. The bullet then exited the palm side of the wrist, above the cuff. Its path left a trail of dark jacket fibers and bullet fragments. Connally's solid gold Mexican peso cuff link was blasted off the shirt and was never recovered. The bullet then entered the front side of the governor's left thigh and burrowed into the muscles. Dr. Gregory removed the most significant bullet fragments from the governor's wrist and gave them to a scrub nurse who handed them to Nurse Audrey Bell. She described the "four or five" fragments as grayish in color and "anywhere from three to four millimeters in length and a couple of millimeters wide." The smallest fragment was about the size of the striking portion of a match, she indicated. The largest piece was twice that size.

Nurse Bell would later point out that they were not able to get all the fragments from Connally's wrist. X-rays would show that some traces were left inside. Bell placed the removed fragments in a small plastic container and put it inside a 3" by 5" manila envelope, the kind typically used for collecting "foreign bodies." She then labeled, sealed, and initialed the envelope. Following protocol, all individuals who handled that envelope after Bell would have added their initials. Bell turned over the envelope to two plainclothes federal agents, one of whom was a "Mr. Sorrels." Forrest Sorrels was the special agent-in-charge of the Secret Service in Dallas. One of the agents who received the envelope gave her a receipt. Again, following protocol, she then handed off the receipt to Parkland Administrator Jack Price. The next day, Bell was interviewed by an FBI agent. But oddly, when she was shown the report the agent filed, it stated that she had only put one fragment in the envelope. The document also stated she had given the envelope to a Texas Ranger, although she was adamant that the person who received it identified himself as a federal employee. Bell's receipt would have verified the chain of possession of the fragments envelope and should have eventually been given to the National Archives. But the receipt was never entered as evidence at the Archives. It seems to have just conveniently vanished. And the fragments never made an appearance at the president's autopsy. In the pages ahead, I will describe a most interesting conversation I had with Nurse Bell years later.

By 4:45 p.m., Connally's surgeries were complete, and he was wheeled to an upstairs recovery room. It would be his base of operations for the state government for the next couple of weeks as his wounds healed, and he fought off blood clots.

X-rays would show that doctors also left a bullet fragment of approximately 1.5 millimeters in size in Connally's femur. It was in an area where it could do no harm, and its removal would have required unnecessary physical damage. In Connally's autobiography, *In History's Shadow* (with

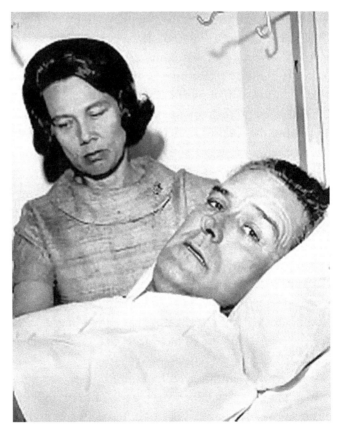

Recovering at Parkland from his multiple surgeries, Texas Governor John Connally is shown with his wife, Nellie (AP Photo/Ted Powers).

Mickey Herskowitz, Hyperion Books, 1994, p. 18), he stated: "The most curious discovery of all took place when they rolled me off the stretcher, and onto the examining table. A metal object fell to the floor, with a click no louder than a wedding band. The nurse picked it up and slipped in into her pocket. It was the bullet from my body, the one that passed through my back, chest, and wrist and worked itself loose from my thigh." Curious, indeed. Hospital engineer Darrell Tomlinson said he found the stretcher bullet and turned it over directly to his boss. The bullet he handled was almost perfectly intact, with no traces of blood or tissue clinging to it. And no nurse was involved. From Connally's passage, one must wonder if the unnamed nurse found his cuff link rather than any bullet.

But Connally was in surgery at that time and would have had to depend on information from Dallas District Attorney Henry Wade, who was waiting for the governor to come out of Trauma Room Two. Almost 30 years after the fact, Wade told a writer with the *Dallas Morning News*: "I also went out to see Connally, but he was in the operating room. Some nurse had a bullet in her hand, and said this was on the gurney that Connally was on...." When the reporter asked if that were the pristine bullet everyone talks about, Wade replied: "I told her to give it to the police, which she said she would. I assume that's the pristine bullet."

There was an unnamed nurse who handled a bullet or at least a bullet fragment. She was in the Connally second-floor recovery room and passed the item to Texas highway patrolman Bobby M. Nolan. Years later, when Nolan was interviewed by assassination researcher Robert Harris, the officer recalled the event well. He had been talking to one of Connally's aides, Bill Stinson. The nurse came over and stated she found a bullet on the gurney, presumably the governor's, Nolan said. She handed him a brown envelope, about 2" by 3" in size. Since it was sealed, he was unable to tell if it was a whole bullet or just a fragment. Nolan initialed the envelope, then turned it over to an FBI agent. Stinson had also told reporters that a bullet had been recovered from Connally's thigh. Soon after the FBI took custody of Nolan's envelope, the official story changed. Now, the material in the envelope was fragments from Connally's wrist instead of the bullet from his thigh. Nolan's initials were still there, but Bell's initials had been overwritten by those of Dallas police Captain Will Fritz. The envelope now included the handwritten words "right arm," which weren't present when Bell handed the envelope to the federal agent. Bell would later tell an investigator that she didn't see her initials on the envelope. For her chain of command to have accepted it, her initials would have had to have been there.

So, we have multiple bullets and fragments popping up in multiple places, like a Feydeau farce with a ballet of gurneys, rather than doors slamming. On a more serious note, we also have what might be considered blatant tampering with evidence. Although ballistic testing would link the fragments from Connally's wrist to the ammunition from Oswald's rifle, the FBI did not test all of the samples it received. Or, I should say, they didn't release the test results if they had them. Did the Bureau already know that the Tomlinson stretcher bullet was fraudulent and that the real Connally bullet came from a second shooter's gun?

Still, all of these loose ends could have been easily tied if Connally had allowed for forensic samples to be taken from his body after death. I even led a charge that requested then–U.S. Attorney General Janet Reno to make a formal request of Nellie Connally for the material. I, or any other forensic pathologist, could have excised the fragments that remained in his body and sent them to a lab for precision ballistic matching. The procedure would have been quick and wouldn't have damaged Connally's flesh if his family wanted an open-casket viewing at his funeral. It would be a final feat of valor in the life of a politician who almost died in one of America's darkest hours—a way to find answers to questions he always raised and an act of respect for the historic record. Alas, Nellie Connally refused the request, and her husband was laid to rest carrying his secrets with him. There would have to be another way to prove that the stretcher bullet was a red herring. And there was. It would be quite the sweet victory.

Three Funerals

After President Kennedy's body arrived back in Washington from its autopsy in Maryland—along with Jackie and Kennedy family members—it was brought to the White House as plans for the Monday's state funeral were solidified. The proceedings were organized by top brass at the Military District of Washington. They found a coffin befitting the majestic occasion; it was made of 500-year-old African mahogany. An honor guard of U.S. Marines escorted it to the East Room where President Abraham Lincoln had laid in repose in 1865. Jackie requested the Library of Congress research the details of Lincoln's funeral, and soon White House upholsterers draped the black cambric, or thin fabric, that was usually used for covering the bottoms of chairs over the windows, mantels, and chandeliers, as was done for Lincoln's wake.

On Saturday, Jackie's Secret Service agent Clint Hill accompanied her and Robert Kennedy for a private viewing of the body. The casket was opened, and Hill backed away to give her and Bobby some personal space as they prayed and cried together. It was the first time Jackie had seen her husband since his death and the first time for his brother. The two placed meaningful items inside the casket. Bobby's gifts were JFK's PT-109 tie tack and an engraved silver rosary his wife Ethel gave him for their wedding. Jackie tucked in a scrimshaw of the presidential seal, cuff links, and personal letters from her and the children. She had Caroline hand-write a card about how much she loved her daddy, and John Jr., added his "X" to his big sister's signature.

Mrs. Kennedy asked Agent Hill to find her a pair of scissors, which he did. He then heard clipping sounds and saw that she had taken a lock of her husband's hair. As much as the skilled morticians worked to restore the president's head and visage, packing his skull with plaster and cotton, he was irreparably harmed. Jackie took a last look at her husband, then turned to Bobby and said, "It isn't Jack." There would be no open-casket funeral.

Two Catholic priests accompanied the casket at all times until the funeral was over. They conducted a Mass that was attended by Kennedy family members and White House aides. Later, several government officials dropped by the White House to express their regards, among them former U.S. Presidents Harry Truman and Dwight Eisenhower. The only other surviving president, Herbert Hoover, was too ill to attend but was represented by his sons.

On Sunday, the president's flag-draped coffin left the White House for a trip to the U.S. Capitol rotunda, 14 blocks southeast. Combined military pallbearers and personnel marched with glorious efficiency, and soldiers carrying flags of the 50 states of the Union lined Pennsylvania Avenue. The casket was carried on a wagon-wheeled, horse-drawn caisson that had previously been used to transport the caskets of President Franklin Roosevelt and the Unknown Soldiers of the Korean and Vietnam Wars. The clip-clops of the horses' hooves and muffled military drums were the predominant sounds. Following the cortege was a riderless horse, with a decorative saddle and a pair of empty boots reversed in the stirrups, symbolizing a great warrior who would ride no more.

At the rotunda, the casket was transferred to the catafalque that was used to display Lincoln's casket. Kennedy was the first Democrat president to ever lie in state at the Capitol and the first president since William Howard Taft's death in 1930. Eulogies were delivered by U.S. Supreme Court Chief Justice Earl Warren and selected politicians. A freezing, steady rain added to the gray atmosphere of the day but didn't stop some 300,000 mourners who waited in line for up to 10 hours for the chance to walk by the closed casket of their fallen leader and pay their respects. Millions more watched the non-stop proceedings on television. Inside the hall, Mrs. Kennedy, holding the hands of her children, maintained her composure. At one point, she and daughter Caroline, who would turn six years old in three days, walked to the casket, knelt, and kissed the flag.

Shortly after the assassination, President Lyndon Johnson told a television and radio audience that Monday, November 25, would be a national day of mourning. He didn't need to announce it. The country—perhaps the world—would be at a complete standstill until the president was interred in his final resting place at Arlington National Cemetery in Virginia. But Jack Kennedy was not the only person buried that day. So were Dallas Police Officer J.D. Tippit and their alleged assassin, Lee Harvey Oswald, who himself had been assassinated the day before. More on that ahead.

Tippit's funeral was held at Dallas' Beckley Hills Baptist Church, and he was buried at the Laurel Land Memorial Park. Hours after Tippit's and Kennedy's deaths, Marie Tippit received separate calls from Lyndon Johnson and Robert Kennedy, expressing their condolences for her loss. She mentioned those at the funeral, but what she didn't talk about—because she didn't know it at the time—was a letter that would arrive in the mail within a few days. It was a handwritten missive from Jackie Kennedy, written after returning from her own husband's funeral, when the weight of suddenly being thrust into widowhood with children was very much on her mind.

The Tippit family received more than 40,000 other communications of support and sorrow, and monetary donations totaling $647,579. The single largest gift was the $25,000 from Abraham Zapruder after he sold his film of the president's assassination. Officer Tippit was awarded the 1964 Medal of Valor from the American Police Hall of Fame and the Police Medal of Honor, the Police Cross, and the Citizens

Traffic Commission Award of Heroism. In 2012, a memorial plaque was unveiled in Dallas at 10th and Patton Streets, where he had died.

A small group of people gathered at Shannon Rose Hill Cemetery in Fort Worth for the burial of Oswald. Dozens of police officers were on hand to provide security, but because the decedent was alleged to have killed their colleague, J.D. Tippit, they declined to carry Oswald's casket to the gravesite. Reporters from the Associated Press and UPI were recruited as pallbearers. No local clergyman would officiate, causing an angry Marguerite to snipe, "So much for Christianity as we know it today."

A non-practicing pastor, Louis Saunders, volunteered and said prayers while Marina, toting infant Rachel, and Marguerite, holding a squirming June, wiped tears from their eyes. Lee's brother Robert was also in attendance, as were federal agents. As the small group departed, Marguerite noticed that the cemetery flag was at half-mast. Oswald didn't exactly rest in peace. Years later, when the question was raised as to whether Oswald, and not an impostor, had been buried, the body was exhumed, confirmed as Oswald's, then reburied in the same cemetery.

President John F. Kennedy's funeral was planned with military precision and helmed by members of the Joint Chiefs of Staff and honor guards. On Monday morning, the white horse-drawn caisson and a Marine platoon escort left the Capitol rotunda for the White House. It would be President Kennedy's final trip home, if only a brief stop. JFK's two brothers, Attorney General Robert Kennedy and Massachusetts Senator Edward "Ted" Kennedy, were driven from the rotunda to the White House with Jackie. There, the group, along with the chief justice of the Supreme Court and the justices, and key State officials and Cabinet members, a chorus of "Danny Boy" was sung.

Then, with Jackie, Bobby, and Ted Kennedy leading the procession, everyone walked four long blocks to St. Matthew's Cathedral. It was the same path Jack and Jackie would take when they would attend Sunday Mass. While Jackie held Bobby's hand at the start of the trek, she soon let go and walked ahead of him, showing the world that she was capable of marching on her own. Approximately one million spectators lined the route, and dozens of news cameras covered every inch of it. The two Kennedy children and the slain president's ailing father, Joseph P. Kennedy, Sr., arrived at the cathedral by limousine.

President Johnson, Lady Bird Johnson, and their daughters Luci and Lynda had been advised not to march in the procession for security reasons, but LBJ insisted they participate. The next day, when he arrived at the Oval Office to spend his first day behind the presidential desk, he found a note from Jackie thanking him for making the walk. While that solemn cortege was taking place, both houses of Congress met to pass resolutions expressing sorrow. The Republican senator from Maine, Margaret Chase Smith, placed a single red rose on the desk Kennedy had occupied when he served in the Senate.

A Catholic requiem Mass was held at St. Matthew's, with 1,200 invited guests. It was officiated by the Archbishop of Boston, Cardinal Richard James Cushing, who had paved the way for JFK's acceptance as a Catholic in national politics. He also performed Jack and Jackie's wedding ceremony, baptized their children, gave the prayer of invocation at Kennedy's presidential inaugural, and officiated at the funeral of their infant son Patrick Bouvier Kennedy. The ceremony was a "low Mass," meaning it was spoken and not sung. The service was concluded with a reading of Kennedy's inaugural address, followed by tenor Luigi Vena singing "Ave Maria," as he did when he performed at the Kennedys' wedding ceremony 10 years before. Hearing the hymn again under such dismal circumstances caused Jackie to sob uncontrollably, the only time she was known to have done so publicly.

Secretary of State Dean Rusk invited representatives from 92 countries to attend the ceremony, the largest gathering of foreign dignitaries in our country's history. Among the 220 world dignitaries were Canada's Prime Minister Lester B. Pearson, Ethiopia's Emperor Haile Selassie I, France's President Charles de Gaulle, Germany's Mayor Willy Brandt of Berlin, Great Britain's Prince Philip, Greece's Queen Frederika, Ireland's President Eamon de Valera, Israel's Foreign Minister Golda Meir, South Vietnam's Ambassador-designate Tran Chanh Thanh, the Soviet Union's First Deputy Chairman Anastas Miyokan, and a retinue from the United Nations that included Secretary-General U Thant and Undersecretary of Political Affairs Ralph Bunche.

Following the service, Jackie and her children stood on the outside steps of the cathedral, with other Kennedy family members behind them. News footage shows various Kennedy siblings and their families. Jackie wore a black suit and low heels, with a black lace mantilla over her head and shoulders. Caroline and John Jr. wore matching above-the-knee pale blue coats, white socks, and red shoes. As the casket passed them, little John—whose third birthday was that day—saluted his daddy.

President Kennedy's burial ceremony was at Arlington National Cemetery in Arlington County, Virginia, across the Potomac River from the Lincoln Memorial. Established in 1864 on an estate once owned by Civil War Confederate General Robert E. Lee, it is the final resting place for distinguished military war veterans, astronauts, government officials, and select citizens, mostly from the United States. Now managed by the Army out of nearby Fort Myer, Arlington's 624 acres contain approximately 400,000 graves. U.S. presidents, even if they don't serve in the military during wartime, have the option to be buried at Arlington, since their presidential duties include being the commander-in-chief of all forces. Still, only one president besides Kennedy is interred there. William Howard Taft, who was not only a president but later a chief justice of the U.S. Supreme Court, was buried with military honors at Arlington after his death in 1930.

Secretary of Defense Robert McNamara and Bobby Kennedy visited the cemetery prior to the funeral and chose a beautiful hillside gravesite that would provide a scenic view of Washington, D.C., and be able to accommodate both a large burial ceremony and many thousands of visitors in the decades to come. The president's friend, architect John Carl Warnecke, would design the memorial. Jackie had one unyielding request: an eternal flame, similar to the one she and Jack had seen at Paris' Arc de

Triomphe in 1961 for the tomb of France's Unknown Soldier. No other eternal flames burned at Arlington. Colonel Clayton B. Lyle and the Army Corps of Engineers were recruited to make the impossibly difficult task a reality. They modified a tiki torch and installed an underground gas line to a propane tank 200 yards away.

Following the Mass at St. Matthew's, the funeral procession crossed the Arlington Memorial Bridge and entered the cemetery grounds just before 3:00 p.m. on what had now become a sunny but crisp autumn day. Jackie Kennedy and the president's family members were in limousines behind the caisson. The Kennedy children did not attend this ceremony. News cameras were staked out at various positions around the cemetery, with pool cameras filming the gravesite for the use of all the networks. An NBC director called the shots. As the casket was carried from the caisson to the gravesite, the Air Force Pipe Band played "Mist-Covered Mountains," and the Marine Band played "Ruffles and Flourishes" and "The National Anthem."

Seated next to the gravesite were Mrs. Kennedy, Bobby and Ted Kennedy, Rose Kennedy, and Eunice Kennedy Shriver. Everyone else stood during the brief ceremony, including the Lawfords and their children. President de Gaulle and Emperor Selassie, in their respective military uniforms, were in the front row of spectators. They and everyone else wearing military garb gestured at the appropriate times. Fifty fighter jets roared overhead in a Missing Man formation, followed by Air Force One. Cardinal Cushing led the commitment rites, then sprinkled holy water on the casket as the pallbearers lifted its American flag. From Fort Myer a 21-gun cannon salute was heard, followed by the traditional rifle tribute at gravesite. Seven soldiers from the Old Guard of the Third U.S. Infantry released three separate volleys of rifle fire. The Army bugler then played "Taps."

The flag was folded and given to Mrs. Kennedy, who then used a candle to light the eternal flame. Following the funeral, Jackie spoke of a conversation she remembered having with her husband. He had said he wanted his family buried together, as President Abraham Lincoln had been when he was laid to rest with his deceased son Willie. Jackie wanted her deceased children to join their father at Arlington, so the JFK burial spot was expanded to a three-acre spread. The Kennedys' daughter who would have been named Arabella and was stillborn in 1956 was disinterred from a plot in Newport, Rhode Island, and son Patrick was disinterred from his site in Brookline. Both tiny caskets were brought to Arlington and reburied near their father. When Jackie died of cancer in 1994, she joined the Kennedy plot. Both Bobby, who was assassinated in 1968, and Ted, who died of brain cancer in 2009, were also buried at Arlington, not far from their brother. Bobby's grave is marked by only a humble white wooden cross.

The design for President Kennedy's permanent memorial was unveiled just before the first anniversary of his death, although it would take time for it to become operational. On March 15, 1967, a consecration ceremony was conducted, with only Jackie Kennedy, President Lyndon Johnson, Senator Robert and Ethel Kennedy, Senator Edward and Joan Kennedy, and a few others in attendance. The president's marker shows a cross and "John Fitzgerald Kennedy 1917–1963." Since then, countless millions of people have paid their respects, turning what used to be a quiet veterans' cemetery into a "must-see" tourist attraction.

It's impossible to know how many people watched President Kennedy's funeral on television, since the method of counting viewers was in its infancy in 1963. The black-and-white live broadcast was estimated to have been seen by 93 percent of all American homes with televisions, and satellites beamed the event to 23 other countries. Numbers aside, the funeral of the 35th president, who was so young and vital and died in such a brutal fashion, left an impact that might be hard to understand for those not old enough to have experienced it firsthand. JFK remains the last U.S. president to have died in office. That his final send-off was organized and executed with such spectacular pageantry on such short notice is a testament to American achievement. Some of the basic plans had been rehearsed in anticipation of President Hoover's demise and were implemented when he died in October 1964. But Hoover's state funeral surely did not have the grand scale as did Kennedy's.

The Zapruder Film

As Dallas dressmaker Abraham Zapruder held his home movie camera to his eye, he expected to see the president and First Lady he much admired. Zapruder held his Zoomatic with one hand and waved at the approaching limousine with the other, hoping to get a reaction from Jack and Jackie Kennedy. He didn't know he was about to capture history's most important piece of film footage. And he certainly didn't anticipate that the footage would make his family millionaires.

Zapruder heard the first gunshot and thought it was a backfire. He kept looking through his viewfinder, pressing the button to record the action. Then he noticed that the president had slumped to the left. "If I had any sense I would have dropped to the ground, because my first impression was that the shots were coming from behind me," Zapruder would tell a reporter, indicating the wooden fence area of the grassy knoll. Then, as the amateur filmmaker saw JFK's head explode, he realized he was witnessing an assassination. Too paralyzed in fear to put down the camera, he kept shooting. As the limousine disappeared from sight, Zapruder shouted: "They killed him, they killed him!"

Zapruder and his receptionist, Marilyn Sitzman, who had been steadying him as he filmed, were stunned. As they made their way back to their office in the Dal-Tex building, they ran into writer Harry McCormick of the *Dallas Morning News*, who asked what had occurred. Zapruder told him the minimum, saying he would give the full story to only a federal agent, so McCormick said he would contact Forrest Sorrels, who headed the local Secret Service office. Back at the office, with McCormick in tow, Zapruder and Sitzman explained their horrific news to the employees. Zapruder's secretary suggested that the local office of the FBI should be notified to tell them about the film footage. Zapruder agreed, and she made the call. While awaiting the FBI, Sorrels soon arrived at the office. Sorrels convinced Zapruder that the official investigation would be greatly enhanced if authorities had copies of the film.

Word soon got out that Zapruder had unique coverage of the tragedy. Another *Dallas Morning News* reporter, Darwin Payne, stopped by the dressmaker's office, asking for publication rights of the footage. Zapruder, his business partner Erwin Schwartz, McCormick, and Sorrels walked to the newspaper's office, but it lacked the proper film-processing capability. They went next-door to WFAA-TV, the broadcast arm of the newspaper. Assistant news director Bert Shipp informed them that WFAA also had no way to process 8-millimeter film, as the station only used 16-millimeter black-and-white footage. He called Eastman Kodak for help, then arranged for Zapruder to do a brief, live interview with the station's program director, Jay Watson. Zapruder was queasy when he explained what he saw, as Schwartz stood on the sideline, holding the home movie camera. Watson announced that the station was in possession of the footage and was working on getting it developed. He then showed Zapruder a photo of the depository and pointed to the sixth floor where he said the gun was fired that killed the president. Zapruder replied that he must have been in the line of fire. Was this just confusion on the part of media trying to understand what happened or a deliberate attempt to convince Zapruder of the direction that the bullets were fired?

Around 2:40 p.m., a Dallas police car drove the group to the Eastman Kodak lab, located near Love Field, and around the same time Lyndon Johnson was being sworn in as the new president. A special viewer was used to assess the film, then it was agreed not to run it again for fear of damaging it. Next, Zapruder and Schwartz were driven to Jamieson Films, where three prints were made for investigators. The men then returned to Eastman Kodak to process the footage and ready it for the projector. By midnight, the film's 26.6 seconds had been viewed by the Zapruder group. Zapruder and Schwartz gave Sorrels two prints, one of which was flown directly to FBI Headquarters in Washington, D.C., and another copy was given to the Dallas police. Zapruder kept the original and one copy, and got sworn statements from the lab workers that they had not made bootleg copies. After consulting with the FBI, Zapruder was assured that all rights belonged to him and that he had the sole privilege of assigning them as he saw fit.

Zapruder went home and tried to sleep. Just before midnight, he got a phone call from Richard Stolley, the Los Angeles editor for *Life* magazine, who had just arrived in his Dallas office. Stolley asked if he could come right over to view the footage, but Zapruder begged off, saying they could meet at Zapruder's office at 9:00 a.m. Stolley arrived at Zapruder's office an hour early, and the men, along with some Secret Service agents, huddled around a film projector in the dressmaker's private office. Zapruder threaded the footage and started the machine, as the men watched in somber silence. Soon, representatives from media agencies, including the Associated Press, UPI, the *Saturday Evening Post*, and others, were allowed in to view the film. Everyone in the room knew that they had witnessed something of unprecedented historic value and that its exclusive rights would be worth a sky-high price.

Dan Rather, the KRLD-TV reporter, was one of those allowed to view the footage, and he spoke about it in a phone call with Don Hewitt, CBS TV News' New York producer, who would go on to create the series *60 Minutes*. Hewitt ordered Rather to sock Zapruder in the jaw, copy the film, and return it after CBS aired it first. The network's lawyers would smooth over everything after the fact, he maintained. But right before Rather embarked upon that ill-advised mission, Hewitt called back to say he had changed his mind.

Since Stolley made the first national contact, Zapruder agreed to hear his pitch first. As the other newsmen exited into the reception area, they yelled at him not to make up his mind until they had a chance to match or beat any offer. Zapruder told Stolley that he wished he hadn't shot the footage, but since he did, he might as well sell it to give his family financial security. One proviso was that the images could not be handled in a sensational fashion. Whoever bought Zapruder's footage would have to keep a tight rein on how it was stored and used. Stolley assured him that *Life* magazine shared that goal and stated that his editor might be willing to pay as much as $15,000 for the exclusive print publishing rights to the 486 frames of film. Zapruder indicated that the offer was nowhere near sufficient. Stolley knew that his competitors outside the door would push any bidding into the stratosphere, so he had to lock up the deal quickly while he had Zapruder's full attention. Stolley called *Life*'s parent company, Time Inc., in New York City. He was granted permission to make a final offer of $50,000.

Zapruder liked *Life*'s reputation and had faith that Stolley and his team would respect the film. Although they both knew the other sources could and would beat the price, Zapruder went with his best judgment. Stolley typed up a rough contract that they both signed, then sneaked out a back door, with the original film. Zapruder kept the remaining print. When representatives of TV or motion picture outlets heard that the magazine's agreement was only for print rights, they besieged Zapruder to sell or license them the footage to run on television or theatrically. Exhausted, Zapruder put off making a deal on that possibility.

Stolley flew his precious cargo to *Life*'s Chicago printing office, where editorial executives viewed the footage to decide which frames to publish. A lab technician accidentally damaged the film in two places, and six frames were removed, leaving splice marks. Stolley then flew with the film to Time Inc.'s corporate office in Manhattan. On Monday, November 25, while the rest of the nation was transfixed by news coverage of Kennedy's coffin on display in the Capitol's rotunda, Stolley screened the footage for his executive publisher, C.D. Jackson. The publisher was so unnerved by the frame capturing Kennedy's head being shot that he said the company needed to obtain full rights to the film, which it would use to keep it off the market, at least for a while. Zapruder turned the negotiation over to Dallas attorney Sam Passman, who insisted on a nondisclosure agreement, citing the anti–Semitism among some locals and fearing for his client's safety. That assured, the two parties reached a new deal of $150,000-plus royalties, which precluded Zapruder from selling off the film and TV rights to any other entity. The money would be paid in six annual installments of $25,000, with the first amount going in full to patrolman J.D. Tippit's widow and children.

To promote the upcoming *Life* issue, United Press International and the Associated Press were allowed to run seven frames of the film in their newspapers around the world. On November 29, the *Life* issue hit the stands, featuring 31 black-and-white frames of the Zapruder film. Two weeks later, the magazine released a special memorial issue with nine color frames. The gruesome head shot frames were not published. Three years later, *Life* published an anniversary issue to reflect public skepticism over the Warren Commission Report. The black cover included the words, "Did Oswald Act Alone: A Matter of Reasonable Doubt," with the color photo of frame 230, showing Kennedy's hands at his throat.

On various occasions, when the FBI asked to borrow the camera to verify the timing, Zapruder complied, and he also participated in a few documentaries. He later donated his camera to Bell & Howell, which later turned it over to the National Archives. Zapruder testified twice before the Warren Commission and took part in a re-creation of the event, once again standing on the pedestal, pretending to film the motorcade. He also testified during the New Orleans trial of businessman Clay Shaw, showing the jury the footage 10 times. In 1970, Zapruder died of stomach cancer. During his lifetime, Zapruder never asked for the return of his original film, which remained in a safe at Time Inc. It was there I was invited to view it in 1966.

On February 14, 1969, KTLA-TV newsman Hal Fishman was the first reporter to air a bootleg version of the Zapruder film but only for the Los Angeles market. Its first national airing occurred on March 6, 1975, when ABC's Geraldo Rivera broadcast the footage on his television program, *Good Night America*. The following month Time Inc. sold the copyright and original film back to the Zapruder family for $1. Zapruder's son, Henry, took control of the film's licensing and rented the footage out for theatrical and television use, earning top dollar.

When the original became too fragile and could no longer be handled, Henry Zapruder gave it to the National Archives in 1978 for safekeeping in its Kennedy Collection. But the family still controlled the copyright. In 1997, the Assassination Records Review Board offered the Zapruder family $1 million for the copyright and original. The Zapruder family attorney counter-offered with $30 million, reasoning that the film rights and possession of the footage should be viewed as a valuable objet d'art. The U.S. Justice Department suggested that the government should just confiscate the film. For two years, the two sides haggled. Then, a federal arbitration panel awarded the Zapruders a payout of $16 million plus interest for the actual footage, with the family still maintaining ownership of the copyright. On December 30, 1999, the family donated the copyright, copies, and photographs to the Sixth Floor Museum at Dealey Plaza.

Other people who filmed key moments of the assassination also monetized their home movies. Mary Muchmore's footage that showed a different angle of the fatal shot was purchased for $1,000 by UPI and ran on WNEW-TV in New York City on November 26. She did not tell the FBI she had the footage, but her family did. When agents interviewed her, she admitted having a camera that day but denied that she used it. In January 1964, the Bureau learned otherwise when UPI published frames in a commemorative book, giving her a credit. Muchmore's footage was later acquired by the Associated Press Television News.

In early December 1963, Orville Nix earned $5,000 from UPI for the copyright and original of his film. The news agency returned the copyright and prints in 1992, but the original was missing. In the 1966 documentary *Rush to Judgment*, based on author Mark Lane's best-selling book of the same name, Nix told Lane that the film he got back was not identical to what he shot. He also said that as he was filming, he was certain the rifle fire came from the grassy knoll but was later persuaded that the bullets came from the book depository. Nix licensed the footage to other outlets over the years, then in 2002, the copyright was assigned to the Sixth Floor Museum.

Oswald Goes Deeper

Prior to the assassination, in February 1962, Marina Oswald was raising an infant daughter and became pregnant with her second child, who would be named Rachel. That summer, her husband landed a job at the Leslie Welding Company in Dallas, but didn't like the work and quit after three months. So, the October introduction of Oswald to Russian émigré George de Mohrenschildt seemed a lucky break for the young family man.

The pairing of the aristocratic Belarusian and the pugnacious Oswald must have raised eyebrows when they were out and about. De Mohrenschildt brought Oswald to some of his anti–Castro meetings in Dallas, then would be debriefed by George's CIA friend, J. Walton Moore. When de Mohrenschildt told Moore he needed help landing an oil lease deal with Haiti's "Papa Doc" Duvalier, the contract was magically finalized. De Mohrenschildt would later say that he assumed it was a nice payback from the CIA for furnishing them with data about Oswald. Individuals like de Mohrenschildt didn't have to be on the Central Intelligence Agency's payroll to derive benefits from its influential executives.

De Mohrenschildt got Oswald a position as a photoprint trainee at the graphic arts firm Jaggars-Chiles-Stovall. Workers found Oswald obnoxious, and one remembered him reading a Russian magazine. After six months, Oswald was fired. Many scholars have wondered whether he got the job there for the access to materials he'd need to create false identifications.

In October 1962, Oswald rented Dallas post office box number 2915 under the alias of "Alek J. Hidell." On the following January 27, he purchased via mail order a Smith & Wesson "Victory" model .38 snub-nose revolver for $29.95, plus shipping and handling. And on March 12, 1963, Oswald bought a weapon that he had seen advertised in the February issue of *American Rifleman* magazine. It was a bolt-operated Mannlicher-Carcano 6.5 millimeter, with a flimsy telescopic sight. Using the phony name "A. Hidell," Oswald wrote a money order in the amount of $19.95, plus $1.50 for shipping and handling, and the rifle was mailed to his post office box. (For anyone believing that Oswald's Mannlicher-Carcano rifle was perfectly capable for the precision firing needed to kill JFK, let me describe a lecture I gave in 1972, at a legal medicine conference in Rome. The attendees spoke English and were fascinated by my presentation, but as I described Oswald's Italian-made World War

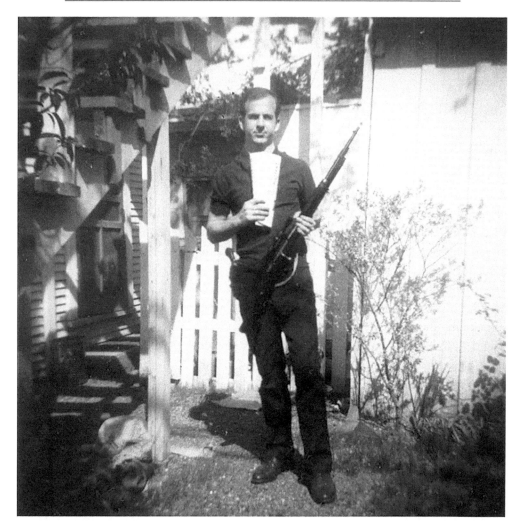

We'll never know Lee Harvey Oswald's motivation in posing for this photograph (House Select Committee on Assassinations).

II–era rifle, there were guffaws from the crowd, many of whom had served in that conflict. When I asked about their reaction, the program chairman explained that the Mannlicher-Carcano was such an unreliable, trashy weapon, it was considered more "an instrument of love than a weapon of war.")

Oswald's political view morphed from backing communism to bashing fascism. He had Marina take a photo of him, holding his new firearms and copies of the radical newspapers *The Worker* and *The Militant*. He signed a print of that photo for de Mohrenschildt: "For George, Lee Harvey Oswald," and dated it April 5, 1963. On the back of the photo, Marina penned in Russian: "Hunter of fascists, ha ha ha." On that day, Oswald moved beyond his normal, belligerent behavior to something more sinister.

Major General Edwin Walker

Army Major General Edwin Anderson Walker was highly decorated and fought in World War II and the Korean War. But in the early 1960s, he fell out of favor with the U.S. government for his ultra-conservative political views while in uniform. In 1961, Walker passed out material from the racist John Birch Society to his soldiers, and there were claims he tried to influence their votes in elections. When Walker referred to President Harry Truman and former First Lady Eleanor Roosevelt as "communist sympathizers," President Kennedy asked for and received Walker's resignation from the military.

Supported by billionaire oilman H.L. Hunt, Walker moved back to his home state of Texas and ran a losing gubernatorial race against John Connally. A fervent segregationist, Walker was arrested in October 1962 for leading a protest against James Meredith, a black student who attempted to enroll in the then all-white University of Mississippi.

Attorney General Robert Kennedy wanted Walker charged with sedition and insurrection and convened a federal grand jury to seek an indictment. He also ordered that Walker be committed to a psychiatric institution for a 90-day evaluation, but after five days, a judge allowed Walker to return home. Five days after the grand jury refused to indict Walker, Oswald bought his mail-order revolver. Walker's anti-communist speeches continued to get a lot of press in Dallas, and, after one in which he urged the U.S. government to get rid of the communist "scourge" in Cuba, Oswald bought his rifle. George de Mohrenschildt and Michael Paine were two particular critics of Walker who expressed their disdain about him to Oswald. Oswald began stalking Walker and taking photos of the general's residence.

On April 5, 1963, Oswald went to Walker's home. He planned to stand on the street and fire his rifle when he saw the general inside. Oswald thought he'd have safe cover because there would be a prayer meeting at a church next door, but when he found the church empty, he postponed his plan. Five nights later, Oswald crouched behind a fence at the rear of the house where he could see Walker sitting as his desk. Oswald fired one shot, at a distance of less than 100 feet away. The bullet hit the wooden frame of the window, and small fragments hit the general's arm and caused bleeding.

A neighbor told police he saw two men run into the church parking lot, then drive off in separate cars. A friend of Walker said that two nights before the shooting, he had seen two men peering into the house's windows. Walker told investigators he didn't see the shooter but spied taillights of a car leaving the area. He even hired private eyes to check it out, but they came up empty.

Oswald had been studying typing three nights a week but quit the class the week prior to the Walker shooting. On April 10, Marina had expected him home after work, but as the night wore on and he hadn't arrived, she became worried. She grew even more concerned when she found an undated note from him to her in a cookbook. The note, in Russian, consisted of directives to Marina in the event he was captured alive after the Walker shooting. He explained the location of the city jail where he would be held. Oswald wanted Marina to collect any newspaper coverage that mentioned him and bring it to the embassy, adding that they would provide her with assistance, as would the Red Cross. He left a small amount of money and wrote that Marina should get rid of his clothing but hold onto his personal papers and military records. He told her the rent and utilities were paid, as well as the rent on a mailbox inside the post office. He furnished the box's key and said that his paycheck would be there soon.

But Oswald wasn't caught that night. Instead, he showed up at home late and "very pale." He told Marina that he had shot at General Walker but wasn't sure if the bullet hit him. He told her he had been planning the attack for two months but refused to give her more information. Marina told investigators that the day after the shooting, when Oswald found out Walker had been only slightly wounded, he expressed regret that he had not killed him. He compared Walker to Adolf Hitler, she said in her testimony to the Warren Commission. A few days later, he showed her a notebook with photos of Walker's home and a map of the area. He told her he had hidden the rifle near some train tracks. The FBI would later confirm the handwriting on the note belonged to Oswald, and, in 1977, when neutron activation testing became available, the Walker bullet was matched to Oswald's Mannlicher-Carcano.

A few days after Walker's sniper assault, the de Mohrenschildts visited Oswald to bring little June an Easter gift. According to George's Warren Commission testimony, he saw Oswald's rifle standing upright in a closet and jokingly asked whether he was the one who had shot at Walker, supposedly eliciting a smile from Oswald. In Jeanne de Mohrenschildt's testimony, she said they all laughed at George's joke and that the day marked the last time she or her husband would see the Oswalds. The de Mohrenschildts' comments undermine what Marina told police about Oswald hiding the rifle outside the home. Marina added that George actually asked Oswald why he had missed the shot. We're left to guess whether this was just lighthearted banter or reflective of some deeper connection between de Mohrenschildt and the Walker shooting. De Mohrenschildt later told his CIA contact Walter Moore about Oswald's part in the attempted assassination and of the signed photo that Oswald had given to him.

Shortly after, Marina and June would move into the Irving, Texas, home of Ruth Paine and her two toddlers. Ruth's marriage had ended, and the women felt they could help each other with childcare. Oswald took a room about 15 miles away, in Dallas, and would visit his family on weekends.

Walker would spend the rest of his life making antagonistic claims against the government, then suing media outlets that disagreed with him. Before he died in 1993 at the age of 66, he had two arrests and served 30 days in jail for fondling an undercover policeman in a public restroom.

Assuming that Oswald was Walker's attempted assassin, did someone give him this mission, or did he think of it himself? Was this event a trial run to test his mettle for an even larger job? If not, what was it intended to prove? Did he have a colleague at the shooting, and, if so, who was it? Unfortunately, these questions were never answered. It would be hard to envision de Mohrenschildt accompanying Oswald on such a mission and running off like some street tough. But it's entirely possible that Oswald had a more "rough around the edges" colleague at the scene. Some scholars believe that second person could have been Jack Ruby. If the Dallas authorities investigated the Walker shooting, they didn't gather enough evidence to make an arrest. Maybe they weren't interested in solving the case.

Oswald in New Orleans

Oswald took an extended stay in New Orleans on April 24, 1963, and got a menial job with the Reily Foods Company in its coffee division. The company's owner, William B. Reily, Jr., was an organizer of the Crusade to Free Cuba Committee, a grass-roots anti–Castro group. Since Oswald's views were favorable to Castro, his employment there didn't last, although Reily cited Oswald's laziness as the reason for his dismissal.

While working for Reily, Oswald wrote to the New York City–based Fair Play for Cuba Committee (FPFC), advising that he wished to open a chapter in New Orleans. He suggested that he would personally pay for a small office rental. His offer was rejected by the Manhattan headquarters, which had no confidence that their message would be warmly received in New Orleans. But Oswald had his own agenda, stating that he had already rented the office space. You might well ask how a man who was perpetually out of work and had trouble supporting his family could afford office space for what seemed like a vanity project, and why. As the self-appointed head and only member of the New Orleans chapter, Oswald also had cards and leaflets printed with the words "Hands Off Cuba! Join the Fair Play for Cuba Committee, New Orleans Charter Member Branch, Free Literature, Lectures, Everyone Welcome!" A special card identified him as chapter president in the name of "A.J. Hidell." Despite Oswald's best attempts to gather steam for his group, no one joined up.

After Oswald's job ended, he stepped up his FPFC activities. On August 5 and 6, he visited a shop owned by Carlos Bringuier, a student leader in an anti–Castro group. Bringuier felt Oswald was trying to infiltrate his organization and sent him packing. On the 9th, the men had a confrontation on a street corner where Oswald was handing out leaflets. They, along with two of Bringuier's pals, were arrested for disturbing the peace. At the police station, Oswald asked to speak to an FBI agent and had an hour-long conversation with local agent John Quigley. Days later, Oswald paid a $10 fine for his arrest.

According to Robert J. Groden's book, *The Search for Lee Harvey Oswald* (Penguin Books, 1995), for which I wrote the foreword, Marina would later tell authorities that she believed Oswald wanted to be arrested because he craved publicity for his cause. She called it "self-advertising" (Groden 73). Marina tried not to criticize Oswald about his political views because he was hot-tempered. He would frequently hit her and once gave her a black eye. She was finding it more and more of a challenge to maintain a peaceful home life with him. She wrote a letter to a former boyfriend in Minsk, telling him that she was sorry she didn't marry him instead of Oswald and complaining that her life was miserable because Oswald didn't love her. But she failed to put enough postage on the letter. It was returned, and Oswald found it and humiliated her by reading it aloud to her. He followed that up with another beating, then cried and told Marina that he did love her.

On August 16, Oswald and two hired associates were passing out FPFC leaflets in front of the International Trade Mart, which moved imported and domestic goods that came through the port city of New Orleans. WDSU-TV, the NBC affiliate, showed Oswald on its news broadcast. The next day he was interviewed on WDSU radio. The host, William Stuckey, arranged for Oswald to debate the Cuban issue with Bringuier and an associate.

Oswald's FPFC office space was at 544 Camp Street in a corner building. The other side of the same building had the address 531 Lafayette Street and housed Guy Banister and Associates, a detective agency run by a former FBI agent. Banister's business had deep ties with the anti–Castro movement. Banister, who died in 1964, was never questioned by the Warren Commission. His brother, Ross, told the House Select Committee on Assassinations that Guy didn't know Oswald but had once seen him handing out his pro–Cuba leaflets. Ross felt Oswald had chosen his office in the building to embarrass his brother. Guy Banister's secretary, Delphine Roberts, had a different take on the intrigue. She maintained that Oswald had visited Banister's office on many occasions, including once when he filled out a job application. Still, the HSCA found Roberts' testimony to be lacking in corroboration and therefore unreliable.

There were also reports that Oswald had been seen with David Ferrie, the former Civilian Air Patrol pilot, and Clay Shaw, a New Orleans businessman. Shaw was a founder and director of the International Trade Mart, where Oswald had been filmed passing out leaflets. Shaw was also involved in efforts to preserve and upgrade historic buildings in the city's French Quarter. More about him later.

Other Oswalds?

Back in Texas now, Lee Harvey Oswald is said to have boarded a bus from Houston to Mexico City on September 26. He supposedly told fellow passengers that he planned to travel to Cuba. Arriving in the Mexican capital on the 27th, he is alleged to have gone to the Cuban Embassy, claiming he wanted to travel through Cuba and go back to the Soviet Union. There are some excellent sources, including author Mark Lane, who believe there was a "second Oswald" who was sent on this mission and others. For one thing, black-and-white photos of the man claimed to be Oswald were taken by surveillance cameras in Mexico City. At the Cuban Embassy, the man in the photo shows a side-view of a much older man with a completely different hairline. The photo taken at the Russian Embassy shows a man who is considerably heftier than Oswald and dissimilar to the man at the Cuban Embassy.

The Cuban Embassy photo was furnished to the FBI by the CIA, via Fort Worth-born David Atlee Phillips, a career CIA officer and chief of all covert operations for the Western hemisphere. In 1963, Phillips ran his empire from the CIA's office in Mexico City, a job previously held by William F. Buckley, Jr., and Buckley's superior, E. Howard Hunt, later known as one of President Nixon's Watergate burglars. Phillips would be in the best position to know what occurred there with Oswald, and he told Lane that Oswald was never there. Could Phillips have lied? And could Oswald have also gone to Mexico but wasn't the individual in the photos? And if Oswald went there, why have no photos of him surfaced?

There was also an Oswald look-alike who took a test drive at a Dallas Lincoln Mercury dealership, bragging loudly that he'd soon have money for a car. The real Oswald didn't drive or have a license, although Ruth Paine had given him a few lessons. And there were several sightings at the Sports Drome Rifle Range in Dallas, where someone purporting to be Oswald engaged in target practice with a rifle, on one occasion shooting at the target for the person next to him. The tradition of spycraft is to spend time rolling out a cover story for operations and agents that need protection. This is not unique to the CIA; it happens with intelligence services in Russia, Great Britain, Israel, and elsewhere. Elaborate legends are crafted to create aliases and backstories for the target. In American parlance, the process is known as "fixing a phony."

Was Oswald given that kind of treatment? I don't know. But in interviews over the years, Oswald's mother Marguerite insisted that her son was used by the CIA in Russia, then reactivated as an agent in mid–1963 with the Agency payroll identity of #110669. She believed he was following orders when he went to New Orleans and posed as a pro–Castro organizer. And she felt he was told to go to Mexico City and try to get to Havana.

But what was the purpose of such a journey? Was he supposed to infiltrate Cuban intelligence, as he tried to do in the Soviet Union, or might he have been told to assassinate Fidel Castro? This was the era when numerous attempts on Castro's life were sanctioned and made by the CIA and their cohorts. Whatever Oswald thought his mission was might have been much different from what his handlers had in mind for him. They would know the "big picture" that he wouldn't necessarily have been privy to. If so, Oswald would have been the "missing link" between the CIA plotters of JFK's assassination and Castro, allowing the Agency to lay blame on our number-one enemy in Cuba. Such an ambitious idea might have resulted in the deaths of both Kennedy and Castro, with Oswald remaining as collateral damage to be dealt with later. If this was the plan, it was not well-executed. Oswald's tourist visa to Cuba was denied until officials at the embassy could reach their counterparts in Moscow. Following days of spats with consulate officials, Oswald was told he was harming, rather than helping, the Cuban Revolution. Oswald's behavior caught the attention of both the KGB and the CIA.

Curtain Rods or a Rifle?

A fter Oswald returned to Dallas and rented the Oak Cliff boarding house room, Ruth Paine's neighbor told her of a job opening at the Texas School Book Depository. The company furnished hundreds of titles of textbooks to area high schools and colleges. Of the seven floors of the building, the second, third, and part of the fourth floors were offices, and most everything else was warehousing. Order-fillers would go to whichever floor the particular books were stored to fill their work orders. There were two side-by-side freight elevators, a staircase, and a loading dock to facilitate the workers. On the street-level first floor was the employees' recreation room, with tables, a Dr. Pepper vending machine, and a refrigerator where they would stow their bag lunches until noontime. The official lunchroom was on the second floor; it had a Coca Cola machine. A sandwich seller would come around in the morning for anyone who didn't bring his or her own food.

At Marina Oswald's request, Ruth called the superintendent, Roy Truly, who told her that Oswald should fill out an application. Oswald met with Truly on October 15, mentioned his need for work and how his wife was almost ready to deliver their second child, and was hired as an order filler. Oswald's job began the next day. It was Monday through Friday, from 8:00 a.m. to 4:45 p.m., with a 45-minute lunch break— he earned $1.25 per hour, a decent wage for the era. Truly told the Warren Commission that Oswald caught on quickly and performed well—and wasn't very social, unlike some of the workers who chitchatted too much. He found Oswald "above average" and someone "who did a good day's work," never missing a day in his weeks of employment.

Nineteen-year-old Buell "Wesley" Frazier was also an order-filler at the depository and had worked there since September. Frazier lived with his mother, his sister, and his sister's family in Irving, three doors away from where Marina and her children lived with Ruth Paine, although he had never met his neighbors. Frazier taught Lee the preferences of different publishers and helped familiarize him with the books and work orders. Frazier offered to drive Oswald to Irving on Friday evening and back to Dallas on Monday morning, which Lee gratefully accepted. Frazier never asked him for gas money, figuring he'd be making the drive anyway, and it would be nice to have someone to talk with. But if conversation was Frazier's goal, he didn't get much from Oswald. The only subject that could get Oswald yakking was when children were mentioned. Frazier's sister and brother-in-law had three little girls, whom Oswald knew from seeing them at the park. When Frazier would talk about his nieces' exploits, Oswald would beam and open up about his own little ones. June was two, and Rachel was just a month old in November 1963.

Oswald told Frazier he had been in the Marines, and when asked about the places in the world he had traveled, Oswald mentioned France, Germany, and Russia—but never volunteered details or mentioned having been posted to Japan. Lee didn't talk about guns, politics, communism, or where and how he had met Marina. Both men would usually pack a brown paper-bag lunch and would often see each other in the second-floor lunchroom during their meal breaks.

On the morning of Thursday, November 21, Oswald asked Frazier if he could get a ride to Irving after work that day. He said he wanted to get some curtain rods from the Paine home that he would bring back to his Dallas apartment. Frazier answered that that would be fine, and at quitting time they both got into Frazier's car. The next morning, as Frazier was having breakfast with his nieces, he spotted Oswald standing by Frazier's car. As both men entered the vehicle, Frazier glanced over his shoulder and noticed a package on the back seat, on the passenger side. It was about two feet long, five to six inches wide, and wrapped in brown paper. He asked Oswald what it was, and Oswald explained it was the curtain rods he had mentioned. The drive to work was typically uneventful. Neither man spoke of the presidential motorcade that would be passing by their place of employment in a few hours. As they got out of the car at the depository parking lot, Frazier noticed that Oswald had not brought a bag lunch on that day, the first time that had ever occurred. Oswald told him he planned to buy his lunch. Oswald had the paper bag tucked under his right arm as he walked toward the workplace. His hand cupped the bottom of the bag, and the top part was under his armpit.

Frazier stated that he saw Oswald here and there in the morning but not after 11:00 a.m. On the sixth floor that day, workers were busy laying an extra layer of plywood to fortify the existent flooring. At noon, Frazier went outside the depository to wait for the presidential parade. The self-described "Texas boy" felt civic pride and wanted to witness the occasion, knowing that Kennedy didn't come to Dallas often. Frazier stood on the steps near the front door with coworker Billy Lovelady and other employees. They watched as the motorcycles first passed by, followed by the president's black limo and the other cars. Frazier remarked to a woman nearby that Jackie Kennedy looked as beautiful as she did in her magazine photos.

When Frazier heard the first rifle shot, he assumed it was a backfire from one of the motorcycles, but when the next shots were heard, followed quickly by people hollering and running, he knew someone had fired at somebody, and JFK was the probable target. He craned his neck to see the last of the cars drive by, as a lady ran toward the building shouting that Kennedy had been shot. Soon police officers were swarming the area, and some went into the depository. A roll call of employees was held outside Mr. Truly's first-floor office. Everyone was present and accounted for, except for Oswald. His absence didn't faze Frazier who figured Oswald might have gone to one of the local sandwich shops, since he hadn't brought lunch.

A police officer made a list of names of the employees and where they were on the premises when the motorcade went by. Afterward, Frazier went into the lunchroom to eat his sandwich, then joined other workers until one of the bosses told them to go home for the day. Instead of driving straight home, he detoured to the Pioneer Medical Center to see his stepfather who was a patient there. On the drive, Frazier turned on the radio and heard that police had closed in on an unidentified male who had lived in Russia. But that scant bit of information didn't make Frazier think of Oswald.

Unbeknownst to Frazier, two members of the Dallas Police Department had already visited his sister's house, searched it, confiscated his shotgun, and learned he was going to the hospital. By the time Frazier arrived, they were waiting for him. Two detectives brought Frazier to a private room and questioned him rather pointedly. They pushed him against the wall and said he was under arrest regarding the president's death. Saying they were taking him to the police station, the officers began to handcuff him, Frazier said that wasn't necessary. He didn't have anything to do with the assassination and would be happy to tell them that in a formal statement. The subsequent interview would go on for many hours. First, they took Frazier's mug shot and fingerprinted him. Then they made him face a wall and told him he couldn't avert his gaze, while they asked him the same questions over and over. Occasionally another team of detectives would replace the original two and repeat the grilling.

Captain Will Fritz entered the interrogation room and leaned into Frazier's face. He waved a piece of paper in front of Frazier and demanded he sign it. The document stated that Frazier had been involved with the assassination. When Frazier refused to sign, Fritz lifted his hand to smack him in the head, but Frazier blocked the shot. Fritz stormed out of the room. The cops never charged him with anything. Frazier told the investigators that no one mentioned Oswald to him after the shooting. When Frazier left the building, he did not know that Oswald would become a target of the police, or that the package he saw that morning contained anything other than the curtain rods he was told were inside. He didn't bother to look for Oswald at the depository for a ride back to Irving, because he assumed Oswald was planning to go to his apartment.

After telling his story to detectives, Frazier repeated it to FBI agents. On March 11, 1964, he was flown to Washington, D.C., to give testimony before the full Warren Commission panel. He was questioned by Commissioner Joseph Ball who wanted him to admit that he knew the package that Oswald had put on his backseat contained a rifle. To try to prove that point, the Commission lawyers made Frazier cut, fold, and wrap similar brown paper into the size and shape of the package he saw that day. Frazier insisted that the Mannlicher-Carcano rifle, even if it had been broken down into two pieces, would not have fit in the small package he saw. Although he only caught a quick peek of it on the car seat, he saw Oswald carrying the package as they walked toward the depository. Had it been a rifle, part of the stock would have stuck up from the package, Frazier said.

Ball also handed Frazier a brown paper bag that two FBI agents had prepared as an Exhibit. Inside was a dismantled Italian rifle, similar to the Mannlicher-Carcano. The Commissioner asked Frazier to stand, hold the bag like Oswald had held his, and—ridiculously—suggested that he ignore the rifle in the bag. But Frazier protested, stating that the packages weren't similar at all. The Ball package was too lengthy to fit under Frazier's armpit, which was even more absurd because they had established that Frazier was a couple of inches taller than Oswald was. And unlike Oswald's package, which topped out at his armpit, the Ball package extended up to the level of Frazier's ear. (Years later, author and JFK historian Josiah Thompson brought a Mannlicher-Carcano rifle to a lecture where he and Frazier were speakers. Thompson separated the rifle's barrel and stock, and put it in a similarly sized paper bag. Just as in the ersatz demonstration before the Commissioners, the rifle's stock was exposed.)

Aware they had a problem area with Frazier's testimony, the Commissioners decided to give it another go. On July 24, the panel's assistant counsel Wesley J. Liebeler flew to Dallas for his crack at Frazier. Perhaps he felt a little "Wesley-to-Wesley" conversation would produce the results the panel needed. But if he were hoping for a "Perry Mason moment" where the witness would admit to lying, he didn't get it. Polite and unflappable, Frazier repeated the same story he had told authorities all along. The questioning was over in about five minutes.

The Commissioners may have lost the battle with him, but they won the war. When they drafted their official account, they detailed Frazier's remembrance—but attributed it to him simply being "mistaken." Frazier was furious when he read the Warren Commission Report and saw how his honest portrayal of facts was not sufficient for the panel. All these years later, he's still adamantly sticking with the narrative he told from the beginning. Frazier says he has no idea how Oswald's rifle got into the building and adds the only person who can be sure about what was in the brown paper package was Oswald.

No one has stepped forward to say he or she planted the rifle on the sixth-floor sniper's nest. By the same token, no curtain rods were found in the depository. But it should be noted that, according to reporters who visited the North Beckley Avenue rooming house where Oswald was a renter, the window in his room had a curtain that was held up by a curtain rod. It's possible Oswald had other plans for the curtain rod, if that's what was in the package. Frazier never discussed the details with Oswald and never went inside his Oak Cliff apartment.

The Murder
of Lee Harvey Oswald

Once my work was finished in Los Angeles, on Sunday, November 24, I flew home to Pittsburgh. All of the assassination coverage of the past two days had made me crave seeing my family. But when Sigrid met me at the airport gate, she told me that Lee Harvey Oswald had been fatally shot by someone named Jack Ruby. She and millions of viewers had seen this awful and historic act happen live on television. When we arrived home and turned on our TV, the black-and-white network film was played again and again. All these years later, the blatant footage remains a paralyzing sight. News directors today, when faced with high-speed chases or situations where a death may occur, switch to other camera coverage, so the public is guarded from seeing something graphic. But in 1963, those protections didn't exist.

Quickly, I learned that Oswald had yet to be formally charged for the deaths of President Kennedy and Officer Tippit. That would happen in a court session in the coming week. Oswald, who had been staying at the city jail at the Dallas Police headquarters, was to be transferred to the county jail, blocks away, which was better suited for a longer stint as he awaited trial.

Police Chief Jesse Curry wanted the press to observe that Oswald had not sustained any injuries while in custody, so a phalanx of reporters lined both sides of the basement corridor. The prisoner would be marched to a waiting armored patrol car for the short trip. Patrol Officer R.C. Nelson, 26, who was usually the partner of Tippit, was on duty that day. While he wasn't present when Tippit was shot, he helped take Oswald into custody at the Texas Theatre. And now he was one of the cops assigned to protect Dallas Public Enemy Number One. A police car drove up to the north entry ramp to the basement as a decoy to confuse the media and ensure Oswald's smooth passage in a different vehicle. Plainclothes officers got into the cruiser, and a lieutenant drove it back to the street, around the block, and then back via the ramp. Its return would have provided the opening for Ruby to also enter the building where he was spotted walking past the decoy car.

Homicide detective Jim Leavelle, who had questioned Oswald about the Tippit shooting, was in charge of the maneuver. He waited for Oswald to put on a black sweater, then cuffed his hands in the front. Oswald wore no bulletproof vest. Leavelle took a second pair of cuffs and attached one manacle to the prisoner's wrist and the other to his own. He told the alleged assassin about dozens of death threats that the police had received about him and joked, "If anybody shoots at you, I hope they're as good a shot as you are." But Oswald assured Leavelle that neither of them had to worry about safety: "Nobody's gonna shoot at me," he said. Those would be his famous last words.

They got into the jail elevator and hit the button for the basement. Leavelle, wearing a light suit and white hat, was on Oswald's right, and another detective was on Oswald's left. Capt. Will Fritz and another officer led the parade, with Oswald and the detectives close behind. The bright lights of the cameras obscured their ability to see for a moment. The unmarked white sedan designated to transport them blasted its horn as it backed up the entry ramp, trying to move the herd of media.

WNEW radio journalist Ike Pappas shouted, "Do you have anything to say in your defense?" and thrust his microphone toward Oswald. But there was no chance for a response. A man in a dark fedora stepped out at Oswald's left front. He held a black .38 caliber revolver in his hand, pointed at Oswald's midsection. It was 11:21 a.m. Leavelle, recognizing the gunman as Ruby, reacted with a jerky motion, trying to move Oswald away, but there wasn't time or room. Another detective in the crowd yelled, "Jack, you son of a bitch, don't!" But Ruby fired once, sending a slug into his target's chest.

The film footage and photographs taken showed Oswald reacting in pain, with witnesses hearing a groan as he slumped over. Officers pulled their own guns and reporters, struggling to get a closer look, blocked the view of the cameras. As Ruby tried to get off more shots, a detective grabbed the gun and stopped him. Numerous cops leapt onto the shooter and brought him to the ground. Ruby looked at them and said, "It's me, it's Jack!" He was handcuffed by Officer Nelson and arrested.

Unconscious, Oswald was loaded into an ambulance, with Leavelle beside him. They sped to Parkland and were rushed into Trauma Room Two, out of deference to the president who had died in Trauma Room One. Dr. Charles Crenshaw was in the trauma room that day, as he had been for President Kennedy two days before. As Oswald was wheeled in, he was "deathly pale" but had a slight heartbeat. The surgeon noted that the bullet had entered Oswald's left thorax and that it could be felt under the skin when the area was palpated. The abdomen was bloated, indicating internal bleeding. The doctors went to work on the patient in much the same way they had worked on Kennedy by giving blood transfusions and Ringer's lactate into venous cutdowns on his leg and forearm. A chest tube was affixed to prevent Oswald's lung from collapsing, and oxygen anesthesia was pumped in.

Once Oswald was stabilized, he was brought via elevator to a second-floor operating room. A federal agent was in attendance, watching quietly, his identity hidden behind a hospital gown and mask. Dr. Malcolm Perry made an abdominal incision from Oswald's sternum to his pubis, releasing a gusher of blood. With Crenshaw wielding a retractor, the bullet was located in the right lateral body wall and removed. It had done a lot of damage, lacerating the aorta and the inferior vena cava—the large vein running from the pelvic area to the heart, receiving venous blood that branched to the spleen, stomach, pancreas, kidney, and liver. All hands were busy, trying to stem the bleeding and repair the damage.

Crenshaw would tell me years later that he was called out of the room to take an important phone call. He couldn't imagine what could be more "important" than what he was doing at the time, but the phone operator made it clear the matter wasn't up for debate. He scrubbed out, then went into the supervisor's room where there was a phone. He identified himself and heard the caller's deep Texas accent. "This is President Lyndon B. Johnson, Dr. Crenshaw. How is the accused assassin?" He told the president that Oswald was holding his own at the moment but that his condition was very serious. Johnson commanded Crenshaw to give the lead surgeons an order—that there should be a deathbed confession from Oswald that witnesses in the room would hear. Crenshaw went back into the surgical arena and delivered the word. But Oswald's body wouldn't cooperate. When his pulse slowed, Perry made another scalpel incision, this time exposing the patient's heart. The doctor who attempted in vain to massage President Kennedy's heart back to life was now performing the same task on JFK's alleged killer. But nothing worked. Not ventricular defibrillation, nor drugs injected right into the heart. Unable to be revived or saved, the now cyanotic Oswald was pronounced dead at 1:07 p.m. There would be no deathbed confession.

Crenshaw said the surgical team was especially dismayed to lose this patient, knowing the implications of the death. If only the ambulance that brought him to Parkland had been equipped with better emergency equipment and more skilled technicians, Oswald might have been resuscitated en route. Today's EMTs would not face the problem those in Dallas encountered on that day in 1963. Dr. Earl Rose, the county medical examiner, immediately performed the autopsy. The cause of death was listed as "hemorrhage secondary to gunshot wound of the chest," and the manner of death was "homicide." As I watched the news accounts of this unbelievable shooting and its aftermath, I felt cheated that there would be no trial for Lee Harvey Oswald.

Who Was Jack Ruby?

Jacob Leon Rubenstein was born in Chicago in 1911 to Polish-born Orthodox Jews, Joseph Rubenstein and Fannie Turek Rutowski, who immigrated to the United States in 1903. Yiddish was the family's primary language, although Joseph could speak a bit of English. He was a carpenter when he worked and an abusive drunk. Fannie had mental issues that led to hospital commitments in 1937 and 1938. The Rubensteins would eventually divorce. Fannie died in 1944; Joseph in 1958.

A middle child with seven surviving siblings, Ruby was a juvenile delinquent who spent time in foster care after his first arrest at 11 for truancy. A psychiatric examination found young Ruby to be "disobedient" and "quick-tempered," especially if anyone called him by his childhood nickname of "Sparky." Although he'd never shy away from a fistfight, he didn't always win them. Ruby's mother, who was illiterate, wanted him to stay in school, but his father considered anything beyond grammar school as pointless. Jack's real education came from the streets, where he hawked horse-racing tip sheets and did favors for the local trash collectors. In his early 20s, he moved to San Francisco and sold newspapers door-to-door. He also worked in Los Angeles as a singing waiter and once served 30 days in jail for selling song sheets he hadn't realized were copyrighted.

At 32, during the height of World War II, Ruby was drafted into the Army Air Force. For three years, he worked stateside as an aircraft mechanic and in 1946 earned an honorable discharge as a private first class. He might have advanced in rank had he not punched out a sergeant who called him a "Jew bastard." Returning to Chicago, he and two of his brothers started a mail order firm, changing their surname to "Ruby." He ran errands for Al Capone's henchman, Frank Nitti, who brought in big bucks from the city's illegal gambling operations. But Ruby dreamed of a career in show business, and the Chicago gangsters were eager to help him expand in exchange for kickbacks. In 1947, Ruby moved to Dallas and worked as a nightclub manager. He learned to take care of the cops who dropped by his establishments off-hours, giving them discounts on liquor and introductions to strippers, although the dancers were barred from having sex with customers. Often depressed, Ruby had a mental breakdown in 1952 and briefly felt suicidal but soon got back on track.

In 1959, Ruby traveled to Havana, Cuba, to visit a close friend named Lewis McWillie, who ran gambling at the Tropicana hotel. That casino and others were operated by Santo Trafficante, Jr., the Mafia boss from Tampa, Florida. The mobster had been briefly jailed by Cuba's new leader Fidel Castro, who wanted to end American influence. Trafficante's goal was to protect his interests by employing people he could trust in case he was taken off the streets again. The potential for skimming huge amounts of cash off the top of the daily gambling proceeds from casinos was too lucrative to abandon. Cuban officials didn't mind if the equipment was rigged to the casino boss' advantage. Trafficante would later admit that he worked with the CIA on efforts to assassinate Castro.

There are no records of meetings among Trafficante, McWillie, and Ruby, but many researchers believe there were ties. A British journalist named John Wilson Hudson, who was detained in the Havana jail at the same time as Trafficante, alleged that Ruby visited the mob boss there and would bring him food from the hotel. Ruby was also said to have been seen with Chicago crime chieftain Sam Giancana, New Orleans kingpin Carlos Marcello, Dallas thugs Joe Campisi and Joseph Civello, and others.

Ruby was politically promiscuous when it came to Cuba. When he was with his Mafia buddies, he was anti–Castro, but he would also make money by running guns from the states to Castro's freedom fighters. After the assassination, a friend told authorities he witnessed Ruby in Texas, loading crates of automatic rifles and handguns onto a boat headed for Havana. A separate source, who was an FBI informant, attested to a similar sighting in Miami. Ruby denied all involvement with gun-running to the Warren Commission attorneys.

By November 1963, Ruby owned the Silver Spur Inn and two strip clubs in Dallas: the Carousel and the after-hours Vegas, which was managed by his sister, Eva Grant. Ruby hired stand-up comics as emcees in-between the dancer sets but warned them not to tell anti–Semitic or vulgar jokes if they wanted to keep their jobs. Wally Weston was one of Jack's regular emcees at the Carousel and helpful when it came to recruiting new dancers. Jack would pitch in to keep the customers in line, once getting part of his finger bitten off by a drunk he was tossing out the door. The Carousel, where Ruby spent most of his nights, was the home for such exotic ecdysiasts as Tammi True, Kathy Kay, Little Lynn, Joy Dale, Toni Rebel, and Peggy Steel, among others. A flashy talent from out of town, Janet "Jada" Conforto, was a featured stripper who'd bring in a crowd of big spenders. The average dancer could take home a stunning amount of money per night. Cocktail waitresses all earned healthy tips.

Although Ruby put his club's earnings into an account at the First National Bank, his own walking-around cash would be stuffed into his coat pockets, usually a couple thousand dollars at a time. He also carried an unholstered gun either tucked in the waistband of his slacks or in an inside pocket of his jacket. Ruby watched his diet and got regular exercise, and seldom drank alcohol or smoked. He read two newspapers per day and liked to listen to the radio and watch westerns on television. Ruby's Dallas apartment had two bedrooms, and he often had someone staying in the spare room, rent-free. There were always dachshund puppies, their mother being Sheba, whom Ruby jokingly referred to as his "wife" and would take everywhere.

Primarily a Democrat, Ruby neither married nor had children but contributed to youth charities. He had platonic relationships with his dancers, and although there were rumors that he might be homosexual, those close to him disputed it when badgered by Warren Commission attorneys to peg him as such. The most direct information about Ruby's sex life came from Ruby himself, during questioning in July 1964, at the Dallas County Jail, when he admitted that if he had married Alice Nichols, a secretary he dated, his life would have turned out better. He met the divorced mother of a young daughter in 1949, and they saw each other for the next several years. At some point, they became engaged but never made any real plans to settle down together. Around 1959, Ruby seemed to lose interest in Alice and stopped calling her for dates.

On the 22nd, Ruby had stopped by the *Dallas Morning News* to place his weekend ads and was there at 12:45 p.m. when news of the assassination broke. He called his assistant at the Carousel and a number of other business associates. Then he called his sister, Eileen Kaminsky, in Chicago, and they both cried on the phone. Around 1:00 p.m., Ruby called Alice, but she was at lunch. The two had not talked for more than a year. She returned his call, and they spoke briefly, and as Nichols testified to the Warren Commission, Ruby seemed very upset that the president had been shot.

Ruby then apparently traveled five blocks to Parkland Hospital where he had the quick exchange with Seth Kantor and was seen by Wilma Tice and radio reporter Roy Stamps. From there, Ruby went to the Carousel to notify his staff that the club would be closed for the next three nights. Then he visited Eva, who had just arrived home after surgery. He told her both the Carousel and Vegas clubs would be closed, no matter how much money they would lose.

Ruby went home to get cleaned up. Around 6:30, he again called Alice and told her he was going to his synagogue. The regular Friday service at Congregation Shearith Israel became a memorial service for the president, according to Rabbi Hillel Silverman. The rabbi reminded the crowd that Kennedy was a man who had fought bravely in all battles but didn't have a chance to fight in Dealey Plaza because he was shot from the rear. Silverman, who had known Ruby for years, said that most of the attendees were either angry or in tears, but Ruby was neither. Ruby stayed at the temple until approximately 10 p.m.

Out of respect for the rabbi, Ruby had taken his gun out of his pocket and hid it behind his car seat while in the synagogue. But when he got back behind the wheel, he returned it to his right trouser pocket. As Ruby drove through the streets of Dallas, he took special note of those nightclubs that remained open, feeling disgust at their owners. He stopped at Phil's Delicatessen, which was across from the Vegas club, and paid for corned beef and pastrami sandwiches on rye bread. He then dropped by the police department, as he thought the homicide detectives would be working late and could use a meal. The officers said they were wrapping up work for the night and turned down his sandwiches, so he gave them to some of the nearby KLIF radio reporters. Ruby blended into the throng of media, and soon Captain Will Fritz and District Attorney Henry Wade brought Lee Harvey Oswald into the hallway and then to a conference room in the basement. Ruby would later state that that was the first time he had ever laid eyes on Oswald. Journalists yelled out questions at the alleged assassin, but Ruby couldn't hear Lee's responses.

In a subsequent press conference, Wade briefed reporters that Oswald was a member of an anti–Castro Free Cuba Committee. Ruby was one of several men present who corrected Wade that Oswald's involvement was with the pro–Castro Fair Play for Cuba Committee. Ruby even set up a phone interview between Wade and one of the KLIF disk jockeys, Russ Knight. Ruby told Knight to ask Wade if Oswald was insane.

After leaving the police headquarters, Ruby dropped by the *Dallas Times-Herald*, where he saw Pat Gadosh who usually placed Ruby's ads. Ruby mentioned the full-page ad that had appeared in Friday's *Dallas Morning News*, accusing the president of subversive activities. Ruby was angry about it, but Gadosh told him not to worry, because there had been a backlash at the paper for running it. Ruby headed home and spoke with his current roommate, George Senator. Ruby was still steamed that the ad reflected poorly on Jews since it stated having been paid for by a "Bernard Weissman." Sometime after 4:00 a.m. on Saturday morning, Ruby, Senator, and Jack's employee Larry Crafard, drove to the billboard, and Crafard snapped three Polaroids of it while Ruby wept. Around 6:00, they dropped Crafard back at the Carousel and went home to sleep.

Ruby awoke around 11:30 a.m. on Saturday and went to Dealey Plaza to see the memorial wreaths that had gathered over the past several hours. He then went to Solomon's Turf Bar and spoke with some of the regulars, showing them the Polaroids of the billboard and stating that someone should do something about it. Ruby spent the afternoon at the Carousel, calling friends to commiserate, including Breck Wall and Joe Peterson, a gay couple that were impresarios at another nightclub. In the evening, he stopped by the Pago club and its owner, Bob Norton, apologized to Ruby for staying open.

On Sunday morning, November 24, Ruby got a call from one of his strippers, Little Lynn, who needed an advance on her pay for her landlord. He told her to go to her local Western Union in Fort Worth, and he would dispatch her $25 from his Dallas branch. He left the apartment, telling Senator he was bringing his dog to the Carousel. Senator would testify that Ruby was pacing and mumbling. Ruby left Sheba in the car when he did his transaction at Western Union, then walked up the street toward City Hall, located on the next corner. Around 11:00 a.m., he noted activity in front of the Main Street ramp to the police department and strolled over. As a police cruiser exited the driveway, Ruby entered and moseyed right into the basement. No one stopped him or said anything to him. Seth Kantor, the newspaperman whose testimony about seeing Ruby at Parkland was discounted by the Warren

Commissioners, was also in the police station basement when Ruby shot Oswald. The award-winning journalist never wavered about his Parkland encounter and was disgruntled that the Commission wasn't interested in exploring Ruby's nefarious connections. Furthermore, Kantor believed a Dallas policeman allowed Ruby into the basement for the express purpose of killing Oswald, although no one was ever charged, and Ruby never admitted having a confederate. Kantor died in 1993.

Ruby entered the history books that Sunday afternoon. As he told investigators, he had been in mourning Friday and Saturday, and the sudden appearance of Oswald in the police basement caused him to lose his senses. Oswald had this "smirky, smug, vindictive attitude," and before he knew it, Ruby was on the ground, and five or six people were on top of him. Ruby claimed he acted impulsively and had no conversations about shooting Oswald with anyone prior to the deed. When asked to explain his animosity toward someone he had said he never met, Ruby cited Oswald's association with communism, adding that although he also didn't know Officer Tippit, he mourned his death, too. But Ruby's main excuse, he said, was that he wanted to spare Mrs. Kennedy from having to come back for a trial.

Soon after Oswald's death, an unnamed TV newsman reported from the police department:

> Murder charges have been filed against Dallas nightclub owner Jack Ruby, and there is considerable speculation as to why Ruby killed Oswald, if in fact it is proven that he did. About the only thing that is clear at this point is that there is not a single police officer in this building who believes that Jack Ruby killed Lee Oswald, if that is proven to be the case, out of patriotic fervor and that if he is proved to have killed Lee Oswald it was for one reason only and that was to seal his lips.

Until documents were declassified in 2017, the public did not learn that a phone call had been made to the Dallas FBI office on the night of November 23, 1963. The unidentified caller said he was a "member of a committee organized to kill Oswald"— and the next day, Oswald was fatally shot. Could Ruby have made the call because he didn't want to carry through with the murder and hoped for increased security for the transfer? We can only guess.

The Next Few Days

Other notable individuals also died on Friday, November 22, 1963, as the news reports reminded us. British intellectual and author Aldous Huxley, best known for the novel *Brave New World*, died in Los Angeles at the age of 69. And Irish-born C.S. Lewis, whose The Chronicles of Narnia is still a prominent children's series, died in Oxford, England, at the age of 64.

Many businesses closed the weekend and Monday in tribute but also because their employees wanted to watch the round-the-clock television news coverage. That's what my wife and I did when we weren't ministering to our babies. David and Danny provided a nice distraction as only a toddler and a newborn could. The world would return to some form of normalcy once Officer J.D. Tippit, Lee Harvey Oswald, and President John F. Kennedy were laid to rest.

President Lyndon Johnson didn't want to seem insensitive by displacing the Kennedy family from the White House and moving in his own family. But Jackie Kennedy understood that must happen and began making plans to vacate the premises within two weeks. Johnson also didn't rush into setting up shop in the Oval Office for official business and continued to use his vice-presidential workplace at the Old Executive Office Building for the initial few days. It was there that he hand-wrote his first two letters as president—to the Kennedy children:

> Dearest Caroline, your father's death has been a great tragedy for the nation, as well as for you at this time. He was a wise and devoted man. You can always be proud of what he did for his country. Affectionately, Lyndon Johnson

> Dear John, it will be many years before you understand fully what a great man your father was. His loss is a deep personal tragedy for all of us, but I wanted you particularly to know that I share your grief. You can always be proud of him. Affectionately, Lyndon Johnson

When news of the assassination broke, Marina Oswald and Ruth Paine watched it on television, spellbound. They were apoplectic when Oswald was named a suspect in the murders of the president and a police officer. Immediately after Oswald's arrest, Dallas police detectives swooped down on Paine's house in Irving to question Marina. Paine provided the Russian/English translation. The cops asked if Oswald owned a rifle, and the women said he kept one rolled up in a blanket in the garage. But when they all went to retrieve it, the blanket was empty.

Officers continued questioning Marina, eventually bringing the women to the police headquarters in Dallas. Marina explained that Oswald had come home on Thursday night with the intention of getting back in her good graces following an argument from the last time they were together. As they folded diapers and Oswald played with his daughters, he tried to talk Marina into moving out of the Paine residence. He said he could find an apartment in Dallas, and the family could live together again. But she wasn't interested. She liked her independence and freedom from his temper tantrums. She and the girls would remain in Irving. After Oswald left for work on Friday morning, Marina discovered that he had placed his gold wedding band and $187 in a small china cup on her dresser. The cup was one of the few things Oswald owned from his grandmother. Marina knew that was all the money he had in the world and felt leaving his ring was a sign that he was giving up on the marriage.

Secret Service and FBI agents joined the investigators and took Marina, her daughters, and mother-in-law Marguerite into protective custody. They would remain in a shabby motel room until the government deemed it was finished questioning them. The last thing law enforcement wanted was the press getting ahold of the Oswald women and suggesting they needed a lawyer. According to Marguerite, on Saturday night, the 23, FBI agent Bard Odum showed her a photograph of a man and asked if she had ever seen him before. She replied she had not. After Oswald's shooting the next day and not knowing the identity of the shooter, she picked up a newspaper at the motel, and on the bottom of the front page was a photo of a man. She told a Secret Service agent that the man in the paper was the same one Agent Odum had shown her the day before. The Secret Service agent told her that was Jack Ruby, the killer of her son.

Ruby was stewing in his jail cell, depressed and refusing to talk to anyone. Dallas County Sheriff J.E. "Bill" Decker felt his prisoner might open up to a friend, so he called Breck Wall, another nightclub impresario who had had a tumultuous friendship with Ruby. Like most of the club owners in Dallas, Wall had shuttered his venue after the assassination. He drove to Galveston, where he saw the news footage of Ruby shooting Oswald. Concerned for Ruby, he drove back to town and hid from reporters. When Decker called, Wall was afraid he was going to be arrested on some phony connection to the assassination and was relieved to learn that the sheriff just wanted his help. Deputies sneaked him into the jail and took him to Ruby's cell. The two pals spent 20 minutes together. Wall was surprised to see that the cell was decorated with telegrams from people thanking Ruby for his patriotic act. Ruby told Breck that the telegrams proved he did the right thing in killing Oswald. Wall didn't see it that way. "Jack, you're not a hero," he said. "You shot the man who killed the president before he could talk." A month later, Ruby sent Wall a letter thanking him for having visited him and noted how crazy it was that the newspapers seemed to have turned against him.

On Monday, the day after Oswald's death, Ruby's roommate, George Senator, stopped by the police station to talk to him but wasn't allowed access. He could see

Jack sitting behind glass and surrounded by officers. Dallas homicide detective Jim Leavelle later transferred Ruby to the county lockup. Ruby told the cop that he feared somebody might gun him down, too. Leavelle replied, "Jack, ain't nobody gonna shoot you," and nobody did. That same day, Jack was visited behind bars by Rabbi Silverman who asked why he had shot Oswald. Ruby replied he did it for the American people and to show the world that Jews have guts. Silverman would visit Ruby occasionally over the years he was incarcerated and noted that the gunman's mental state seemed to deteriorate over time. At one point, Ruby screamed at the rabbi to cower under a table, because someone was pouring oil on the Jews and trying to set them on fire.

The Warren Commission

With President Kennedy's funeral over and Washingtonians back to work, much consideration was given to finding answers. While FBI Chief J. Edgar Hoover would be in charge of the criminal investigation into the president's assassination, key figures within both the U.S. House of Representatives and the U.S. Senate discussed conducting their own probes. Hale Boggs, the Democrat House majority whip from Louisiana, even drafted a resolution, and Senator James Eastland, the Democrat from Mississippi who served as the Judiciary Committee chairman, started organizing a team.

Almost immediately, President Johnson's advisers began telling him that these competing groups would be a bad idea. A more efficient way to go would be for LBJ to appoint a blue-ribbon committee that would take charge of the investigation. It should consist of members of the House and Senate, both Democrats and Republicans, along with other dignified men in and out of government. Names were kicked around, and Johnson became comfortable with the plan. He just had to run it by Hoover, the one man to whom he always deferred. It's impossible to overstate the power that Hoover held in his position as the country's top law enforcement official, and his imprint on the Warren Commission was a prime example.

Many Americans who lived through the Watergate scandal believe that secret taping of Oval Office phone calls began with President Nixon. Not true. JFK and LBJ both recorded hundreds of hours of phone calls there, and those from Johnson's office in the wake of Kennedy's death outline the formation of what would become known as the Warren Commission. These calls and transcripts can be found at mary-ferrell.org.

On November 29, LBJ took a 20-minute phone call from Hoover. Johnson told the G-man that although he'd prefer if Hoover's assassination report could just be filed without a challenge, there were factions in the House and Senate that wanted to do their own studies, which would be difficult to rein in. Hoover agreed that the scattershot approach would be a "three-ring circus." Johnson's solution, therefore, would be to appoint a high-level panel to evaluate the FBI account, and he proceeded to cite some of the names he and his colleagues had earmarked as the committee members. Most of the men named were familiar to Hoover, and he gave his approval, although he cautioned about those people he found to be too friendly with the press. Johnson mentioned that he had been informed that Hoover's deputy associate director, Cartha "Deke" DeLoach, would be designated to assist Johnson's Commission, and he praised Hoover's knack for choosing such good workers. DeLoach was the number-three person at the Bureau, just under Clyde Tolson, Hoover's top deputy.

Hoover explained that an initial report he had planned to present to Johnson would be delayed as his staffers ironed out the details. They were trying to verify a potential Oswald sighting in Mexico City in mid–September, where the alleged assassin was said to have received $6,500 from the Cuban embassy before returning to the United States. The CIA was also investigating this angle and would relate, the next day, that the story was a lie by someone hoping to get favors from the U.S. government. Johnson inquired whether the FBI had turned up any prior connection between Oswald and Ruby, and Hoover replied they had not. Hoover filled him in on Ruby's background as a "shady character" who liked to hang out with police officers.

In a worried voice, LBJ asked how many shots were fired at JFK and whether any were intended for him. The director told him three shots were fired at Kennedy, who was the sole target. Ballistics, he said, proved that all the shots came from Oswald's rifle. The telescopic lens, which Hoover had himself looked through, "brings the person as close to you as if they were sitting right beside you," so there was no doubt that the shooter had the proper victim in his sight. He added that any rumor of more than one shooter was eliminated when the FBI replicated Oswald's three shots by firing his rifle in the same amount of time used to shoot JFK. Hoover maintained that JFK was shot by the first and third shots, and Connally got hit by shot #2 when he turned to see what was happening. This led LBJ to repeat that if Connally hadn't gotten in the way, the president would have taken all three shots.

Hoover mentioned that he had sent a Russian-speaking agent to tell Marina Oswald she could stay in the United States if she cooperated with the investigation, but he wasn't sure how much valuable information she might have. Johnson asked questions about Oswald's work, Officer Tippit, and general issues, all of which Hoover answered. After they discussed a $25,000 offer by the press to purchase a photo of Clint Hill climbing atop the Kennedy limo, the subject turned to whether the president's car should be armored. Hoover stated yes and revealed that he had four bulletproof cars at his disposal in different parts of the country. Johnson seemed stunned to hear this, as if realizing how vulnerable he was to a similar attack as that which befell JFK. Hoover suggested that Johnson should also step up security at his ranch in Texas. Do these things quietly, he advised. The call ended as Johnson flattered the older man, saying: "You're more than the head of the Federal Bureau, as far as I'm concerned. You're my brother and personal friend and have been for more than 25 or 30 years. … I've got more confidence in your judgment than anybody in town."

Later that afternoon, President Johnson announced the creation of his Commission. He issued Executive Order No. 11130 "to ascertain, evaluate, and report upon the facts relating to the assassination of the late President John F. Kennedy and the subsequent violent death of the man charged with the assassination." Investigative powers would be controlled by the FBI, with local help from the Texas Court of Inquiry. A report of the conclusions would be written and issued to the president, "to the American people, and to the world" at the conclusion of the Commission's work. Two weeks later, on December 13, Congress would adopt a joint resolution to authorize the Commission and its members, or any agencies or personnel they designate, to administer oaths and affirmations, examine witnesses, and receive evidence.

There were a few hectic hours leading up to LBJ's public declaration as he tried to wrangle a chairman for his Commission. He chose Earl Warren, the chief justice of the U.S. Supreme Court. Warren, born in 1891, was a Republican who had served as California's governor before joining the high court in 1953. He knew the dueling calls of justice and politics, and felt those disciplines would be undercut by the president's Commission, which would need to eventually form a unanimous opinion on the matters at hand.

Johnson had Attorney General Bobby Kennedy make the first pitch, but Warren rebuffed him, not realizing it wasn't an "offer" but a "demand." Then over the phone and in person with Johnson, Warren refused the appointment multiple times. LBJ wouldn't let Warren ditch the duty. He told the chief justice of Hoover's story about Oswald taking Cuban money in Mexico City. The lives of 40 million Americans would be at stake from a nuclear holocaust, he insisted, if Khrushchev were to be blamed for an assassination he had nothing to do with. Finally, a tearful Warren agreed to helm what would be called the "Warren Commission." The next day, when the Oswald story was found to be untrue, it was too late for Warren to back out of his chairmanship. He died in 1974.

Johnson was equally persuasive with the other members of the panel, refusing to take no if they cited objections. He even completed his press release of the announcement before he got all of the parties onboard. Johnson was an earthy, cradle-to-grave politician who knew how to cajole, threaten, or browbeat to get his way. With this Commission, he achieved his dream team whether the participants liked it or not. Serving under the chief justice were these six members of the Warren Commission, in alphabetical order:

- Hale Boggs (1914–1973), Democratic U.S. representative from Louisiana and House majority whip
- John Sherman Cooper (1901–1991), Republican U.S. senator from Kentucky
- Allen W. Dulles (1893–1969), director of the Central Intelligence Agency until 1961 when JFK fired him and author of the 1963 book *The Craft of Intelligence*
- Gerald Ford (1913–2006), Republican U.S. representative from Michigan and House minority leader (and later 38th president of the United States)
- John J. McCloy (1895–1989), former president of the World Bank and chairman of the board of directors of Council on Foreign Relations, and
- Richard Russell, Jr. (1897–1971), Democratic U.S. senator from Georgia.

The general counsel for the Commission was J. Lee Rankin, the former U.S. solicitor general. Rankin would make the final edits on the material for the Commission's report. The assistant legal counsel included Francis William Holbrooke Adams, Joseph A. Ball, David W. Belin, William T. Coleman, Jr., Melvin A. Eisenberg, Burt W. Griffin, Leon D. Hubert, Jr., Albert E. Jenner, Jr., Wesley J. Liebeler, Norman Redlich, W. David Slawson, Arlen Specter, Samuel A. Stern, and Howard P. Willens. There were additional lawyers, clerks, court reporters, and secretaries, including fact-checker Stephen G. Breyer, who is currently a U.S. Supreme Court associate justice.

The Warren
Commission Report

By the fall of 1964, I was swimming with the big fish in my medical and legal career in Pittsburgh and elsewhere. I held the post of assistant district attorney and medical adviser in the Allegheny County district attorney's office and served as the acting chief of laboratory and pathology services at two local hospitals. I had also taken on duties as owner/director of the Pittsburgh Pathology and Toxicology Laboratory and was a clinical instructor in legal medicine at the University of Pittsburgh.

I very much enjoyed teaching and lecturing, and did so at a number of professional groups and societies, including the Law-Science Academy of America and the University of Texas School of Law, as well as at engagements throughout the country and abroad. I was also a Fellow of the American Academy of Forensic Sciences (AAFS), the "ne plus ultra" organization for forensic scientists.

My wife Sigrid and I were busier than ever with our burgeoning family. Our son David was almost 2½, our son Danny was 1, and we were just months away from the arrival of our third son, Ben. (Our daughter Ingrid would come along in 1968.) And I was still serving as a USAF captain, on inactive reserve, for the Medical Corps.

One of the joys of my job at the prosecutor's office was interacting with experts from the crime lab, including its director, Charles A. McInerney. The lab had only been established a few years before and, under Charlie's guidance, was always adding new "toys" in the form of acquiring the cutting-edge tools crime-solvers needed to crack cases. I always liked getting calls from Charlie to rush to the lab and see the latest scientific discovery that would help prosecutors put bad guys behind bars or free someone wrongly charged. He would also be a good audience for me to discuss aspects of forensic pathology that might be from the news, rather than from cases my office was handling. We shared a passion for these topics. And, as you shall see, our bonding over the Kennedy assassination would send my career into a stratosphere I could never have imagined.

On September 24, 1964, the Warren Commission presented its 888-page final report on the Kennedy assassination to President Johnson. The blue clothbound book was published by the U.S. Government Printing Office. Three days later, copies were made available for purchase to the public. The report was sold for a nominal

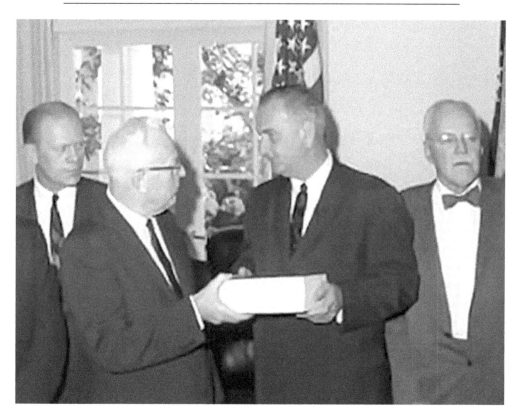

The Warren Commissioners hand over their report. The 26-volume set of interviews and evidence would follow later. *Left to right:* **Rep. Gerald Ford (R–MI), Chairman Earl Warren, President Lyndon B. Johnson, and former CIA Director Allen W. Dulles (Robert J. Groden collection).**

fee at every newsstand and bookstore in the country and quickly became a best seller. I bought two copies: one for posterity, and the other I marked up with ink and paper clips as I read it. In two months, the GPO would publish a 26-volume set of all the raw material that was synopsized for the book.

The report's table of contents showed there were eight chapters and 18 appendices (including one appendix with footnotes). Biographical briefs on the commissioners were included, along with the mission statement, press releases, and procedures for questioning witnesses. The table of contents also included a summary of the activities in Dealey Plaza on November 22, 1963; biographical information about Lee Harvey Oswald and Jack Ruby; Oswald's finances and trip to Russia; Oswald's murder, and Ruby's polygraph. Notes from Parkland Hospital detailed Kennedy's, Governor Connally's and Oswald's treatment there, and JFK's autopsy report. There was content about the avenues pursued to determine if JFK's assassination was the result of a conspiracy, data on previous historical presidential assassinations and attempts, as well as a view of how the Secret Service did its job to protect our leaders. Throughout the text were numbered footnotes, which were listed toward the end of the book and would correspond to pages within the 26 volumes. A nine-page index closed out the book, with an alphabetical listing of each of the 552 witnesses who gave testimony or depositions within the 888 pages.

The Warren Commission Report concluded that Oswald, acting alone, shot the president and wounded Governor John Connally, firing three bullets from the sixth floor of the Texas School Book Depository building. The stated evidence proved that Oswald also killed Dallas policeman J.D. Tippit. And the book stated incontrovertibly that Dallas nightclub owner Jack Ruby fatally shot Oswald and that the two men did not know each other before Ruby's impulsive action.

The best minds in the country had investigated the matter and found that Oswald was simply a violent misfit, with no previous connections to any intelligence agencies. Americans could rest assured that there was no conspiracy within our government or acts of war from any foreign entities. Not only was this very thorough book issued but, in the interest of full disclosure by our leaders, the entire work product of the commissioners would also be available soon. It would include transcripts of all the testimony and every exhibit. I pored over each page of the initial report, considering it a delicious appetizer for the full banquet that lay ahead. How very lucky we citizens were to have such openness by our governmental agencies. Imagine how the communist countries of Russia, Cuba, or Vietnam would propagandize such an earth-shattering event to make themselves look good. Their leaders can read our book and learn how business is conducted in the Land of the Free!

I relished each word of the 888 pages. It was like no other book I had ever read, a curious blend of governmental curtness, along with juicy personal narratives on the individuals highlighted. I dropped everything, closed the door, and settled into a comfortable chair until the entire tome was devoured.

From my perspective as a forensic pathologist, I was primarily interested in what was said about the president's autopsy and the facts surrounding the shooting. So, I was a bit dismayed when I realized how little content on these matters was present in the book. Pages 85–96 was a section entitled "The Bullet Wounds" and covered the injuries to Kennedy and Connally. "Treatment of President Kennedy" consisted of pages 53 to the top of page 56. The balance of that page described Connally's treatment. The report's index only referred to Kennedy's three autopsists on three pages: 86, 88, and 89.

Appendix VIII, pages 516–537, consisted of handwritten or typed medical reports from the Parkland doctors who tried to save JFK's life: William Kemp Clark, Charles J. Carrico, Malcolm O. Perry, Charles R. Baxter, Robert N. McClelland, Fouad Bashour, and Marion T. Jenkins. Pages 531–535 were the accounts about Governor Connally from Drs. Robert Shaw, Charles Gregory, and Tom Shires. And pages 536–537 reproduced Shires' statement about Oswald's death. Appendix IX, on pages 538–546, consisted of President Kennedy's autopsy report and supplemental report. There were no autopsy photos, drawings, or X-rays. And Appendix X, on pages 547–597, was expert testimony regarding the gunshot wound and ballistics experiments, making the case that Oswald was JFK's only shooter. I comforted myself with the thought that perhaps the extended 26 volumes would more deeply cover the medical angles. But for these 10 months I had been waiting since the assassination for some specific coverage on Kennedy's death, at least now I had a starting point.

The President's
Autopsy Report

S ince the assassination, I—and, I'm sure, many other medical examiners and reporters—had requested access to President Kennedy's autopsy report, to no avail. We were told it was kept secret by the government for reasons of "national security." Given that the chief suspect, Lee Harvey Oswald, was dead, that suggested to many observers that there could be other individuals who might yet be indicted. Otherwise, why not release the report?

But now that the Warren Commission book was available to the public, it was clear that the government experts had laid all blame for the assassination on Oswald, and only Oswald. As I read through the medical and autopsy information, I learned what happened after President Kennedy's body left Dallas. The Warren Commissioners interviewed all the Parkland Hospital doctors, as well as the doctors who performed JFK's autopsy at the National Naval Medical Center in Bethesda, Maryland.

Because there was so little content, I read the autopsy pages again and again, my temper heating up more with each pass. I debated with myself whether the upcoming 26 volumes would expand on the information in this book and eventually weighed in on the side that the purposefully minimal descriptions would likely be all they were going to give us. If it were critical to understanding, it would be in this report. And that made me both puzzled and angry. What would possess the autopsists from writing less than what they certainly had to know?

On March 16, 1964, the Commission heard testimony from Dr. James J. Humes, the lead autopsy doctor. His autopsy report was entered into evidence as (Commission Exhibit) CE-387. President Kennedy's "full" autopsy report was six pages in length. CE-391, a three-page supplemental document on his brain, was also included. Compare that to the autopsy report of Senator Robert Kennedy, which is 65 pages and discusses his head and body wounds in depth. All of these accounts can be found online.

In my career as a forensic pathologist, I have performed autopsies on thousands of gunshot victims, and I assure you the reports I wrote on each were thorough and as lengthy as necessary to accurately describe the scientific findings. During the writing of this book, I conducted a procedure on a homicide-by-gunshot case, which yielded a document of 24 pages without the investigative scene description that would have made it longer. Yet, the president of the United States, a murder victim with a fresh, almost intact body to examine, received an autopsy protocol that was cut-rate and wholly inadequate!

President Kennedy's six pages also included his general physical description; the "clinical summary," which recapped the information about the day's events; numerous typos; and plenty of room for the titles and signatures of the three doctors who performed the procedure. Were I one of them, I would not have wanted my name on this document. Whereas the pathological diagnosis of the cause of death was noted as a "gunshot wound, head," there was no subsequent finding of the manner of death. Although we might presume that the president died from a homicide, it was not spelled out in the report. Perhaps these doctors wanted to believe that Kennedy committed suicide.

Autopsy number A63–272 was identified as that of "Kennedy, John F.," "President, United States." The decedent was described as a 46-year-old Caucasian male, measuring six feet and a ½-inch tall and weighing approximately 170 pounds. He was described as "muscular, well-developed, and well-nourished." His eyes were blue, and his hair was reddish brown and described as "abundant." His teeth were in "excellent repair."

Three physicians were named as being responsible for the procedure: the chief prosector, Commander James J. Humes, and his assistant, Commander J. Thornton Boswell. Lieutenant Colonel Pierre A. Finck was also listed. All three were attached with the U.S. Medical Corps, with the first two from the U.S. Navy. Dr. Finck was brought to the Bethesda morgue from the Armed Forces Institute of Pathology, although that was not mentioned on the document. (I later obtained the manual for AFIP's autopsy protocols for that time period, and, at 79 pages, it is appropriately complete. Surely, Finck would have known about that manual and perhaps even had a hand in writing it. One wonders how he justified that the president's autopsy report was only six pages long, when the steps for conducting a proper postmortem examination was 13 times greater in length.)

Kennedy's autopsy report noted that he was pronounced dead on November 22, 1963, at 1:00 p.m. CST, and that the autopsy was performed that evening at 8:00 p.m. EST. The narrative stated that Kennedy was riding in an open car in a motorcade during an official visit to Dallas, Texas, and mentioned where he was sitting in relation to Mrs. Kennedy and Governor John Connally and his wife. It describes the car as moving at a slow rate of speed down an incline into a freeway underpass, on its way to the Dallas Trade Mart where the president was to deliver an address. Three shots were heard, and the president "fell forward bleeding from the head." The same gunfire "seriously wounded Connally," it was stated.

That same paragraph mentioned Bob Jackson, the *Dallas Times-Herald* photographer, who said "he looked around as he heard the shots and saw a rifle barrel disappearing into a window on an upper floor of the nearby Texas School Book Depository Building." But Jackson didn't make that comment to the autopsy doctors or even the doctors at Parkland. This was strictly information the report's authors gleaned from

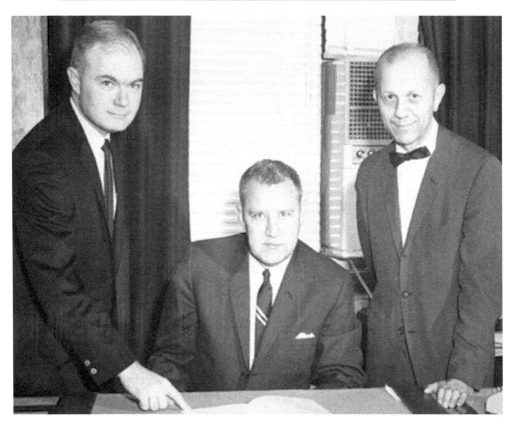

The Bethesda autopsy doctors. *Left to right:* Navy Commanders James J. Humes and J. Thornton Boswell, and Army Lieutenant Colonel Pierre A. Finck (Robert J. Groden Collection).

an article in the *Washington Post*, which ran the day after the shooting. Why would the authors of this autopsy report cite an unverified observation from a newspaper photographer? If a photograph of Jackson's claim existed, he would have published it, and his account would have had been quite compelling. But no photograph was ever produced. Jackson would later win the Pulitzer Prize for his photograph of Jack Ruby shooting Lee Harvey Oswald, but I contend that a photo showing a rifle sticking out from the alleged shooter's window would have rivaled that career triumph. In the absence of such a photo, his comment deserves no special weight beyond what anyone else in Dealey Plaza might have said. Yet, his was the only remark included in the autopsy document.

The report goes on to describe that after the wounding of the president and the governor, the car was driven to Parkland, where the president "was attended by Dr. Malcolm Perry." A telephone conversation with Dr. Perry on November 23 recounted his observations about what he saw and did when the president was in his emergency room. From the report (with my explanations of medical terms in parentheses):

Dr. Perry noted the massive wound of the head and a second much smaller wound of the low anterior (front) neck in approximately the midline. A tracheostomy (surgical opening of the neck into the trachea, to assist breathing) was performed by extending the latter wound. At this point bloody air was noted bubbling from the wound and an injury to the right lateral (side) wall of the trachea was observed. Incisions were made in the upper anterior chest wall bilaterally (on both sides) to combat possible subcutaneous emphysema (air getting into tissue beneath the skin). Intravenous infusions of blood and saline were begun and oxygen was administered. Despite these measures cardiac arrest occurred and closed chest cardiac massage failed to re-establish cardiac action. The president was pronounced dead approximately thirty to forty minutes after receiving his wounds.

The narrative concludes by stating that the remains were transported via the presidential plane to Washington, D.C., and subsequently to the Naval Medical School, National Naval Medical Center, Bethesda, Maryland, for the postmortem examination. By the time the autopsy began, Kennedy's body was beginning the process of rigor mortis, the natural stiffening of the muscles that sets in after a person dies, becoming fixed after about eight to 12 hours and lasting for 24 to 36 hours before diminishing. There was a minimal amount of livor mortis of his back, the purplish discoloration from blood pooling due to gravity, and there was an early stage of algor mortis, or the cooling of the body temperature after death. The pupil of his right eye measured 8 mm (millimeters) in diameter, and the left pupil measured 4 mm. (This is a common phenomenon from a gunshot or severe head injury.) There was also swelling and bruising to the inner portion of his left eyelid, near the bridge of his nose. There was clotted blood on the external ears, but otherwise the ears, nostrils, and mouth were "unremarkable."

In the upper right posterior thorax (back of the rib cage), just above the upper border of the scapula (shoulder blade), there was a 7 by 4 mm oval wound. This wound was located 14 cm (centimeters) from the tip of the right acromion process (top of the shoulder) and 14 cm below the tip of the right mastoid process (bony prominence at the base of the skull, behind the ear). (A centimeter is one hundredth of a meter and equivalent to .3937 of an inch. A millimeter is one thousandth of a meter and equivalent to .03937 of an inch.)

In the low anterior neck at approximately the level of the third and fourth tracheal rings was a 6.5 cm-long transverse wound with widely gaping irregular edges. At the anterior chest wall in the nipple line were bilateral 2 cm-long recent transverse surgical incisions into the subcutaneous tissue. The one on the left was situated 11 cm cephalad (toward the head) to the nipple, and the one on the right was 8 cm cephalad to the nipple. A wound measuring 2 cm in length was situated on the antero-lateral (front-side) aspect of the left mid-arm. Situated on the antero-lateral aspect of each ankle was a recent 2 cm transverse incision into the subcutaneous tissue. (The chest, arm, and leg incisions were from the Parkland doctors trying to send fluids through his bloodstream.) There was an old, well-healed 8 cm abdominal incision (from previous surgical removal of his appendix). Over the lumbar spine in the midline was an old, well-healed 15 cm scar (from previous back surgery). Situated on the upper antero-lateral aspect of the right thigh was an old, well-healed 8 cm scar.

As is customary, a surgical incision down the chest in the shape of a "Y" was made to examine the internal cavity and organs. A scalpel provided a deep cut from shoulder to shoulder diagonally down the chest, and then down the abdomen to the pubic bone. The skin, muscle, and soft tissues were separated, and the rib cage and neck areas exposed and opened. The thoracic cavity was deemed "unremarkable," with the organs in their normal positions and no leakage of pleural fluid. The lungs were of normal weight, size, and color. A bruised area at the top of the pleural cavity was noted, corresponding to a 5 cm diameter area of purplish red discoloration and increased firmness to palpation at the top of the right upper lobe. Recent hemorrhaging was revealed into the pulmonary parenchyma (bronchial passages). The heart's pericardial cavity was of normal size, weight, and appearance but contained approximately 10 cc (cubic centimeters; a bit more than two teaspoons) of straw-colored fluid. There were no abnormalities to the pulmonary artery or valves and just moderate amounts of postmortem clotted blood in the cardiac chambers. The organs of the abdominal cavity were all in their normal positions, with no leakage of fluids. The appendix was surgically absent. Its scar left minor adhesions where the cecum (peritoneal pouch) joined the ventral (lower) abdominal wall.

The report notes that except for the skull wounds, there were no significant gross skeletal abnormalities. In the section titled "Missile Wounds," two defects were noted: the head wound and a wound to the right back. I will paraphrase passages as they appeared in the autopsy report (I have corrected various typos):

1. There was a large irregular defect of the scalp and skull on the right involving chiefly the parietal bone (top of the skull) but extending somewhat into the temporal (lower side) and occipital (lower rear) regions. In this region, there was an actual absence of scalp and bone, producing a defect which measured approximately 13 cm in greatest diameter. From the irregular margins of the above scalp defect, tears extended in stellate (star-shaped) fashion into the more or less intact scalp as follows: (a) From the right inferior (lower) temporo-parietal margin anterior to the right ear to a point slightly above the tragus (rounded, lengthy external opening of the ear). (b) From the anterior parietal margin anteriorly on the forehead to approximately 4 cm above the right orbital ridge (brow bone). (c) From the left margin of the main defect across the midline antero-laterally for a distance of approximately 8 cm. (d) From the same starting point as c. 10 cm postero-laterally (rear-side). Situated in the posterior scalp approximately 2.5 cm laterally to the right and slightly above the external occipital protuberance was a lacerated wound measuring 15 by 6 mm.

   In the underlying bone was a corresponding wound through the skull which exhibited beveling of the margins of the bone when viewed from the inner aspect of the skull. Clearly visible in the above described large skull defect and exuding from it was lacerated brain tissue which, on close inspection, proved to represent the major portion of the right cerebral hemisphere. At this point, it was noted that the falx cerebri (sickle-shaped fold of the fibrous membrane that covers the top of the brain) is extensively lacerated with disruption of the superior sagittal sinus (large vein at the top of the head, beneath the skull). Upon reflecting the scalp, multiple complete fracture lines were seen to radiate from both the large defect at the vertex (top of the head) and the smaller wound at the occiput (back of the head). These vary greatly in length and direction, the longest measuring approximately 19 cm. These result in the production of numerous fragments which vary in size from a few millimeters to 10 cm in greatest diameter. The complexity of these fractures and the fragments thus produced tax satisfactory verbal description and were better appreciated in photographs and roentgenograms (X-rays) which were prepared (although not reproduced in the Commission's report).

The brain was removed and preserved for further study following formalin fixation. Also received as separate specimens from Dallas were three fragments of skull bone that, in aggregate, roughly approximate the dimensions of the large defect described above. At one angle of the largest of these fragments was a portion of the perimeter of a roughly circular wound presumably of exit which exhibited beveling of the outer aspect of the bone and was estimated to measure approximately 2.5 to 3.0 cm in diameter. Roentgenograms of this fragment revealed minute particles of metal in the bone at this margin. Roentgenograms of the skull revealed multiple minute metallic fragments along a line corresponding with a line joining the above described small occipital wound and the right supra-orbital ridge. From the surface of the disrupted right cerebral cortex (outer layer of brain, associated with higher brain functions) two small, irregularly shaped fragments of metal were recovered. These measure 7 by 2 mm and 3 by 1 mm. These were placed in the custody of FBI agents Francis X. O'Neill, Jr., and James W. Sibert, who executed a receipt therefore.

2. The second wound presumably of entry was that described above in the upper right posterior thorax. Beneath the skin there was ecchymosis of subcutaneous tissue and musculature. The missile path through the fascia (connective tissue) and musculature cannot be easily probed. The wound presumably of exit was that described by Dr. Malcolm Perry of Dallas in the low anterior cervical region. When observed by Perry, the wound measured "a few millimeters in diameter." It was extended as a tracheostomy incision, and thus its character was distorted at the time of autopsy. However, there was considerable ecchymosis of the strap muscles of the right side of the neck and of the fascia about the trachea adjacent to the line of the tracheostomy wound. The third point of reference in connecting these two wounds was in the apex supra-clavicular portion (above the collar bone) of the right pleural cavity (lung sac). In this region, there was contusion of the parietal pleura and of the extreme apical (uppermost) portion of the right upper lobe of the lung. In both instances, the diameter of contusion and ecchymosis at the point of maximal involvement

measured 5 cm. Both the visceral and parietal pleura were intact overlying these areas of trauma.

The report stated that black-and-white and color photographs had been taken and exposed but not developed. Unlike today when people have the means for instant photography, in 1963, it was a process of a few steps. The undeveloped photos were placed in the custody of U.S. Secret Service Agent Roy H. Kellerman, who executed a receipt. Kellerman executed another receipt when he took custody of the undeveloped full-body X-rays and three small bone fragments.

Let me break down the autopsy report's summary. For clarity, I will present the statements from the document, then add my commentary. These are not thoughts I had when I first read the material or even for a period of time afterward but represent how I feel now:

> It is our opinion that the deceased died as a result of two perforating gunshot wounds inflicted by high-velocity projectiles fired by a person or persons unknown.

Certainly, the headshot was lethal. But the other gunshot did not cause much internal damage and was not necessarily fatal. Within five minutes of being shot, the president was rushed to Parkland Hospital, and doctors went to work on him immediately, which would have improved his chances of survival. I concur with the use of the word "persons."

> The projectiles were fired from a point behind and somewhat above the level of the deceased.

This one sentence is a direct contradiction of the medical evidence and numerous witness statements. It puts into play every action of governmental conspiracy that followed and may even reveal the mechanism for prior planning of the assassination. To maintain their story, the powers that be needed a solo shooter to be in a high window of the Texas School Book Depository. Any other proof of a second shooter or bullets coming from another direction would be quashed.

> The observations and available information do not permit a satisfactory estimate as to the sequence of the two wounds.

The report's authors wrote this sentence before they heard what Dealey Plaza witnesses observed and long before the Zapruder film made clear that the neck wound came first. So, although the statement was true at the time it was written, it should have been amended in a supplemental report that factored in the new information.

> The fatal missile entered the skull above and to the right of the external occipital protuberance. A portion of the projectile traversed the cranial cavity in a posterior-anterior direction (see lateral skull roentgenograms) depositing minute particles along its path. A portion of the projectile made its exit through the parietal bone on the right carrying with it portions of cerebrum, skull and scalp.

Through no fault of the autopsy doctors, it would be revealed later that they were prevented from adequately tracking the trajectories of either bullet. While they probed the holes by inserting their fingers up to the first or second knuckle and with a metal rod, they were not allowed to explore beyond that or create an incision that would reveal the wounds' depth. This is a stunning piece of news. None of the doctors would disclose the name and/or rank of the person who gave them that order or whether the individual was from the military or a civilian.

> The two wounds of the skull combined with the force of the missile produced extensive fragmentation of the skull, laceration of the superior sagittal sinus, and of the right cerebral hemisphere.

By the report's own definition, there was only one skull wound. The other wound was substantially lower and should not be mistaken for a head shot. That said, I allow for the possibility that Kennedy could have sustained other wounds not noted here.

> The other missile entered the right superior posterior thorax above the scapula and traversed the soft tissues of the supra-scapular and the supra-clavicular portions of the base of the right side of the neck. This missile produced contusions of the right apical parietal pleura and of the apical portion of the right upper lobe of the lung. The missile contused the strap muscles of the right side of the neck, damaged the trachea and made its exit through the anterior surface of the neck. As far as can be ascertained this missile struck no bony structures in its path through the body.

This passage states that the defect to the president's back was an entrance wound, which exited out the right front of his neck. This was substantiated by photographs and drawings that were later released. Although the entrance wound would change its position on the back over the years, depending on who was talking, it remained a small, round wound.

> In addition, it is our opinion that the wound of the skull produced such extensive damage to the brain as to preclude the possibility of the deceased surviving this injury.

Yes, as I stated above.

> A supplementary report will be submitted following more detailed examination of the brain and of microscopic sections. However, it is not anticipated that these examinations will materially alter the findings.

True, and that would also apply to what was in the 26 volumes, as we would soon discover.

There is most often a difference in appearance of an entrance wound and an exit wound. As a bullet goes into flesh, it produces a small hole. As it moves through tissue and/or bone, the bullet expands and tumbles, leaving a greater hole when it exits. Dallas, Texas, was and is "gun country," where people enjoy their 2nd Amendment right to own and use firearms. Ergo, doctors at Parkland Hospital have vast experience with gunshot wound victims.

Usually, first impressions of eyewitnesses are the most credible. In the press conference that occurred shortly after the president was declared dead, two of the surgeons described the events in Trauma Room One. Dr. Malcolm Perry was the attending surgeon and vascular consultant on duty, and Dr. Kemp Clark was the chief neurosurgeon. It was Perry's job to try to save the unconscious president's life, who he says was "nearly dead" and unlikely to survive when he arrived in the emergency room. Still, Perry began resuscitative measures, which included assisted respiration with oxygen and an anesthesia machine, and administering blood and fluids. An electrocardiograph monitor detected the slightest of heartbeats, which soon stopped. Ignoring the endotracheal tube that was down the president's mouth, Perry began his tracheostomy procedure. With his scalpel, he expanded the small round hole at the front of Kennedy's throat and inserted a tracheotomy tube and flange.

On three separate occasions during the press conference, Perry described the bullet wound in the throat as an "entrance wound." He said it was on the "mid line" of the neck and "below the Adam's apple." Asked which way the bullet came, he answered, "It appeared to be coming at him." It was later learned that Perry was phoned at home that night by a local Secret Service agent named Elmer Moore, who explained that the doctor had to have seen an exit wound in the throat and berated

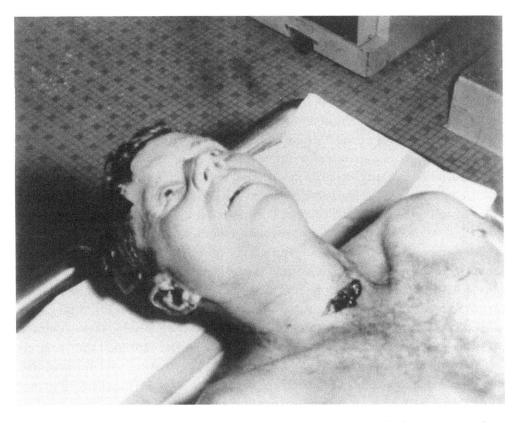

Parkland doctors inserted a breathing tube into a throat exit wound, leading some people to believe it was an entrance point (Wecht Collection).

him for holding an opinion that would cause the government trouble. The next day, Dr. Perry complained about the phone call to Audrey Bell, the chief operating room nurse who, years later, would describe the doctor's anguish to me. Perry, she said, expressed concern to Bell that his professional status would suffer if he didn't change his story. Soon after, he began publicly modifying his observation of the throat wound as being "either an entrance or exit wound" and got progressively annoyed when asked about the matter. Dr. Perry died of lung cancer in 2009.

At the Parkland press conference, neurosurgeon Clark recounted that he came into the room only after Perry had begun the tracheostomy, so he didn't see the throat wound. He was there to evaluate Kennedy's head wound, which he described as a "large" and "gaping." He stated that a missile had "gone in or out of the back of his head, causing extensive lacerations and loss of brain tissue."

The doctors did not roll over Kennedy's body for a full inspection, so they didn't know about the bullet that had entered his back and exited his throat. Drs. Robert McClelland and Charles Crenshaw arrived in the trauma room together after the endotracheal tube had been inserted but before the tracheostomy procedure. McClelland and another doctor helped ease in the tracheotomy tube, while Crenshaw was busy inserting a catheter near the president's ankle to transport fluids to his brain and organs. After all the doctors left the emergency room and the nurses and an orderly prepped Kennedy in the coffin, Crenshaw came back for one last look. He pulled down the sheet that covered the slain president's head, noted that all the tubes had been removed, and got his first and only glimpse of the throat wound. The scalpel incision that Dr. Perry had made had closed on its own, as if the tracheostomy had never happened, but the small bullet hole was still visible. Based on that, Crenshaw determined that the throat wound was an entrance and that the bullet exited through the wound in Kennedy's head. Despite being presented with evidence to the contrary over the years, Crenshaw never abandoned that belief.

As detailed in Douglas P. Horne's compelling five-volume book set, *Inside the Assassination Records Review Board* (self-published in 2009 and still available online), by the afternoon of the 22nd, Dallas authorities and the U.S. government agreed that three shots were fired by one person from the book depository. At this point, no one was aware of a shot that slightly wounded a car salesman named James Thomas Tague, who was standing on Main Street by the triple underpass. As the motorcade approached, Tague heard what he later described to the Warren Commission as "a very loud firecracker" followed by two similar sounds. When he realized they were gunshots, he ducked behind an abutment, as the motorcade sped by. Tague ventured out to see people and cops running around, and one person explained that the president's head had exploded. Tague told a sheriff's deputy that he had felt something sting his face, and the officer replied there were blood drops on his cheek. Together they found a fresh bullet mark on the curb and agreed that a tiny concrete chip had broken loose and ricocheted upward to hit Tague's right cheek.

The president's autopsy concluded around 11 p.m. on the 22nd. Before they left the morgue, FBI agents James Sibert and Francis O'Neill, Jr., heard Dr. Humes say that two shots had hit JFK, one to his high-shoulder and the other to his head—and both were fired from behind and above him. The two agents departed, and then something happened that changed everything.

It was not until the next morning that Humes made a phone call to Parkland Hospital's Dr. Malcolm Perry, who advised him of a gunshot wound to the president's throat. That forced the autopsy doctors to conclude that Kennedy was hit by three bullets instead of two. Richard Lipsey, an aide to Philip C. Wehle, the commanding general of the Military District of Washington, D.C., would tell investigators that he overheard the three autopsists, shortly before they left the morgue, state that Kennedy had been shot by three bullets, with no mention of Connally's wounds.

Humes went home and on the next day—Saturday, November 23—wrote a first draft of his autopsy report, presumably reflecting the new information. But as Humes would later testify, he wrote a new report on the following day, the 24th, after burning his original report and handwritten notes in his home fireplace. He claimed that the original paperwork had the president's blood on it, but I think that's bullshit. It should have been included in the master file, regardless of its condition. I believe his motivation was that his original observations did not comport to the "new reality" he was convinced to communicate. Burning that first draft was wholly unprofessional in a murder case that would presumably go to trial. A routine question I get from opposing counsel in homicide trials is "Do you have any notes that are not part of your testimony?" If I were to ever answer that I had burned some paperwork, I would be ripped apart. So Humes' conduct was inappropriate and inexcusable.

Horne theorizes that someone higher up the chain of command at Bethesda reviewed the report's first draft and called Humes to remind him of Connally's wounds. Because the government was married to the idea of "one assassin, three shots," the number of shots to Kennedy then had to be reduced to the two that the FBI agents had heard. Now, the story would be that JFK was shot by bullets one and three, with Connally shot by bullet two. Horne believes that the new draft of Humes' report was the first one to be signed. This draft explained the throat wound as having been caused by a bullet fragment from the head shot. Remarks made in a top-secret report by Warren Commission general counsel J. Lee Rankin in an executive session provided evidence for Horne's assertion. This document later went missing. But quickly another factor interceded to require a rewrite. Within a day or two of the first executed draft being prepared, authorities who were studying the Zapruder film realized that the throat wound came before the head shot. So much for the bullet fragment scenario. A new autopsy report would have to be written. By December 11, the second version was signed by Drs. Humes, Boswell, and Finck.

On December 6, 1963, a supplemental report was written by Dr. Humes. Signing the document were the commanding officer of the U.S. Naval Medical School, Captain J.H. Stover, Jr., and the commanding officer of the U.S. Naval Medical Center, Admiral Calvin B. Galloway. Copies of the report, along with black-and-white and color negatives, were supplied to the White House physician, Rear Admiral George G. Burkley, who also took receipt of the original photos. The supplemental report was an examination of President Kennedy's brain. The weight of a typical adult human brain is about three pounds, or 1,360 grams. JFK's was on the upper register of that scale at 1,500 grams—and that's after a great portion of it was blown away.

The right cerebral hemisphere of Kennedy's brain was found to be "markedly disrupted." There was a long laceration down the parasagittal plane, "approximately 2.5 cm to the right of the midline, extending from the tip of the occipital lobe posteriorly to the tip of the frontal lobe anteriorly. The base of the laceration is situated approximately 4.5 cm below the vertex (highest point) in the white matter." Above the laceration was a considerable loss of cerebral cortex substance, the brain's gray matter associated with higher brain functions such as controlled movement, learning, and memory. The parietal lobe, at the top of the brain, was particularly affected. The margins of the laceration were jagged and irregular, with other lacerations extending into various directions. Damage to the corpus callosum, the neural fibers that connect the brain's hemispheres, was significant. The left cerebral hemisphere was intact but with considerable hemorrhaging associated with the right side's injury.

The missile that hit Kennedy's head disintegrated completely. This would indicate a frangible, soft-tipped, or hollow-nosed bullet. More than 40 tiny lead fragments trailed through the right cerebral hemisphere and embedded into the interior of the skull. Most were about the size of the nib of a pen, but the largest was the size of the nail of an adult's little finger. But the neck wound didn't have that same trail of detritus. According to the Warren Commission, it was consistent with the bullet that hit John Connally, a full metal jacketed bullet that did not lose much mass and ended up in pristine condition on his stretcher at Parkland Hospital. The single-bullet premise has that missile course in and out of JFK's back and neck, into the governor's back and out his chest, into and out of his wrist, and into his thigh. Seven points of flesh and bone contact for one bullet. And that's not counting Connally's jacket and shirt fabric and knocking off his gold cuff link. And the government claims this wondrous, one-of-a-kind bullet exited from Connally's thigh basically intact. However, it would be some time before I would come to understand that the single-bullet theory was a hoax.

Kennedy researcher Howard Donohue wisely points out that this would indicate different ammunition was used to shoot Kennedy and Connally. And he's right. What kind of professional assassin would load up his rifle with at least two types of ammunition? And, by the way, at the time of James Tague's Warren Commission testimony—July 1964—authorities had not collected or analyzed the chipped curb by the underpass, but at Tague's insistence, they did so the following month. Forensic testing at the FBI lab determined that no embedded copper residue was present on the curb—and their report stated that the bullet that hit it could not be linked to an "unmutilated military full metal jacketed bullet," such as the one recovered from

Connally's stretcher. To any reasonable person that alone would be proof of a second shooter, but logic and truth were in short supply in this investigation.

Kennedy's brain had been removed at the Bethesda autopsy and put into a formalin solution so it would harden. After about two weeks, it would have been ready for examination. First, it would be analyzed as a whole, then dissected coronally. Parallel slices are made at regular intervals at about ¼ to ½". Then, representative sections are submitted for preparation of microscopic slides. But, according to the report, this was not done. The document stated: "In the interest of preserving the specimen coronal sections are not made." Instead, representative sections were used. In the interest of doing a full and complete autopsy, the entire brain should have been examined. If this were a matter of "giving respect" to the decedent, it would seem the victim was short-changed instead of honored. That would not be my final complaint about the handling of President Kennedy's brain.

Another mysterious absence in Kennedy's autopsy report was a corresponding toxicology screening, a pro forma procedure for any death investigation. In the interest of doing a competent, thorough report, samples of the deceased's blood, urine and tissues are sent to a toxicology laboratory that will screen for the presence of alcohol and licit or illicit drugs at the time of death and for days prior. Including these results is imperative, even if the cause of death is clearly not related to drug or alcohol ingestion. Was an exception made because this patient was the president and deserved special consideration? I have never seen this addressed in this case, but from my perspective, the accuracy of the official record outweighs any concerns for privacy. Were the tests performed and simply not revealed, or not requested at all? One could argue that the White House and the press corps were well-experienced in covering up medical details of our leaders, from preventing photos showing Franklin D. Roosevelt in his wheelchair after polio took its toll to Ronald W. Reagan's onset of Alzheimer's disease during some of his last years in office. When they died, their autopsy reports—if indeed, they were autopsied at all—and toxicology screens were not made public. But neither of them died in a traumatic event that required an autopsy. Kennedy did, which is why a toxicology data should have been included.

Kennedy had many significant medical conditions, going back to his spinal injury as a teenager. When he was shot in Dallas, he was wearing a back brace under his clothing. The autopsy doctors had every right to request a look at his full medical records, which were easily available through Dr. Burkley and Bethesda's National Naval Medical Center, JFK's treatment facility for any physical issue. This could have been easily accomplished since Dr. Burkley was present at the autopsy, which was performed at Bethesda.

Kennedy had Addison's disease and hypothyroidism, or abnormally low thyroid production. Addison's withers the adrenal glands, which generate adrenaline and other hormones. Symptoms can include sluggishness, muscle weakness, weight loss, light-headedness, nausea, sweating, and mood swings. Yet, there was no indication of adrenal deficiency mentioned in the president's autopsy report. Two boxes to show that the right and left adrenal glands were reviewed should have been marked with Xs but were blank. Tuberculosis accounts for about 20 percent of the Addison's cases, and the rest are autoimmune in origin. When Addison's became a campaign rumor in 1960, JFK's doctors issued a statement that he did not have tuberculosis, and the matter was dropped. But he collapsed twice due to the disease: once in a parade and the other time on a congressional visit to Great Britain. The president was first diagnosed with Addison's in the 1940s. It can run in families. His sister Eunice had it, and his son John Jr., had Graves' disease, which is the basis of hyperthyroidism.

Steroids were part of JFK's regular drug regimen throughout his presidency. He took 25 micrograms (mcg) of liothyronine, a synthetic thyroid hormone, twice daily. Add to that a daily dose of 10 milligrams (mg) of hydrocortisone and 0.1 mg of fludrocortisones, and 2.5 mg of prednisone twice daily. To combat weight loss and the gonadal atrophy associated with steroid usage, he took 10 mg of methyltestosterone daily. And to treat diarrhea, he took diphenoxylate hydrochloride and atropine sulfate, as needed. He also took 500 mg of vitamin C twice daily. And, according to a 2013 book called *Dr. Feelgood*, by authors Richard A. Lertzman and William J. Birnes (Skyhorse Publishing), Kennedy was a secret user of methamphetamines. The book describes a celebrity doctor, Max Jacobson, who had invented an injectable formula for giving people energy and curing pain. So familiar was Jacobson around the White House, where he also supposedly treated Jackie, the Secret Service dubbed him "Dr. Feelgood."

The doctor's formula consisted of vitamins, enzymes, animal placentas, and hormones, with a dollop of methamphetamine. He administered Kennedy's initial treatment right before the historic first debate against Richard Nixon. Hours before the televised event, JFK's voice was a mere whisper, and he was suffering from extreme lethargy. "Jacobson plunged a needle directly into his throat and pumped methamphetamines into his larynx," the authors wrote. Kennedy was revitalized within minutes and handily won the showdown. The authors stated that Kennedy flew Jacobson on Air Force One to a Vienna summit where the president was to speak with Nikita Khrushchev, not long after the Bay of Pigs crisis. Kennedy, whose back was causing him woe, got a megadose of the doctor's formula, but it wore off before his meeting. Kennedy asked for another dose, but Jacobson advised against it because there would be a serious crash when the drugs wore off. Kennedy prevailed by convincing Jacobson another shot would be good for America.

The Lertzman and Birnes book asserted that Jacobson injected Kennedy with the drugs four times a week. Bobby Kennedy warned his brother that the potion might be harmful, but JFK replied, "I don't care if there's horse piss in there as long as it makes me feel good." On a 1962 visit to Manhattan's Carlyle Hotel, Jacobson accidentally gave too much of the potion to the president, leading to what the authors call a psychotic break. Kennedy peeled off his clothes and ran naked and delirious through the hotel's hallways, doing cartwheels, until his Secret Servicemen safely rescued him.

Jacobson's practice continued to thrive for the next decade, until the *New York Times* published an expose on him, causing him to eventually lose his medical license. He died in 1979. If Kennedy had methamphetamines in his system when he died, a toxicological screen would have revealed the information. Perhaps that's why the testing wasn't requested or made public.

The Warren Commission's
26 Volumes

When the Warren Commission's 26 volumes were released in November 1964, I went to Pittsburgh's Carnegie Library, the only nearby location that had the blue clothbound books. For the next couple of weeks, I became a regular visitor at the library as I flipped through the 20,000 pages and reviewed the material. The first thing I noticed was the absence of an index at the back of the final volume. But then as I paid attention to the overall structure, I learned something that will dash a long-held belief on the part of many Warren Commission critics. The first five volumes include narrative and transcripts of testimony that were heard in Washington, D.C. The next 10 volumes include transcripts from those people who were in Dallas, New Orleans, and elsewhere. Toward the back of volume 15 is a 48-page alphabetical index of people who gave testimony or whose names were mentioned in the 26 volumes. The remaining 25 pages of that volume is a listing of the Commission exhibits, which includes photographs and drawings. A rumor began long ago that the 26 volumes had no index, citing this as proof that the government was in cover-up mode. But the index is there; it is just very incomplete—I would later learn there were many individuals who should have been listed but weren't—and should have appeared at the end of volume 26.

Reading through the 26 volumes was exhausting yet exhilarating. While my main purview was the material that pertained to the president's cause of death, I couldn't resist plowing through the entire set of volumes in order. I wanted to have a comprehensive sense of what the Commission did and how its members arrived at the conclusion I already knew they had reached from reading the report. I didn't see any of the commissioners, staff members, or even the witnesses making the media rounds, so the material was the only insight into what they went through. The panel and staff spent all of these months assembling this unique historic document, and I needed to honor their work by reading the whole megillah.

The task of the Commission, at least ostensibly, was to gather testimony and depositions from a variety of witnesses and log exhibits into the official record. When the members and their staff began meeting, their first order of business was to familiarize themselves with the materials that had been prepared by the police, FBI, CIA, and other governmental agencies, as well as news accounts. Only then would they be ready to start hearing testimony. The parameters would cover general areas: the basic facts of the assassination, Lee Harvey Oswald's motivation and background, possible international conspiracies involving Oswald in Cuba and Mexico, Oswald's death and any links beforehand to Jack Ruby, whether the Secret Service's performance was adequate, and how this assassination compared to those of other U.S. presidents. So, once the panel began its work, there was no interest in evaluating any other potential suspects in JFK's murder—Oswald was the sole target.

Each area of inquiry would include a legal team with a senior and junior member. Depending on each team's background and expertise, its lawyers would conduct the primary questioning of a particular witness. The process of hearing testimony turned out to be an odd mixture of formality and informality. Each witness was sworn in at the top of his or her session and asked to raise one's right hand and "tell the truth, the whole truth, and nothing but the truth, so help me God." All of the testimony was chronicled by a court reporter taking notes in shorthand, which were later typed up. Chairman Earl Warren and the other Commissioners would listen as the testimony proceeded, sometimes interrupting with questions of their own. As I read through the volumes, it became obvious that the seven panelists were not in attendance during all of the testimony. Although the members were the designated "triers of fact," they were free to come and go, with their entrances and exits noted in the transcripts. Can you imagine a criminal or civil court trial taking place with the judge stating for the record that he or she had an appointment and telling the lawyers to carry on anyway? That's what happened here. When the members did ask questions, they were usually on point, except for those of Allen Dulles, who would sometimes go off on unrelated tangents about his CIA career.

According to Walt Brown, who has a Ph.D. in history from the University of Notre Dame, taught history at Ramapo College of New Jersey, and has encyclopedic knowledge of the Kennedy murder, Warren Commission testimony was not heard in a courtroom. Instead, several locations were employed. In Washington, D.C., much testimony was conducted at the Veterans of Foreign Wars building, around the corner from the U.S. Supreme Court. As witnesses entered the building, they would pass through the lobby where Exhibits from the hearings could be seen. Prior to giving testimony, clever observers might gather from those poster-board visuals the direction the panel was headed on a specific topic. The room used for testimony was wired by the FBI "for security reasons." It's unknown what those reasons were, but presumably the electronic work would have allowed FBI liaison Deke DeLoach to listen in on the testimony from the comfort of his office at Bureau headquarters.

The preponderance of the testimony was heard in Dallas, either at Parkland Hospital or the office of the U.S. attorney. Some witnesses were questioned by staff lawyers only in New Orleans or other cities. I don't know whether the FBI also wired those other rooms. The Warren Commission sessions were not conducted in secrecy, and witnesses were not instructed to never discuss their testimony afterward, as occurs in grand jury proceedings. The lawyers knew that all testimony would be reproduced in full and made available to the public upon the termination of the Commission's work. Although the sessions were closed to the public, in some cases, witnesses who worked for the same entity—such as the Bethesda autopsy doctors and some of the FBI agents—were called in together. They would each be questioned separately but were able to hear their colleagues' responses—and, presumably, adjust their own answers.

If hearings of this historic importance were to occur today, reporters with live television camera crews and citizens with cell-phone cameras would be camped out on the steps of the buildings, letting the world know when each witness was giving testimony. On TV and radio news programs and Internet forums, there would be much conjecturing beforehand about what he or she might say. And as the witnesses left the premises, they'd be followed to their cars and asked how their session went. Then there'd be a new round of media debate about what might have been said, based upon how long a person was inside the hearing room. News crews would make tempting offers to get critical witnesses' exclusive stories, and if the individuals weren't famous before they walked in and gave testimony, their names and faces would soon be front-page news. Instant media stars would be born, with the most telegenic and glib ones called upon in the future to give commentary on news stories unrelated to the JFK assassination. Perhaps one or two would connect so well with the public, they'd be offered an ongoing spotlight in the form of their own interview or reality program. That's the world we live in today!

But in 1963, the media were more restrained or, if you'd prefer, just not curious enough. They didn't realize the clout they had to ask questions and demand answers. They accepted that the Warren Commission had its job to do, and the press would find out what happened when it was told. It helped that there was no publicly available schedule of witnesses published to tip who was giving testimony on what day and time, and at which location. So, although the Commission's sessions weren't "secret," per se, its members still enjoyed a virtual press blackout as it conducted its business. Looking back, I wish the press had been more aggressive, but at the time it didn't occur to me to challenge the way things were. I, and everyone I knew, was satisfied to wait until this auspicious Commission furnished its report. I actually didn't expect to find that much earth-shattering news in it. From where I sat, having read and watched and listened to everything the professionals were telling us, Lee Harvey Oswald shot the president, and some angry nightclub owner shot him in retribution. People pretty much expected that the Warren Commission would confirm what we already knew.

There was no mandated amount of time allotted for the Commission to do its work. It was agreed that with the imminent end-of-the-year holidays wreaking havoc with everyone's schedules, the proceedings would start in early 1964. And so, on February 3, testimony began with the panel's first witness: Mrs. Lee Harvey Oswald. Marina Oswald, her two children, and her mother-in-law Marguerite Oswald were flown to Washington, D.C., for her session. Marguerite's testimony followed. According to Marina's transcript, the commissioners present were the chairman, Chief Justice Earl Warren; Senator John Sherman Cooper; Representative Hale Boggs; Representative Gerald R. Ford; and former CIA director Allen W. Dulles; along with their general counsel, J. Lee Rankin. Marina's attorney, John M. Thorne, was there, along with two Russian-language interpreters. Warren opened the session by advising Marina of the mission of the proceedings and pledging to protect her rights "in every manner." She could consult with her attorney at any time, and at the end of her questioning, her team would be furnished with a transcript of the session. They would be able to make any necessary changes or clarifications. This process would also be available to all of the subsequent witnesses.

Attorney Rankin conducted Marina's session. Although her questioning would extend over four days, the schedule was not particularly uncomfortable. There would be a few hours of testimony in the morning, a long lunch where she would be brought back to her hotel to feed her children, then another two hours or so of testimony in the afternoon. There would also be morning and afternoon refreshment breaks. This was the schedule that the commissioners and lawyers adhered to, as

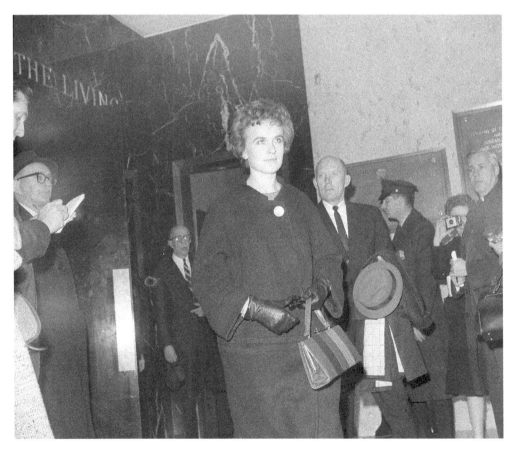

On Feb. 3, 1964, Lee Harvey Oswald's 22-year-old widow, Marina, was the first witness to testify before the Warren Commission (Associated Press/Byron Rollins).

witnesses came and went. Some who gave testimony or depositions were only questioned for a few minutes, just long enough to establish for the record what the Warren Commission lawyers needed them to say. When witnesses tried to add material that the attorneys felt was immaterial, they would be shut down and limited in their responses.

Arlen Specter:
A Worthy Opponent

Reading the transcripts made me relate to these witnesses as people instead of as one-dimensional figures I had gleaned from news footage or photographs. It also gave me keen awareness into the Commission attorneys who were conducting the sessions. One was a fellow Pennsylvanian with whom I would have a decades-long, tangled relationship. Arlen Specter was a Yale Law School graduate who, in 1964, worked as an assistant district attorney in Philadelphia. A Democrat, he enraged his party chiefs the next year when he decided to parlay his notoriety from the Warren Commission into a run for his boss' job as district attorney. Impervious to charges that he was "Benedict Arlen," he switched his affiliation to Republican and won the election, an office he would hold for two terms until he was defeated. He had unsuccessful bids for U.S. senator in 1976 and Pennsylvania governor in 1978, then ran again for U.S. Senate in 1980 and won. He served in that capacity until 2011, although he switched back to the Democratic Party in 2009. In both 2004 and 2010, he asked if I would endorse him, even though I've been a lifelong Democrat and even served as the Allegheny County Democratic Committee chairman between 1978 and 1984. But Specter's views on issues were sufficiently moderate enough to win my endorsement—his 2004 campaign was the only time I ever crossed a party line. He had a 59-year marriage with his wife Joan, and they raised two sons in their hometown of Philadelphia.

Specter's main responsibility on the Warren Commission was to handle the medical testimony. But, on so many occasions, his questioning of witnesses would fall short of the kind of competent inquiries I would have liked. It was maddening to read transcripts where Specter failed to nail down basic information of probative value. At first, I couldn't figure out if he were simple-minded or purposely avoiding opening doors that could lead to inconvenient testimony. As I read on, I determined it was the latter option. He knew exactly what he was doing to negate the process of finding the truth. Nowhere was this more acute than when he was questioning the autopsy doctors and didn't bother to ask the Bethesda doctors why *they* were chosen to perform the single most critical autopsy in American history instead of a forensic pathologist with vast experience in analyzing gunshot wounds. Or to establish the typical protocols for any gunshot wound autopsy, or to account for their differences from what the Parkland doctors saw, or to request the names and ranks of the individuals who seemed to guide their work in the Bethesda morgue. And on and on....

Drs. James Joseph Humes, J. Thornton Boswell, and Pierre Antoine Finck all sat in the same room during their Warren Commission questioning. Navy Commander Humes, the senior pathologist at the National Naval Medical Center, was up at bat first. This was my first occasion to read the in-depth biographical information and expertise of these autopsists and, as it was from their own mouths, it was rather astounding. Humes made clear that his specialty was not specifically *forensic pathology*. Here's a snippet of his questioning by Specter:

> SPECTER: Have you been certified by the American Board of Pathology?
> HUMES: Yes, sir; both in anatomic pathology and in clinical pathology in 1955.
> SPECTER: What specific experience have you had, if any, with respect to gunshot wounds?
> HUMES: My type of practice which, fortunately, has been in peacetime endeavor to a great extent, has been more extensive in the field of natural disease than violence. However, on several occasions in various places where I have been employed, I have had to deal with violent death, accidents, suicides, and so forth. Also, I have had training at the Armed Forces Institute of Pathology, I have completed a course in forensic pathology there as part of my training in the overall field of pathology.

Although none of the photos or X-rays of the president were published in the 26 volumes of the Warren Commission, Humes stated that sets of both were taken before the autopsy began. He testified that he and his colleagues were unsure whether the Commission would have access to the actual photos, so they asked a Navy medical illustrator to make schematic pencil drawings of what they verbally described. The artist didn't even work from the photographs, which would have given him more precise measurements. He just translated the general idea of what the three doctors told him about the wounds. You might argue that, with the state of photography back then, it took some time to develop the films into prints, and you'd be right. But there was no rush to have the drawings done in time for when the autopsy report was written. Then there were still many months between the report and the publishing of the 26 volumes, during which the illustrator could have worked at a comfortable pace to produce accurate drawings for the official record. And if you want to argue that the photographs were too sensitive to be included in the publicly-released 26 volumes—a point I would agree with—there would be nothing amiss with the three doctors bringing them in to show the commissioners, with the proviso that the material not be disseminated. But far be it for Specter to find fault with the very rough descriptions of the president's injuries by the doctors who handled his deceased body.

After being sworn in by Warren, Boswell was turned over to attorney Specter. His questioning took less time than it would take to cook a soft-boiled egg. Here is the full transcript of his testimony:

> SPECTER: Will you state your full name for the record, please?
> BOSWELL: J. Thornton Boswell, Commander, Medical Corps, U.S. Navy.
> SPECTER: What is your profession?

BOSWELL: Physician.

SPECTER: And where did you obtain your medical degree, please?

BOSWELL: At the College of Medicine, Ohio State University.

SPECTER: And what experience have you had in your professional line subsequent to obtaining that degree?

BOSWELL: I interned in the Navy and took my pathology training at St. Albans Naval Hospital in New York. I was certified by the American Board of Pathology in both clinical and pathological anatomy in 1957 and 1958.

SPECTER: And what is your duty assignment at the present time?

BOSWELL: I am the Chief of Pathology at the National Naval Medical School.

SPECTER: Did you have occasion to participate in the autopsy of the late President Kennedy?

BOSWELL: I did.

SPECTER: And did you assist Dr. Humes at that time?

BOSWELL: Yes, sir.

SPECTER: Have you been present here today during the entire course of Dr. Humes' testimony?

BOSWELL: I have, sir; yes.

SPECTER: Do you have anything that you would like to add by way of elaboration or modification to that which Dr. Humes has testified?

BOSWELL: None. I believe Dr. Humes has stated essentially what is the culmination of our examination and our subsequent conference, and everything is exactly as we had determined our conclusions.

SPECTER: And are you one of the three co-authors of the autopsy report which has been previously identified as a Commission Exhibit?

BOSWELL: Yes, I am.

SPECTER: All the facts set forth therein are correct in accordance with your analysis and evaluation of the situation?

BOSWELL: Yes.

SPECTER: And specifically, as to the points of entry and points of exit which have been testified to by Dr. Humes, do his views express yours, as well?

BOSWELL: They do, yes.

SPECTER: Dr. Boswell, would you state for the record what your conclusion was as to the cause of death of President Kennedy?

BOSWELL: The brain injury was the cause of death.

SPECTER: And in the absence of brain injury, what, in your view, would have been the future status of President Kennedy's mortality, if he had only sustained the wound inflicted in 385? (Note: Commission Exhibit 385 is a rough, hand-drawn image of the president's back wound.)

BOSWELL: I believe it would have been essentially an uneventful recovery. It could have been easily repaired, and I think it would have been of little consequence.

SPECTER: Those are my only questions, Mr. Chief Justice.

Lieutenant Colonel Pierre A. Finck's testimony came next and lasted just a tad longer than Boswell's. Perhaps long enough to cook a *hard*-boiled egg. Finck was the Army pathologist who had performed approximately 200 autopsies early in his career, including "many" from military-related gunshot deaths. Specter and some of the Commissioners asked Finck about the differences between an entrance wound and an exit wound. Rather than just having everybody stipulate that a bullet enters and leaves a small hole, while its exit hole is larger, Finck spoke about other cases that proved this point on a variety of different body parts. He even brought a simple chart that he had prepared prior to the president's death as a tool for classes he taught. It consisted of a very rudimentary drawing that showed what was labeled as a "perforating missile wound of the skull." Arrows pointed out the trajectory of a bullet going in small and coming out large.

When Specter asked Finck if one bullet could have gone through the president, then continued on to go in and out of Governor Connally's body, Finck answered:

> On the basis that if we assume that this is one bullet going through President Kennedy's body and also through Governor Connally's body, the reduction of velocity would be of some extent after passing through President Kennedy's body, but not having hit bones, the reduction in velocity, after going through President Kennedy's body, would be minimal.

But, as I would come to understand later, bones *were* hit! The single-bullet idea they're advocating here is the very essence that states there was only one assassin. It presupposes that one bullet went into Kennedy's back, exited the front of his neck, re-entered into Connally's back, pierced the right lung, broke four inches of the fifth anterior rib, exited from the front of his chest, re-entered the back of his wrist, shattered the distal end of the radius—one of the two long bones from the elbow to the wrist—re-entered the governor's left thigh, then fell out onto a stretcher at Parkland, where it was allegedly recovered still in pristine condition.

Attorney Specter had no interest in exploring that dichotomy. And for the rest of his career, he would adopt the single-bullet theory as his favorite theme in defending the Warren Commission Report and its conclusions. All logic and reason were stubbornly discarded as he embraced the implausible and held on for dear life. Finck's testimony concluded with him hewing to the party line that the president was shot from behind and above, and that no exploding bullets were used. He also confirmed that his findings matched those of the other two autopsy doctors and that they had not had any disagreements on the case.

I debated Specter more times than I can count over the years: on television and radio, at JFK conferences, even at state bar events that had nothing to do with the assassination, but we were both there and always ready to scuffle. In truth, it became a bit like the Battle of the Titans or something you'd see on a professional wrestling card. We knew our roles in the debate and never wavered in doing everything possible—short of throwing chairs—to win the crowd to our side. He was quick and brilliant, and could argue vociferously, despite always being on the wrong side of the debate, to my mind. It was simply impossible for him to counter my presentation of the scientific evidence. He was left with no choice but to criticize conspiracy-minded citizens and act as if demanding honesty from our government was somehow shallow or un-American. It reminded me of a great saying taught in law schools, authored by someone whose name has been sadly forgotten. It goes: "When you have the law on your side, pound the law. When you have the facts on your side, pound the facts. When you have neither the law nor the facts going for you, pound the table." Specter was an excellent table pounder.

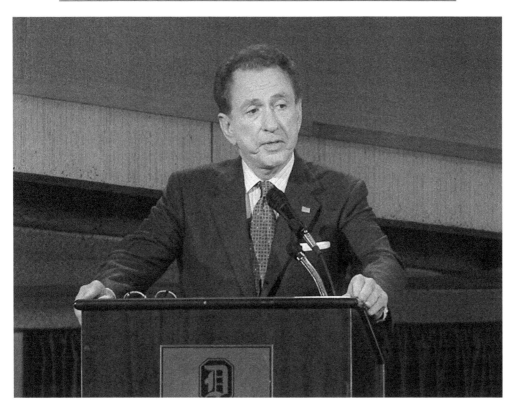

Even though we often sparred, I invited Warren Commission lawyer Arlen Specter to lecture at the 40th anniversary symposium at the Cyril H. Wecht Institute of Forensic Science and Law, at Duquesne University (Wecht Collection).

As a lawyer, he was an adamant advocate for his client, the U.S. government. As a politician, he was a moderate who voted against gun control and in favor of many social issues. I admired how he always supported Israel, and, more than once, when we were in each other's city, we would take the other to lunch at the local deli. As long as we didn't talk the Kennedy case, we'd have pleasant discussions. Knowing how intelligent he was, I always wondered how he could buy into the load of malarkey he was pushing with the single-bullet premise. One day, after an especially strenuous debate, we shared an elevator to the parking structure. On the way, other passengers departed until we were the last two left. I turned to him and gently said, "You don't really believe that, do you?" He shrugged and dismissed my query with a wry smile. I believe he was boxed into sticking to his script even though it made no sense.

I've often wondered how I would fare if I had been in Specter's position. Any law school or debating class student has been given the assignment of arguing both sides of a case, often finding the language to convey ideas that one would never person-ally subscribe to. If I had to argue the single-bullet hypothesis, I would probably do as Specter did. There would be no other way to address it. But frankly, I would never be in that position. I've never encountered a situation where I had to conform to some institutional idiocy in order to retain my job, thank God. But if I had to abandon logic and serve up the single-bullet theory to the world, I would have quit my job. There are many fewer embarrassing ways to feed my family than to mislead the public about something of such crucial historical importance. Specter's career blossomed because he did the government a favor. Or maybe his silver-tongued facility was so powerful, he convinced himself. I just can't understand how an otherwise bright man could sign off on something that could be so easily scientifically disputed.

Beginning in 2006, Specter embarked on a whole new career—as a stand-up comic. Despite the chemotherapy treatments he was receiving for the lymphoma that would eventually end his life, he never lost his sense of humor. In 2007, he competed for the Funniest Celebrity in Washington and came in second. He'd videotape his comedy club appearances, studying what worked and where he could improve, using the same kind of shrewdness that served him well as a lawyer and Warren Commission interrogator. You can find him delivering his routines on YouTube. Specter died on October 14, 2012, at the age of 82. I sent a letter of sympathy to his family and have missed his presence at JFK events.

My Lecture at the American Academy of Forensic Sciences

A s I finished reading the 26 volumes of the Warren Commission's hearings and exhibits, I noticed that there was a significant commonality with the initial report: the medical evidence and testimony was engulfed by many other facets of the investigation. Sometimes the sheer minutia was laughable. Did I really need to see a photo from 1949 of Lee Harvey Oswald's dog, Blackie? Or to spend almost two pages learning about the ill-fitting dentures of Jack Ruby's mother, back in 1938? Unless Fannie Rubenstein's mouth problems led her to come back from the dead and slay our president, I didn't see the reason for including this filler material. There were many other items that could and should have been deleted. Perhaps, I thought at the time, the Commission wanted to include everything, so it couldn't be criticized for unfair editing. But as I learned from Specter's skillful avoidance of uncomfortable areas, the way to shape witnesses' testimony to a favorable outcome would be not to ask tough questions in the first place. And it would be a while before I learned how deficient the Commission's work was.

For more than a year I studied the volumes, debating aspects with old and new friends who were as fixated about gathering information as I was. Like me, my crime lab colleague, Charlie McInerney, was also a member of the American Academy of Forensic Sciences and would be one of the program chairs for the annual conference in February 1966. He told me that the upcoming AAFS conference would include a full-day General Scientific session about the Warren Commission Report. Everyone who attended the meeting would be invited, an audience of a couple thousand forensic scientists. McInerney explained that he was putting together a panel of experts in various fields to analyze the case from angles that would include forensic pathology, criminalistics, questioned documents, jurisprudence, and psychiatry. He asked if I'd be interested in making the forensic pathology presentation. Of course, I readily said yes. Not only did his question make my day, but it set my life and career on a trajectory that hasn't slowed down now more than 50 years later.

The meeting was at the Drake Hotel in Chicago on February 25. A harsh blizzard meant fewer attendees ventured outside, leading to an even greater turnout for us. My fellow presenters and I had a captive audience, and we entranced them with our speeches about all aspects of the report. When I gave my talk, all hell broke loose.

There were FBI agents in the audience who were AAFS members. They didn't like my take on the case, as I made various criticisms of their agency and other law enforcement entities. But this was early on in my investigation, so I barely even broached the farce of the single-bullet idea. All I had to go on was the Warren Commission's work, which was enough to begin poking holes in the government's story. I simply brought up the obvious questions that any reasonably educated person would ask after reading through the 26 volumes. I concluded my speech by saying that despite the missing pieces in the Commission's report, there was not sufficient evidence for me to reject the overall findings. Aside from the glares from the FBI agents, my presentation was wildly successful. I got a standing ovation and spent the rest of the week-long conference being treated like a rock star. My week's schedule overflowed with breakfasts, lunches, and dinners with seriously fascinated experts who wanted more details and my opinions.

One moment at that conference really stood out in my memory and is more significant to me today than it was back then. Pierre Finck, the Army forensic pathologist called into the Bethesda autopsy room as an afterthought and who arrived after the autopsy had commenced, told me during a private breakfast meeting at the conference that he was extremely unhappy with the handling of the autopsy proceedings. "You cannot believe what it was like," Finck told me. "It was horrible. Horrible! I only wish I could tell you about it." Unfortunately, I never got more details out of him because I was mobbed by other attendees, and Finck slipped away. Over the years when I tried to reconnect with him and get him to elaborate on his experience, he refused, once even stating that he had never made such a comment to me. But I know what I heard, and I've never forgotten it.

With the delivery of my paper finished, I believed my brief inquiry into the Kennedy assassination to be over. I returned to Pittsburgh, expecting to put all of this behind me. Sigrid congratulated me on my new status and swollen ego, then requested that I roll up my sleeves and help her bathe our three sons.

A number of interesting developments arose as a result of my assassination speech. For one thing, I became a force to contend with among my colleagues at AAFS. Immediately thereafter, any topic I wanted to present would be given a key position on the schedule and the best audience. I joined the AAFS executive committee, and, in 1971, the membership elected me president of the Academy. At 40, I was the youngest person to hold that year-long office, a distinction I believe I still enjoy decades later.

Through interviews and articles, news of my AAFS address filtered out to the public and led to a number of contacts from people who would soon form a nascent Warren Commission critics' brigade. A 38-year-old New York lawyer was the first to phone me. I had never heard of Mark Lane, but he explained his background. Upon his honorable discharge from the U.S. Army and graduation from Brooklyn Law School, he began his career as an attorney for mostly indigent people who needed defense counsel for criminal matters. A strong supporter of the civil rights movement, he staged fundraising concerts with folk musicians and fought the House Un-American Activities Committee. He helped found the reform movement of the Democratic Party and caught the attention of notables such as Eleanor Roosevelt, John and Robert Kennedy, and Martin Luther King, Jr. His political contacts opened doors for him to enter that realm where he served as an executive assistant to a U.S. congressman and, in 1961, one term as a member of the New York State Assembly. He could have continued in politics but trying court cases was more fulfilling for him.

Lane believed we shared common views about JFK's assassination, so I settled in for what would turn out to be the first of many long discussions, over the phone and later in person. Lane told me he had met President Kennedy on a few occasions but didn't know him well. Nonetheless, he applauded Kennedy's progressive views, as did I. On November 22, 1963, Lane was at the Manhattan courthouse, preparing for a pre-trial hearing for a jailed prisoner scheduled for the afternoon. On the lunch break he walked past a grocery store where people were gathered around a radio, crying. That's how Lane learned that the president had been shot in Dallas and would likely die of his injuries. He ran back to the courthouse's media room, where people were awaiting more details. Soon, a *New York Times* journalist gave everyone the bad news that Kennedy had died. Lane finished his hearing and, as he left the courthouse, a judge he knew asked what he thought of Lee Harvey Oswald as the lone suspect. Mark stated that he didn't know many details at that point. The judge advised him to keep an open mind, since some news reports said that Kennedy had sustained an entrance wound to his throat, an impossibility if Oswald was behind and above the president. That *was* a quandary, Lane agreed, and they pledged to pay attention to what would promise to be an interesting trial.

Like everyone else in America, Lane was engrossed by the perpetual TV and radio coverage from Dallas. As he explained, he didn't like the glut of media indicating that the legal case against Oswald was a fait accompli. A defense attorney with 10 years' experience, Lane knew the hazards of pre-trial publicity for a criminal defendant. Many of his clients had been railroaded by negative portrayals by police, prosecutors, and the media, and he knew that could impact a fair shot from a jury. On Sunday, when he saw Oswald assassinated at the police station, while 70 officers were on duty and supposedly protecting him, Lane broke into a cold sweat. There would be no trial for this defendant now. And the accused died without even having a lawyer helping him, even though he requested one.

Even more unsettling to Mark was a subsequent press conference where Dallas County District Attorney Henry Wade said Oswald was JFK's sole assassin and also guilty of patrolman J.D. Tippit's death. Wade listed 15 reasons for his conclusions, some of which Lane felt contradicted known facts of the case. When the *New York Times* published Wade's theories, Lane sat down and crafted his own counter-brief. Before he knew it, he had written a 10,000-word article, asking that people dispassionately examine the evidence instead of just accepting what was being spoon-fed to them. The article asserted that Oswald's guilt had not been established and ended with a plea for a temporary suspension of certainty while the case was being investigated. But finding an outlet for his article was a challenge, Lane said. While he assured magazine executives that he wasn't stating that Oswald was innocent, the very idea of dissent seemed treasonous to publishers, including those who had previously welcomed his op-ed pieces. Lane felt the public needed to read what he had written, so he even offered to let the outlets run the brief without payment. Still, there were no takers, including at the *New York Post*, which was then one of the city's most liberal newspapers.

Lane's article ended up running in a radical, leftist, independent weekly newspaper, the *National Guardian*, on December 19, 1963, and sold so many copies that extra press runs and a special pamphlet were ordered. The *New York Times* finally wrote a story about the story, but no other publication would acknowledge it. While the American press seemed dedicated to ignoring Lane's piece, it got major attention around the world, including Italy, Mexico, and Japan. Lane mailed a copy of the article to me, and I was very impressed by it.

By the time the Warren Commission was gearing up to hear testimony, Lane was contacted by Oswald's mother, Marguerite. He didn't know her but learned she had read his article. Marguerite said that he was the only attorney to publicly state that her son should not be condemned as a murderer, since he had been denied a trial by his peers. Then she asked him to represent Oswald's interests to the Warren Commission. So, Mark contacted the commissioners, asking to cross-examine witnesses and be allowed to find more witnesses who could offer a more complete view of Oswald's activities. As much as Lane was desperately intrigued by working on Oswald's behalf, Marguerite couldn't afford to pay him at all, even for reimbursement of expenses. That provided a conflict, considering that Lane's law practice consisted of impoverished defendants and one corporate client who kept the wheels turning—but that client didn't want Lane distracted by the Kennedy case, and they ended up parting company. Although the *National Guardian* had sent Mark an unexpected check for $100, such a windfall wasn't enough money to justify him abandoning his law practice. Still, Lane threw caution to the wind and jumped into the Kennedy assassination full time.

Marguerite could not be controlled when it came to speaking out to the press, especially when she announced her belief that her son was an agent for the U.S. government. Although Lane would come to agree with this contention many years later, at the time he could see no proof of it and found her statements inflammatory and unproductive to gaining public sympathy. So, Lane and the alleged assassin's mother drafted an agreement that he would represent Oswald but not Marguerite and that she would appear before the Commission without his assistance or presence. The agreement contained a clause that if Lane's investigation proved that Oswald was, indeed, guilty, he could state so publicly. Only because Oswald was dead could that clause be written, as it is forbidden for any defense attorney to take that position for a living client.

Lane spent the next 15 months living like a student as he took on the defense for his reviled, deceased client. Armed with courage and a prodigious commitment, Lane threw himself into learning every facet of the case. Shortly before the Warren Commission Report was released, he was filmed for hours by a CBS news crew and told that nine minutes' worth of footage would appear on the next evening's Walter Cronkite broadcast. It never aired. Lane did, however, embark on a lecture tour that helped spread his views, especially throughout Europe. He also formed a group that paid for a modest Manhattan theater where he would give regularly scheduled speeches on the subject.

Dorothy Kilgallen, a star writer with the now-defunct *New York Journal-American*, became an ally. Since she feared that their phones were being tapped, they called each other from public phones, using the code names "Miss Parker" and "Mr. Robinson." Kilgallen shared a scoop with Lane, giving him an early look at Jack Ruby's testimony to the Commission before it was released to the public. Her own newspaper was reluctant to run it until she pledged personal responsibility for any legal fallout. Kilgallen wouldn't tell Lane or anyone how she had obtained the transcript. When questioned by the FBI, she stayed mum but made the point that it had not come to her through John Daly, who was then the director of the Voice of America. Daly was also the host of *What's My Line?*, a popular CBS weekly quiz show on which Kilgallen appeared as a panelist. This was a significant since, since Daly's wife, Virginia, was the daughter of the chief justice of the U.S. Supreme Court, the Warren Commission's capo di tutti capi, Earl Warren.

Lane sent a copy of his article to Warren, requesting appointment as Oswald's legal representative. Two weeks later, Commission counsel J. Lee Rankin wrote back thanking him for the communication and stating that his request would be given "appropriate consideration." But soon, Rankin wrote that the panel had decided that it would not be "useful or desirable" to permit an attorney who was representing Oswald to have access to investigative materials or participate in hearings. Later, and oddly, the Commission appointed Walter E. Craig, the president of the American Bar Association, to be Oswald's attorney. Craig had initially rejected the appointment, but after the *New York Post* and other news outlets praised the idea, he went forward, although he hardly did anything but lend his name to the proceedings. He wasn't the advocate for Oswald's defense that Lane would have been.

The Commission called Lane to testify about what he had learned during the time he had represented Oswald. Lane had made audio recordings of assassination and Tippit witnesses, but although interesting, in a legal venue the recordings would be considered hearsay as he had no firsthand knowledge of what happened in Dallas. Warren questioned Lane and made clear that he was still not recognized as Oswald's legal representative, despite the agreement with Oswald's mother.

During Lane's questioning, he referenced a November 14, 1963, meeting he had heard about that was attended by J.D. Tippit and Bernard Weissman, the sponsor of the vitriolic anti–Kennedy ad that ran in the *Dallas Morning News* on the day of the assassination. A third person was at the meeting, Lane stated, but he would not give the name in a hearing that would be made public. Lane insisted on a private executive session to provide the sensitive information and, when that was granted, told the panel that the third person was alleged to be Jack Ruby. Because Ruby was awaiting trial for Oswald's murder, Lane felt the need to respect his rights. Despite the need for protecting Ruby's name, it was revealed in a transcript sent to Lane for his comments, in an envelope that was not marked "classified." The envelope was opened by Lane's secretary as just another piece of mail she handled for him.

Lane was also repeatedly followed and harassed by FBI agents and given grief by immigration authorities when he returned from flights abroad. He told me he felt that, in particular, Warren, Rankin, and Gerald Ford treated him as a defendant they were prosecuting for some crime. If the commissioners were really interested in thoroughly investigating the deaths of the president and the patrolman, they would benefit from having a devil's advocate on the panel. Lane's treatment was proof that the Commission was only formed to promote a foregone conclusion that blamed Oswald for both murders.

Those early days of speaking with Lane left a big impression on me. For the first time, I was discussing this massive case with someone as unabashedly obsessive as I was about it. He knew the content of the 26 volumes as well as I did, and our conversations seemed the intellectual equivalent of playing tennis at Wimbledon. As we spoke of how he contacted the Commissioners and petitioned being a part of the proceedings, I realized I could do a similar thing about the autopsy information. I wouldn't contact the Commission, however. My target would be whoever was in charge of the materials at the National Archives. Why should I be frustrated about the paucity of information about the autopsy facts when there had to be someone, somewhere, with more data than made it into the 26 volumes? If there was nothing to hide—and at that point I didn't even really consider that would be the case—why not allow an independent and qualified observer to look at the materials? Lane encouraged me to fire off a letter, which I did. Still, it would take more years and many more letters before I was allowed the privilege to review the autopsy files.

It took Lane several months to write his book, *Rush to Judgment*, and even longer to find a publisher after representatives of the CIA warned publishing houses to stay away. After it was turned down repeatedly by many major entities, the hardcover edition came out in England in October 1966 (Holt, Rinehart, and Winston) and went to the top of the best-seller list, eventually getting worldwide publication. The next year's release of the paperback edition also topped the charts, and the book has not been out of print since. Lane went on to write more books on the Kennedy assassination and other cases, and continued to be fearless as a lawyer and critical thinker. We remained friends until his death from a heart attack on May 10, 2016, at the age of 89.

A reminder to younger readers: Back in the mid–1960s, we had telephones for communication but not answering machines or cell phones. Offices did not have fax machines, and only fairly large operations had Telex machines for intra-branch correspondence. Documents and letters were typed and sent through the mail. There were no personal word processors, home computers, desktop printers, or emails. Electric typewriters were just coming into play, with many offices still using manual ones with whatever font came with the machine. Photocopiers had been invented but were not in wide use, so if people wanted copies of documents, they had to type on an original piece of paper, with carbon paper underneath leaving inky blue reproductions that would easily smear. Many times, people did not strike copies of documents and had to mail their originals. One reason it took Lane so long to secure a publisher was because he had to mail his original manuscript, then wait for it to be reviewed and returned, holding his breath that it would come back intact.

Consider all of that as I tell you about Sylvia Meagher, who contacted me after my AAFS lecture. In 1966, Sylvia was a 45-year-old New Yorker who worked as a research analyst at the United Nations World Health Organization. Born Sylvia Orenstein, she was married to a poet who had been her teacher when she attended Brooklyn College. They remained married, even though she told me they lived separate lives. Sylvia and I had several phone conversations, and I visited her once in Manhattan. She had been reviewing the 26 volumes of the Warren Commission and taking copious notes. She had a two-pronged mission: to provide the volumes with a proper index that the original crafters chose not to offer and to keep track of the plentiful inconsistencies and misrepresentations throughout. Sylvia's method of doing this was via typed 3 × 5" index cards that were color-coded and kept in numerous shoe boxes. To say that Sylvia was organized just doesn't do justice to her herculean effort. As I mentioned earlier, there was an index at the tail of volume 15 of the report, but until I began speaking to Sylvia, I hadn't realized how inept it was. Sylvia's view was that the 20,000 pages deserved an index that was wide-ranging. Could I imagine, she asked, "if the *Encyclopedia Brittanica* were published with its contents unalphabetized, untitled, and in random sequence?"

Whereas I had read through the volumes and made notes about the autopsy and other areas, Sylvia pored over every line, cataloging each individual who was named and all the facets that were covered. That gave her a tremendous databank of not only what was in the work but also the significant omissions. Whereas I was more willing to let pass the slipshod writing, she was downright offended at the incompetence and told me she thought it demonstrated "irrefutable dishonesty and terrible bias." And she was right!

Sylvia knew Lane and was up to date on his struggle to get his article and book into the marketplace, and when I asked if she planned to publish her information, she said she hadn't decided. She adamantly believed Oswald was framed as the assassin and that the true killers were a cabal of anti–Castro exiles. But Sylvia wasn't trying to blaze a trail as an investigative journalist. She simply saw a pronounced need and decided to be the one to fill it. At some point she was persuaded to go public with her observations. Sylvia released the 152-page *Subject Index to the Warren Report and Hearings and Exhibits* (Scarecrow Press, 1966). It immediately became an indispensable guide to everyone who was reading the volumes and dashed any confidence readers had in the Warren Commission's infallibility. If that were Sylvia's only contribution to American history, it would earn her a place of honor among scholars and citizens. But her contributions were just beginning.

In December 1966, *Esquire* magazine published Sylvia's article, "Notes for a New Investigation." With this, she fired off a warning to the Warren Commissioners that their job was unfinished. She outlined numerous witnesses who should have been called to testify but were ignored and highlighted what they would have to say for the record. She also listed a variety of witnesses who gave seemingly endless testimony about things that had no bearing on the case and discovered a number of areas in which the Commissioners should have ordered testing or further research. Her *Esquire* piece provided the basis for her 1967 masterpiece, *Accessories After the Fact: The Warren Commission, the Authorities, and the Report on the JFK Assassination* (Bobbs-Merrill). The hardcover edition was a best seller, and over the years it has been republished in paperback and e-book form. In 1980, Sylvia and coauthor Gary Owens wrote *Master Index to the J.F.K. Assassination Investigations*, which includes the Warren Commission and the House Select Committee on Assassinations volumes. Sylvia questioned everything and with good reason. In our conversations, she even stated that she wouldn't put it past the government to have phonied up the autopsy photographs and X-rays to suit their "lone nut" scenario. There was no way to prove it at that time because the materials had not yet been released, but I would reflect back on her comments in years to come and appreciate how prescient they were. Sylvia died in 1989 at the age of 67, but her work will always be considered an encyclopedia of the assassination.

The Warren Commission Report testimony has endured as a point of interest to a later generation as well. Beginning in 2003 and continuing for a number of years, film director/writer Mark Sobel crafted a documentary titled *The Commission* that used popular actors to perform actual dialogue from the report's transcripts. The stars of this very fascinating project included Edward Asner, Martin Landau, Sam Waterston, Martin Sheen, Joe Don Baker, and Corbin Bernsen. The black-and-white film had the feel of newsreel footage of the era and included snippets of President Kennedy's speeches. The film won an IFP Award for Best Narrative Feature.

The Zapruder
Film Screening

As Sylvia Meagher became known in the burgeoning assassination research community, she befriended many like-minded authors, lawyers, and experts. It was a renaissance of people helping each other with their projects and sharing information as their collective skepticism of the government's position on the case grew. Many of these bright people contacted me in Pittsburgh, and when I visited New York City, I would spend time hearing about their latest provocative developments.

In 1966, I had left the Pittsburgh District Attorney's office for full-time postings as a forensic pathologist. I continued to keep my state bar membership but was pleased to switch my attention to morgue work and testifying as an expert witness in court hearings and trials. In addition to my duties as director of the Pittsburgh Pathology and Toxicology Laboratory, I became the associate pathologist and associate director of laboratories at nearby St. Clair Memorial Hospital. I continued as a lecturer at the Law-Science Academy of America and added duties as a clinical instructor of both legal medicine and forensic pathology at the University of Pittsburgh School of Medicine. My professional memberships now expanded to include the Pennsylvania Academy of Science, Pittsburgh Academy of Medicine, Pittsburgh Medical Forum, American Association for the Advancement of Science, Pan-American Medical Association, and the Pennsylvania Association of Pathologists and co-chairmanship of its Legislation Committee.

That year, I received a phone call from someone who would become—and remains—a cherished friend. Dr. Josiah Thompson, whose close associates call him "Tink," said he had heard about my American Academy of Forensic Sciences lecture and was impressed. Tink had been exchanging information with Sylvia and others about the Kennedy matter and was writing his own book about the assassination.

Tink served in the U.S. Navy on Underwater Demolition Team 21 and led the beach reconnaissance team in Beirut, Lebanon, receiving commendations for these operations. He earned a B.A., M.A., and a Ph.D. in philosophy at Yale University. He studied at England's Oxford University, Austria's University of Vienna, Denmark's Copenhagen University, and would later go on to Germany's Goethe Institute in Munich. His postgraduate honors included an American-Scandinavian Foundation fellowship and a Fulbright Travel grant and, later, a John Simon Guggenheim Memorial Foundation Fellowship. Tink had been a teaching assistant, then an instructor, of philosophy at Yale, and was at the time an assistant professor of philosophy at Haverford College, just outside of Philadelphia. He would go on to become a tenured professor there until his retirement in 1978. He would also become one of the world's great scholars on Søren Kierkegaard, authoring several biographies and reference works about the 19th-century Danish philosopher. In the late 1970s, Tink would turn his skills toward a career as a private investigator in California. Today, Tink works as a defense team investigator on high-profile criminal and civil cases around the world—but, back then, it was his vast knowledge about the Kennedy case that captured my attention.

In October 1966, Tink had been hired by *Life* magazine as a special editorial consultant for its various articles on the assassination, a position he would hold for more than a year until his book was released. In the lead-up to the third anniversary of the president's murder, the magazine planned to release more photographic evidence than it had previously published and relied on Tink for his critical perspective. The November 25 issue, entitled "Grounds for Reasonable Doubt," was the much-heralded achievement and remains a collector's "must have" on the case.

In preparation for that issue, Tink asked if I could fly to New York City and review the 8-millimeter film that Abraham Zapruder had shot in Dealey Plaza. At that point I had only seen the selected still-frames that were published in the press. *Life*'s November 29, 1963, issue had featured 31 small black-and-white photos, several of which were from the Zapruder film. Others included the Kennedys earlier in the day, the limousine after the assassination, shocked bystanders, JFK's casket being offloaded at Andrews Air Force Base, etc. Seven of the Zapruder frames had also appeared in the Associated Press and United Press International newspapers to promote the *Life* issue. Two weeks later, *Life* had released nine color frames from the Zapruder film. Even though those accompanying articles had made clear that the president's head had practically been blasted off by gunfire and that the Zapruder film showed everything, the graphic images had not been made public. So, when Tink asked whether I would be interested in seeing the film and all of its frames, I said yes. Truth be told, if I had to crawl on my belly the whole way there, I would have done so without complaint!

By the mid–1960s, *Life* had the largest circulation of any weekly publication in the world. Founded in 1883 as a lightly topical weekly, it was bought in 1936 by publisher Henry "Harry" Robinson Luce, who already owned *Time* and *Fortune* magazines. Harry developed an interest in journalism in boarding school, then went on to Yale College and joined the Skull and Bones, an undergraduate secret society whose members would grow into the elite caste of government and industry, enjoying solid ties with the U.S. intelligence community. A workaholic editor-in-chief, Harry's bankroll and prestige were boundless as he influenced what Americans thought about politics, business, athletics, culture, and public policy.

In 1935, Harry divorced his first wife and married Clare Boothe, a future two-term Connecticut congresswoman and former managing editor of *Vanity Fair* magazine. She convinced her husband to acquire *Life* and turn it into a photo-journal with snappy captions, while letting *Time* cover more hard-edged reportage. The Luces were the ultimate journalistic power couple, with Clare authoring many of the articles under Harry's bylines to avoid charges of nepotism. They didn't care who got the credit so long as they carried their vision of the world to the masses—and that vision was a politically conservative one. In 1952, President Eisenhower appointed Boothe Luce as U.S. ambassador to Italy. In 1959, Ike named her to head the Brazilian embassy, but by then, she was such an outspoken and polarizing figure, she resigned after four days without having visited the country.

Neither Harry nor Clare were fans of President Kennedy. Although ardent Republicans, they attended events at the White House and once stormed out after getting into a spat with JFK over his handling of matters in Cuba. The jingoistic duo wanted a harsher stance against communism, and when Kennedy refused to increase the budget for anti–Castro exiles, the Luces subsidized at least $250,000 on intelligence-gathering raids by commandos in speedboats. Harry retired as editor-in-chief for Time Inc., in 1964, but the right-slanted precedents he established remained during the post–Kennedy era. Harry died in 1967; Clare died 20 years later.

At the time of Kennedy's death, *Life* magazine was being edited by C.D. Jackson who, as I mentioned earlier, had supervised the purchase of the Zapruder film from the Dallas dressmaker who shot it. Jackson, then 61, had been working with Harry Luce since 1931. Simultaneously, Jackson worked with the Office of Strategic Services (OSS) during World War II, specializing in psychological warfare and propaganda. He served as President Eisenhower's special assistant on the discipline. As the OSS morphed into the CIA, Jackson was a liaison between the intelligence office and the Pentagon. He had a close friendship with Allen Dulles when the spy chief headed the CIA, and it continued after Dulles was fired by JFK and later became a member of the Warren Commission. Jackson not only published frames from the Zapruder film but also bought the exclusive rights to Marina Oswald's story for his magazine.

On that day in 1966, I met Tink at the Time & Life Building in Manhattan. Some executives from *Life* were present, as well as Sylvia Meagher. Another attendee was a fledgling Republican congressman from New York, Theodore R. Kupferman, who was a Columbia Law School graduate and taught at New York Law School. He served on the local city council before winning his congressional seat in 1966 where he would remain until 1969. He then became a justice of the New York State Supreme Court until 1996 and died in 2003. Kupferman may not have shared Kennedy's political persuasion, but he was anguished by the assassination. He publicly criticized the Warren Commission and proposed that a special committee review the Commission's work and conclusions. He wanted to reopen Rep. Hale Boggs' resolution on the assassination that had been shut down when President Johnson appointed the Commission. Unfortunately, there was not enough interest on Capitol Hill at that time, but it was a valiant goal and one that would eventually come to the fore.

The Zapruder film had been kept in a climate-controlled vault under lock and key. We were ushered into a large room that had a movie projector screen and chairs. We took our seats and were handed 486 11-by-15-inch photographs representing each frame of the 26.6-second film. We were able to study in extreme detail the facial expressions and body movements of the four passengers in the presidential limousine's backseats, along with the driver and navigator, and the spectators who lined the street to watch the motorcade. The sense of history from those still images was humbling and powerful. But nothing compared to what followed when we were screened the actual 8-millimeter silent film. Brief though it was, it packed a wallop. We watched it again and again, sucking in our collective breath the first few times, leaving us almost unable to speak. Subsequent viewings allowed us to see specific elements, even being able to have the footage stopped and shown again so we could critique various parts.

As we watched the film, we discussed what had been written by the Warren Commissioners. The panel was steadfast in its belief that Lee Harvey Oswald was the sole shooter and that he fired from the sixth-floor window of the Texas School Book Depository building. The high and rear angle, they maintained, allowed Oswald to fire his rifle three times into Kennedy's back and head as the limousine drove down Elm Street toward the overpass. Three shell cases were discovered on the floor near the supposed assassin's perch.

At first, federal authorities reported that President Kennedy had been shot with the first and third bullets, and that Governor Connally had been hit with the second. But the Zapruder film didn't fit that scenario and caused the government to scramble for another explanation. There simply wasn't enough time for Oswald to have shot the gun, reloaded, fired again, reloaded, and fired for a third time, in those crucial few seconds. Even the world's greatest marksman would have trouble trying to pull off such a skillful display and, in the Marines, Oswald was a mediocre shooter. Factor in the moving target and Oswald's unreliable bolt-action rifle, and the Warren Commission knew it had a problem that would become only too obvious to anyone who viewed the Zapruder film. Out of that dilemma came the revelation that Kennedy and Connally had both been hit by bullet number two—the single-bullet theory.

Although I had come to seriously discount that notion by this point, seeing the Zapruder film underlined its fantasy. If the same bullet struck both Kennedy and Connally, then why did the film show the president reacting to his injuries immediately upon impact but the governor taking approximately 1.5 seconds before he reacted to being hit? If a person is shot in the upper right back by a bullet that pierces a lung, breaks a rib, shatters the wrist bone, severs a nerve, and lodges in the thigh, he or she would have an instantaneous reaction. Yet, Connally did not. If Oswald fired from the depository, this bullet would have penetrated JFK's upper back and exited his neck, traveling from back to front, from right to left, and at a downward 17-degree angle. For this same bullet then to have struck Connally in the right part of his back behind his armpit, the bullet would have had to make a complete stop in midair for 1.6 seconds after exiting Kennedy's neck, taken an acute turn to the right for 18 inches, stopped again, and turned downward at an angle of 27-degrees before entering Connally's back behind the right armpit. Without this impossible turn, the bullet would most probably have passed over the governor's left shoulder. You do not have to be a forensic pathologist or a firearms expert to know that bullets travel in a straight line and do not make horizontal and vertical turns in midair like a roller coaster.

Furthermore, in frame 230 of the Zapruder film, Connally's right wrist and hand were clearly visible. Each finger was easily identifiable as he held his large white Stetson hat. However, the Warren Commission's reconstruction of the events stated that more than a second before this frame, the magic bullet had already shattered his wrist and severed the radial nerve. This is one of the nerves that enable the thumb and index finger to grasp objects. Yet in the film, he sat there with absolutely no evidence of pain on his face and his hand firmly gripping his hat. At the end of our screening, we spectators were unified in calling the single-bullet concept scientifically absurd. Arlen Specter's brainchild to try to promote a false scenario was not only implausible, but it was also insulting. This shameful lie demonstrated how far the federal government would go to make the facts fit the portrait it had painted. We told the people from *Life* that the government's position was outrageous. Then we thanked them for allowing us to view the footage and left the office.

We weren't sure what *Life* was going to do with our information but found out when the third anniversary issue hit the stands on November 25, 1966. Inside the issue was a photo of Connally at his home in Austin, bent over a photography light table and using a magnifying glass to inspect the stills that one of the editors had shown him. The magazine chose a cover that reflected the skepticism we had conveyed on our office visit, as well as the public distrust of the Warren Report. In the upper left-hand corner in a red rectangle was the magazine's title: *Life*. The rest of the background was black, with the following gold lettering in the center: "Did Oswald Act Alone?" A smaller font of white lettering read: "Amid controversy over the Warren Report Governor Connally examines for *Life* the Kennedy assassination film frame by frame." And in uppercase, large-font letters, the words: "A MATTER OF REASONABLE DOUBT." The color photo image was frame 230 from the Zapruder film, showing President Kennedy clutching at his throat area, Jackie looking at him, and Connally looking straight ahead and holding his Stetson hat.

The next year brought the release of Tink's book, *Six Seconds in Dallas: A Micro-Study of the Kennedy Assassination* (Bernard Geis Associates/Random House), for which I wrote an appendix. Tink's tome zeroes in on the critical timespan between the first and third shots. It also scrutinizes the mass of evidence (photos, physical evidence, witness interviews) accumulated by the FBI during its probe of the shooting and comes to conclusions diametrically opposed to those of the Warren Commission. Its reconstruction of what happened in Dealey Plaza has become the most plausible alternative to the official government scenario and served as a backbone for research for the House Select Committee on Assassinations.

Other early books worth reading include Harold Weisberg's *Whitewash: The Report on the Warren Report* (1966, Dell Publishing) and *Whitewash II: The FBI–Secret Service Coverup* (1967, Dell), Edward Jay Epstein's *Inquest: The Warren Commission and the Establishment of Truth* (1966, The Viking Press), Léo Sauvage's *The Oswald Affair: An Examination of the Contradictions and Omissions of the Warren Report* (1966, World Publishing Company), and Robert Sam Anson's *"They've Killed the President!": The Search for the Murderers of John F. Kennedy* (1975, Bantam Books). All justifiably became best sellers and whetted the American public's appetite for answers to this heart-wrenching mystery.

The Jack Ruby Enigma

On November 24, 1963, after Lee Harvey Oswald died at Parkland Hospital from a gunshot to the gut, the shooter, Jack Ruby, was charged with murder by Dallas sheriff's officers. Secret Service Agent Forrest Sorrels visited Ruby in his cell but was sent packing when local defense whiz Tom Howard arrived. Ruby told him the same story he would stick to for the rest of his life—that his act was impulsive and done to spare Mrs. Kennedy the pain of a trial.

Howard spent several hours with his client, then told the press that many people wrote letters of praise for Ruby's deed, adding his own view: "I commend what he did. I think he ought to win the Congressional Medal of Honor for it, and a lot of good American citizens think he did exactly the right thing in shooting down this communist." He added that any criticisms were from cranks with warped minds who wanted to keep Ruby from getting a fair trial. Despite Howard's valiant effort, he was soon fired after Ruby's brother, Earl, in Detroit persuaded another lawyer to take the case.

Ruby's next defense attorney was Melvin Belli, a 56-year-old legal eagle who was better known in civil court circles rather than criminal ones. He agreed to take Ruby's case pro bono, seeing as he was wealthy enough from representing movie stars, including Errol Flynn, Tony Curtis, and Lana Turner, plus mafia figures like Mickey Cohen. Belli earned the nickname "The King of Torts" after his mastery in personal injury cases brought him multi-million-dollar judgments. His office in San Francisco's Barbary Coast district was rumored to have been a Gold Rush–era bordello. A Jolly Roger would be hoisted on its roof, and a signal cannon would fire off two blasts whenever swashbuckling Belli celebrated a trial victory.

I experienced firsthand some of Belli's creative derring-do in the courtroom in the mid–1960s when he hired me as an expert witness in a couple of his medical malpractice cases. That was not a popular field at the time, with many attorneys refusing such cases because they feared going up against insurance companies. Not Belli, though. The first time I visited his scenic hilltop home, I noticed that the bathroom had a bidet, with a marble plaque over it. Its inscription was: *res ipsa loquitor*, which is Latin for "the thing speaks for itself." That's a doctrine of law that states that everything would have been fine if the defendant hadn't screwed up. For example, if a patient with an infected leg goes to a surgeon who amputates the wrong leg, the plaintiff's counsel would have the client show the still-infected leg—and his other, empty pant leg—to the jury. Thanks to that surgeon's error, the patient now has double his problem: *res ipsa loquitor. Ca-ching!* is the sound of the huge award the jury would find for the plaintiff. And double *ka-booms!* would be heard that evening on Belli's office roof.

Belli's advocacy was brainy and scientific yet somehow homespun. He knew how to push the boundaries for the jurors, re-creating graphic crime scenes and engineering mechanisms, and even introducing human skeletons, autopsy evidence, and photos of bloody victims. Today, those dramatic elements are a normal part of big-league trials, but in the old days, it was mind-blowing. I felt privileged to watch him work.

Belli was a larger-than-life character who married six times and divorced five times, and died of pancreatic cancer in 1996, at the age of 88. He was also an author and an actor in movies and on TV. It is said he earned $600 million from his legal career. But in 1995, after he represented 800 women in a successful landmark class-action lawsuit against breast implant manufacturer Dow Corning, the company filed for bankruptcy, necessitating Belli to do the same when he couldn't pay his expert witnesses. I was not one of his witnesses in that case, but had I been, I would have torn up my invoice if it would have helped him out.

The State of Texas vs. Jack Ruby would be heard by Judge Joe B. Brown for Criminal District Court Number 3. Dallas County District Attorney Henry Wade would be the chief prosecutor, aided by Assistant District Attorney Bill Alexander. Due to the global media interest, the proceedings would be held in a large, 194-seat courtroom. Next door, a second courtroom would serve as a pressroom, with scores of phone lines and teletype machines. An advertising agency worked with the judge on a pool system inside the main courtroom for media attendees, saving a few seats for the general public.

Bond hearings were heard in December 1963 and January 1964, but Ruby was denied bail, to no one's surprise and for his safety. Because Belli was not licensed to practice law in Texas, he brought in a local legal heavyweight. Joe Tonahill, 50, was one of the founders of the Texas Trial Lawyers Association and knew his way around both criminal and civil cases. He was popular with juries, other attorneys, and even opposing counsel. Attorney Phil Burleson was also onboard.

In February, Ruby's defense team argued that the trial needed to be moved out of Dallas County, which was too prejudicial toward their client. The judge not only turned them down but also scheduled the trial for the end of that month. The case would be tried as "murder with malice," with a possible penalty of death in the electric chair. Most criminal defendants enjoy getting a "speedy trial," which is one of the rights secured to them by the Sixth Amendment of the U.S. Constitution. Defendants often demand it in hopes they will get their matter before a jury before the prosecution has its side ready to go. But in this case, where Ruby had far more to gain by waiting until some of the dust settled, there was no reason to rush to trial. When I spoke about that to other lawyers and Kennedy assassination experts, we were in agreement that it was an odd and risky choice. Perhaps the thinking in Dallas was that the community needed to complete this task before it could begin to heal. There was a lot of animosity toward the Big D as the city that killed America's president.

Belli and Tonahill hired three noted psychiatrists to evaluate Ruby's mental state before determining a defense strategy. They decided that their client was legally insane, and when Ruby stepped into the police department basement, amidst the flashing lights from the reporters' cameras, it set off "psychomotor epilepsy" that resulted in his shooting Oswald. That was the defense they presented in the 23-day trial. The jury didn't buy it. Jurors deliberated only two hours and 20 minutes before Ruby was found guilty of murder with malice; on March 14, 1964, he was sentenced to death. Cameras were allowed in the courtroom to capture the verdict, with jury members unanimously raising their hands when asked by the judge if that was their decisions. The room exploded, with reporters pushing and jumping on top of the furniture to get better views.

News footage showed Ruby being ushered out of the courtroom as Belli yelled, "Don't worry, Jack. We'll appeal this and take it out of town." Then Belli addressed reporters. "I hope the people of Dallas are proud of this jury that was shoved down our throats," he snarled. "Every Texas jurist knows this thing was the greatest railroading kangaroo court disgrace in the history of American law. ... When I think we're coming into Holy Week and Good Friday, to have a sacrifice like this, I think we're back 2,000 years. And the blight that's on Dallas with those 12 people who announced the death penalty in this case—they'll make this a city of shame forevermore."

We armchair observers wondered whether the legal strategy was to blame. Was hiring a civil court pro like Belli a sound move when a hard-core criminal defense attorney might have fared better? And what if Belli had not presented the mental defense and instead argued that Ruby's patriotism and a rush of emotion had resulted in the lethal gunplay? Is it possible that such a plea, even from someone as resoundingly despised as Ruby was, might have brought a "murder without malice" conviction? That would be similar to manslaughter and would earn a maximum prison sentence of five years. We also questioned the wisdom of Ruby not taking the stand to testify in his own defense. But later, after I read his testimony to the Warren Commission, I realized that he would not have played well to the jury—as you will see.

Decades later, some of the jurors were interviewed by the Sixth Floor Museum's Oral History Project. Two said they preferred the prosecutor's style. "Henry Wade was just a rough old lawyer, tough, rough, and pretty proud of himself. ... He could chew Belli up in a minute," said one. Another added: "Henry Wade was very businesslike. He didn't fool around. He, as they say today, told it like it is. I had high regard for Henry Wade." The ad agency director who assisted the judge had a negative view of San Francisco's finest. "When Belli came in, he looked like he had got off a stagecoach because he had this red velvet briefcase," she sniped. "A carpetbagger, that's what he looked like. And then he had on this cape and it had some kind of a velvet collar, and I think it was lined with red, the cape. And it was just Dracula or something. It was very flamboyant. ... He was just full of himself." Apparently, she never heard that her homeboy Tonahill was pretty colorful himself, known for driving around in a red Lamborghini truck worth about $100,000.

After Ruby's conviction, Belli turned the case over to appellate ace Sam Houston Clinton, Jr. Staying on were Tonahill and Burleson, who were joined by local counsel Emmett C. Colvin, Jr. New to the team were noted defense attorneys Sol Dann of Detroit, William M. Kunstler of New York City, and Elmer Gertz of Chicago. A motion to the Texas Court of Criminal Appeals was filed immediately. You can learn Belli's views of the case in a book he wrote with Maurice C. Carroll, *Dallas Justice: The Real Story of Jack Ruby and His Trial* (David McKay Publications, 1964).

On June 7, 1964, members of the Warren Commission and staff traveled to the Dallas County Jail to question Ruby. It was probably the most memorable interview any of them would conduct. Chief Justice Earl Warren was the main interrogator, with Rep. Gerald Ford backing him up. General Counsel J. Lee Rankin was present, along with assistant counsels Joseph A. Ball and Arlen Specter. U.S. Secret Service agent Elmer W. Moore was there, along with Leon Jaworski and Robert Storey of the Texas attorney general's office, local assistant district attorney Jim Bowie, and Dallas Sheriff J.E. Decker. Tonahill was on hand as Ruby's counsel, and there also was a court reporter.

From the moment the three-hour procedure began, Ruby was talkative and in charge. Even before he was sworn in, he started asking for a lie detector test and/ or truth serum, so the panel would know what he was going to tell them was accurate. Warren assured him that such a test could and would be arranged, but they weren't prepared for it now. The current session would just be him answering some questions. Ruby replied with a monologue of how Belli didn't really know him and wouldn't let him talk at trial, and how he was in his predicament because he got carried away emotionally and had a spotty background in the nightclub business. Then he asked the flummoxed jurist: "Am I boring you?" After finally being sworn in, Ruby began another long monologue about events the night before the assassination: his buying ads at the newspaper and awareness of the parade the next day. Over the course of his testimony, Ruby referred to Kennedy eight times as "our beloved president." Continuing on to hearing the news about JFK's shooting, he discussed crying as he made phone calls to family and friends, visiting his sister and rabbi, deciding to close his club through the weekend but being angry that other clubs would stay open, and seeing Oswald at the police department only three feet away from where he was standing as he delivered his sandwiches.

The first chance for Warren to speak was when Ruby asked: "Is there any way to get me to Washington?" He said he needed to go there to take the lie detector test, which his attorney refused to allow. Warren informed him that Tonahill had indeed indicated Ruby's willingness to take a test in a letter two months before, but that the panel decided it could happen at a later time. For now, it just wanted to get Ruby's statements on record. That begat another monologue where the Texas tornado described his friends at radio station KLIF, the Bernard Weissman ad that made Jews look bad, and a cop who dated one of his dancers. Ruby asked Warren if he was sounding "dramatic" or "off the beam," to which the chief justice said no, praising him on his good recall. Then Ruby made another pitch to go to Washington and indicated that his lawyer was a liar who thought he acted with premeditation when he shot Oswald. He produced a letter Joe Tonahill wrote and struggled to read it, prompting Warren to take the eyeglasses off his own face and hand them to Ruby. Nothing in the letter proved Ruby's claim about his lawyer, but Ruby wasn't listening to reason. He then became angry at the Commission for not questioning him before his trial, causing Warren to tell him that they didn't want to prejudice matters and had no ulterior motives.

Another monologue followed, with Ruby talking about his love for JFK and ending with having Tonahill and the sheriff tossed from the room. Ruby told Warren that both of their lives were in danger in Dallas and they should go to Washington. Ruby hinted that he might not live another day to give further testimony and that he needed to reveal "the truth of everything and why my act was committed, but it can't be said here." He had to talk to people "of the highest authority" who would give him the benefit of doubt, followed by a polygraph test. Ruby never gave specifics about what information he had. Warren explained that neither he nor his Washington-based colleagues were law officers who could protect Ruby on such a trip. When the nightclub denizen said his information was "too tragic to talk about," Warren countered that the panel took Mrs. Kennedy's testimony two days' prior, inferring that if anyone had known tragedy, it was she and she still spoke to them.

Ruby now went into overdrive, talking about Chicago, the Jews, and his great sympathy for Mrs. Kennedy. He also mentioned that his family was in danger from the John Birch Society and General Edwin Walker, and that he was set off by seeing the Sunday newspaper mentions of Jackie and Caroline. In response to questions, he replied that he didn't know Oswald or J.D. Tippit and said he wasn't a criminal, gangster, goon, or communist; had never been in jail; and wasn't at Parkland after JFK's shooting. Near the end of the session, Ruby stated: "You can get more out of me. Let's not break up too soon." But with Warren's promise that Ruby would get the chance to be polygraphed, the testimony was complete. Warren had remarked that he was due back on the Supreme Court the next day, and I will guess that once he and the others got onboard the plane eastward, they ordered tall, stiff drinks. Not mentioned in the record was whether the chief justice reclaimed his reading glasses.

On July 18, almost six weeks after Ruby's testimony with Warren, some members of the Commission and others held a second session at the Dallas County jail. This time Ruby would get his wish for a polygraph test. Warren stayed away, so Specter led the proceeding. Joe Tonahill and Clayton Fowler were there as counsel for Ruby, while a local psychiatrist observed. A Dallas assistant district attorney, Bill Alexander, and the county's chief criminal deputy were also present, along with two FBI agents who were both polygraph operators, and a court reporter.

Before Ruby entered the room, Specter established the ground rules. As is typical, all polygraph questions would be discussed with the subject prior to hooking him up and getting his "yes" or "no" answers on the record. Control questions of a general nature would also be asked amidst the more pointed questions, in order to measure physiological differences. There would be a series of questions, with breaks in-between. During the pauses, the entire group could be present, but once the polygraph portions began, only Ruby, Specter, the two operators, and the court reporter would remain. Ruby would sit facing the wall to minimize distractions. Tonahill stated for the record that when he and Belli entered the case in December 1963, they insisted Ruby take a polygraph examination to see if there was a connection between him and Oswald or if there had been a conspiracy. Ruby had denied both premises and was eager to take any test. Tonahill explained that he made numerous requests to the FBI to conduct the procedure, but one never occurred, causing Ruby to physically lash out at him. Ruby's psychiatric team had unanimously told the lawyer any results might be faulty since Ruby was not of sound mind, didn't know right from wrong, and was an emotional wreck. But Tonahill reasoned that, given Ruby's agitated state, he might actually suffer mentally without the test. And he added, if convicted, an appellate court might overturn the verdict because of Ruby's willingness to undergo the exam. Such musings didn't seem to impress Specter who simply replied that the test was Ruby's idea, not the Commission's—and with that, the game was afoot. When Ruby entered the room, he alluded to the brawl he had had with Tonahill where the lawyer's pants were torn, and his leg was injured. Then Ruby politely asked the attorney to leave the room and requested that the prosecutor stay. Tonahill remarked: "Let the record show that Mr. Ruby says he prefers Bill Alexander being here during this investigation, who is the assistant district attorney who asked that a jury give him the death sentence, to myself, who asked the jury to acquit him, his attorney."

Ruby advised those in the room that he wanted the results of his test to be released to the public as soon as possible. He was then sworn in by Specter and averred that he was in fine health and on no medications. The polygraph operator described the process to him. As the FBI agent put the Galvanic Skin Response monitor on Ruby's fingers, he noticed a finger was missing; Ruby told him he had lost it in an altercation at his club. A standard blood pressure cuff was hooked to Ruby's upper arm to chronicle changes in his blood pressure, heartbeat, and pulse rate. And a rubber tube was placed around his chest to monitor his breathing pattern. The procedure lasted nine hours, with 13 series of questions asked on the polygraph. There were no changes in any of the statements Ruby had previously given, except he did admit to having served 30 days in jail long ago for selling copyrighted songs, but said it was not a felony conviction. He stated "no" when asked the very general questions of whether he had labor union or underworld influence or was induced by anyone to carry out the shooting of Oswald. He answered "yes" when asked if he considered himself a "100% American patriot" and whether he had told the complete truth. No bombshells, no surprises. It's fair to say the exercise was a waste of time for everyone in the room, except for Ruby who got his wish, courtesy of the absentee Warren.

The fact that Ruby gave testimony while hooked to a polygraph machine made the news, although the results were not revealed. I wondered why his attorneys had allowed him to take the test but didn't understand that it was Ruby's demand until I read a brief description of the test in the initial Warren Commission Report. The full transcript of the proceedings appeared in the 26 volumes. The final paragraph in the initial report read: "Having granted Ruby's request for the examination, the Commission is publishing the transcript of the hearing at which the test was conducted and the transcript of the deposition of the FBI polygraph operator who administered the test. The Commission did not rely on the results of this examination in reaching the conclusions stated in this report." It wasn't a matter of whether or not Ruby passed his polygraph test. The Warren Commission published all of the testimony without taking a stand on its veracity.

After Ruby returned to his cell, one last person gave testimony to Specter at the request of Ruby's two attorneys. William Robert Beavers was the psychiatrist who had observed Ruby's question preparations and had previously met with the inmate some nine or 10 times since his incarceration. Beavers was a staff psychiatrist at Parkland Hospital; an assistant professor of psychiatry at the University of Texas Southwestern Medical School; a consultant at the state mental hospital; and a member of the appropriate local, state, and national associations. Beavers stated that when he first met with Ruby, the inmate was in a psychotic depression, with auditory hallucinations and delusions. Ruby said that due to his crime, his family was being abused, and Jews were being massacred. The psychiatrist testified that he had observed, and been told by the jailer, that sometimes Ruby wanted to seem delusional, but if called on it, he'd get angry. Ruby's polygraph session proved that he understood the questions and answered them appropriately, with a sharp memory, said Beavers. He added that the polygraph session was probably a good idea for placating Ruby, although it might not have any actual value to investigators.

Tonahill was allowed to question Dr. Beavers and wanted to know why Ruby seemed to despise him while favoring the prosecutor who wanted him to be executed. The doctor surmised that was because the defense attorney had a mandate to delve into the possibility of Ruby being part of a conspiracy, whereas the prosecutor never opened that door. But Beavers suggested that unpredictability was part of Ruby's mental condition and shouldn't be taken in a personal way. Tonahill pointed out that Ruby had exhibited suicidal behavior, including ramming his head into his cell wall and trying to push a finger into an electric socket, but Beavers stated that was all part of the disease.

Beavers stated that he was one of five forensic psychiatrists who examined Ruby post-conviction, in anticipation of the appellate court granting him a new trial. All five doctors—Beavers, John T. Holbrook, Robert Stubblefield, Emanuel "Emek" Tanay, and Louis Jolyon "Jolly" West—agreed that the inmate would benefit from a sentence served in a mental institution where he could get care and medication, rather than in a prison, facing the death penalty. Of the five, only Beavers gave testimony to the Warren Commission. Of these doctors, the only one I would come to know in future years was Tanay, who would be an expert witness on numerous well-publicized cases, including kidnapped heiress-turned-revolutionary Patty Hearst, child slayer Andrea Yates, serial killer Ted Bundy, and others. We both worked on the defense of Sam Sheppard, the physician charged with murdering his wife, and I found Tanay to be a compassionate psychiatrist. He was well-regarded in his field, was a Distinguished Fellow of the American Academy of Forensic Sciences, and spent considerable time helping veterans in his hometown area of Detroit. He was also a Polish Holocaust survivor who supported Jewish causes. He died of cancer in August 2014 at the age of 86.

West's successes as a pioneering forensic psychiatrist were blemished by controversy. According to a statement by Alan Adelson, an attorney representing Earl Ruby, West was the last psychiatrist to have examined Jack Ruby. Adelson brought him in after Ruby's conviction in preparation for the appellate ruling. Adelson and West had extensive conversations in Detroit and Dallas, and West also testified during a probate court hearing over the disposition of Jack Ruby's will. In interviews with West, Ruby supposedly told the doctor that he was surprised his brother Earl was still alive because he thought he would have been annihilated during the Holocaust.

Prior to West's work as a university professor and his private practice, he served in the USAF Medical Corps, studying brainwashing, false confessions, sleep deprivation, and torture techniques used by our wartime enemies upon our enlisted personnel and pilots. In the early 1970s, he would advocate opening a center at the University of California at Los Angeles to study "interpersonal violence," which included surgical implanting of brain electrodes to affect personality. Notwithstanding fervent support from then–California Governor Ronald Reagan, there was massive public protest, and West's program was cancelled. For decades, from the 1950s forward, the psychiatrist also allegedly had a long-standing contract with the CIA and held a top-secret clearance. Working on a series of "off the books" operations, West devised sinister experiments that included LSD and other psychoactive drugs, biological warfare, mind control, hypnosis, hallucinations, dissociation, and suggestibility, often on unsuspecting patients. The administrators of these programs were assisted by the military, major academic institutes, and the pharmaceutical industry. And, significantly, the work was done with the knowledge and encouragement of the CIA, including Allen Dulles when he was director and Richard Helms, who was the deputy director of the agency's clandestine division and, later, was promoted to CIA director.

At an appellate hearing before Judge Louis Holland on September 9, 1965, Ruby was flanked by his attorneys Sol Dann and Elmer Gertz. A brief YouTube search will show a clip where, despite his counsels' attempts to silence him, Ruby insisted on speaking to the media in the room. "I know what I'm doing," he snarled, then continued: "The Warren Report never gave me the true authenticity. When I requested a polygraph test, there was a little, small article, in small type, that stated 'Due to the fact that Mr. Ruby's—we cannot divulge the results of it.' Why they held back the answers and give the results, whether they're true or false, that's for you to find out." Ruby turned to Dann and said, "Sol, I insist on getting this out. Will you let me please do this? I want to get this out, please." Then he continued to a reporter: "They never released the results of my polygraph test. That was deleted from the Warren Report. Why was that deleted? I don't know why. I insisted on the polygraph right from the beginning. As a matter of fact, certain questions I created and originated, that they would ask me at the time. They spent nine hours with me at the time, and yet the finality—the finality of the results of the test, they stated, they refused to divulge the answers that I had given, whether true or false, due to my mental condition."

In a second short film clip from the same court hearing, Ruby added: "The world will never know the true facts of what occurred, my motives. The people had—that had so much to gain and had such an ulterior motive for putting me in the position I'm in—will never let the true facts come aboveboard to the world." A reporter asked: "Are these people in very high positions, Jack?" and Ruby answered: "Yes." The footage then showed Ruby leaving the courtroom and walking in the hallway. To a reporter, he stated: "I want to correct what I said before about the vice president. ... When I mentioned about Adlai Stevenson, if he was vice president there would never had been an assassination of our beloved President Kennedy." The newsman replied: "Would you explain again?" And Ruby answered: "Well, the answer is the man in office now."

We can only surmise what Ruby meant when he said them. We can proffer that his reference to the "man in office now" is about President Johnson and that Ruby is inferring that if Stevenson, and not Johnson, had been Kennedy's vice president, there would not have been an assassination. But there's no way to fill in the blanks to form a coherent theory on Ruby's part. In Ruby's testimony to the Warren Commission, he claimed that right-wing forces, from the John Birch Society to General Edwin Walker, were a threat to his family's safety—but he didn't elaborate, and no one on the panel asked him for an explanation.

On October 5, 1966, in a unanimous opinion, the Texas Court of Criminal Appeals ruled that Judge Joe Brown had deprived Ruby of a fair trial. Presiding Judge William Arthur Morrison wrote: "It is clear from a careful study of ... the record of this case that the trial court reversibly erred in refusing appellant's motion for the change of venue." The appellate court also pointed out discrepancies in the trial testimony of Dallas police Sergeant Patrick T. Dean, one of the jail officers assigned to guard Ruby, who was in solitary confinement. Dean said that right after the arrest,

Ruby told Secret Service agent Forrest Sorrels that he decided to kill Oswald on the night of the assassination when he first spotted him, which would have indicated premeditation. But Sorrels testified that Ruby never made such an admission. Dean also told the court that, some 40 minutes later, Ruby commented that he shot Oswald to prove that "Jews had guts." Although that utterance might have again proved premeditation, the appellate panel found that it should not have been admitted in trial because it was not a spontaneous statement, which allows for comments made very close in time to a defendant's arrest.

A new trial was set for February 1967 in Wichita Falls, a city approximately 140 miles northwest of Dallas. But the defendant wouldn't make it to his retrial. On December 9, 1966, Ruby was admitted to Parkland Hospital with pneumonia. Tests came back the next day showing he had cancer in his lungs, liver, and brain. He never left the hospital and died on January 3, 1967, taking his secrets with him. He was 55 years old. On his deathbed, Ruby gave one last taped interview to his attorney Elmer Gertz, while his brother Earl observed. If the men hoped to get Ruby to make any changes to what he had insisted on the record over the years, they would be disappointed. The gunman again stated that he walked down the police station ramp without incident and that everything was "in such a blur" until the officers wrestled him to the ground. He denied knowing Oswald or being aware that he was to be moved through the basement at that time, and that he only shot him because he had been emotionally upset since JFK died. The only new thing that Ruby added to the conversation was that he had a sore rectum.

I've been asked many times whether I believe Ruby was injected with some sort of "fast-acting cancer-causing drug," or cancer cells themselves, by people who wanted to silence him permanently. My answer has always been the same: *Not a chance*. First, I have never heard of a fast-acting, cancer-causing drug. Perhaps some evil genius has created a potion, but in the more than 60,000 death cases I've investigated, I've never encountered any such substance. But even back in 1963, if there were a researcher with knowledge and experience in biomedical weaponry, and who had access to Ruby, would any possible gain from dosing and killing him be worth the risk of being caught in the act?

Second, Ruby's primary cancer was in his lungs and spread outward to his organs. At autopsy, Ruby's brain, alone, had 15 tumors. All of that takes an amount of time to manifest and could mean he didn't have regular doctor visits when the symptoms first arose. Whether that was before JFK's assassination or during his time in jail, I can't say—but no doctor testified or was mentioned as having treated him for anything prior to his hospitalization.

Third, although Ruby was not a smoker, he spent a lot of time in his nightclubs during a time when people smoked like chimneys. Ruby's lung cancer might well have been from secondhand smoke. Of course, sometimes people who are nonsmokers and never around smokers develop and die of lung cancer. It's a pernicious disease.

Fourth, no one needed to stop Ruby from talking because he had no intention of doing so. Ruby's overweening desire was to control the spotlight that was on him, while making sure it did not shine on anything he wanted to keep in the dark. He got into his mind that he could pass any polygraph test and likely expected that would affect the way the public, and hopefully a new jury, would see him. Whether that was arrogance or ignorance, or both, I don't know. But it actually worked, to a degree.

What would have happened if Ruby had gotten a new trial? Would his new lawyers have proffered the mental defense, as Belli had? The first jury didn't accept it, but a second jury might have. The unanimous opinion of Ruby's psychiatrists indicated that his emotional and mental acuity went downhill during the time he was incarcerated, and these five doctors were prepared to testify to that. As before, if Ruby were incapable of making cogent points in front of a jury, it would not be in his best interest to put him on the stand. Therefore, arguing that he was mentally ill and stating that he reacted impulsively when he shot Oswald would probably have been the wise course for his legal team. Ruby seemed to bristle at suggestions that he had a mental illness yet was capable of playing that up when it served him. If his first conviction and death sentence had been upheld, or if his second trial were to end with the same results, there would be fireworks as his execution date approached. There is always a debate when a condemned killer with a low I.Q. or mental defect faces execution, and, due to the notoriety of Ruby's case, there would have been protestors around the world. Would such a legal and public outcry have stopped his date with destiny?

Despite attempts to link Ruby and Oswald before November 24, no concrete evidence was produced that could help either side at trial. That's not to say it couldn't have been developed, had the Warren Commission dug in to get to the bottom of such rumors, instead of issuing a cursory query that turned up nothing. For a panel whose chief interest was in shutting off avenues that could reveal a conspiracy, they put little effort into trying to connect the two men. It's entirely possible there was no relationship between Ruby and Oswald prior to their fatal meeting in the police basement. Whether Ruby was working on his own or at the behest of someone pulling his strings, knowing Oswald was not a requirement.

I have often thought about what might have inspired Ruby to shoot Oswald. With all of his police connections, he could have learned about the scheduled date and time to move Oswald into the basement. And from the cops' point of view, seeing Ruby there among the press reporters wouldn't have been unusual. With that backdrop, Ruby would have been the ideal person to commit a hit on the inmate, if that's what happened. But what might have provoked him to do it?

As he testified to the Warren Commissioners, Ruby was having money woes. He owed thousands of dollars in back taxes to the Internal Revenue Service, had recently borrowed money from a friend to make payroll, and had told another pal he needed money to open a new cabaret. Bad finances are a frequent motivator for criminal activity. What if someone came to Ruby with the order to commit the murder, in exchange for money or some sort of compensation? Since there was no way for Ruby to shoot Oswald and escape, Ruby would have known he'd be arrested and tried. But he might have been assured that, if convicted, the combination of his legal all-stars and precarious mental state would net him a brief jail term. He would then be released, with a pot of gold waiting and a new life ahead. Or, just as easily, he could have been threatened to kill Oswald or be killed himself. Ruby complained about his family's safety, attributing threats that were made to him by right-wing forces. Maybe there were threats, but maybe they didn't come from any political extremists.

Any amateur detective might have wondered, "Gee, could the Mafia have steered Ruby's actions?" Was Ruby talking about underworld crime figures when he referred to "the people with the ulterior motive for putting me in the position I'm in"? Apparently, the Warren investigators weren't that inquisitive. Ruby testified that he had no organized crime connections, and the Commissioners signed off on his response, just like that! The members knew Ruby's background, which was rife with shady alliances that were worth exploring. His Chicago hometown was where he first became acquainted with gangsters and illegal gambling. In the 1960s, that city's mob boss was Sam Giancana, some of whose men sponsored Ruby's move to Dallas and entrée into the nightclub business—an enterprise that operates primarily on a cash basis, with the potential for profit skimming and kickbacks. A few years before Kennedy's death, Ruby admitted going to Havana, Cuba, where he visited a pal who ran a casino owned by Santo Trafficante, Jr., the Mafia chieftain from Tampa, Florida. There were alleged sightings of Ruby with New Orleans crime boss Carlos Marcello, among others. Each of these Mafia dons had great animus toward JFK and might have benefited from his death, along with that of Oswald. Yet, the mighty Warren Commission dropped the ball when it decided not to use its vast subpoena power, and unlimited time and resources, to probe possible affiliations between Ruby and the Mafia.

Could such chicanery have been a directive from FBI Director J. Edgar Hoover, who barely recognized the Mafia's existence, lest it disturb his fun at the mob-run racetracks and casinos he frequented? Hoover was getting regular updates from his deputy director, Deke DeLoach, who was the Commission liaison and likely listened in to all of the testimony as it was piped into his office at FBI headquarters. It's clear to me that the motivation behind Ruby's murderous deed was not properly researched by Warren and his boys. There would be other investigations down the line that would bring Ruby's connections into better focus. But even still, and to this day, Jack Ruby remains an enigma.

Assassination Nation

After JFK's assassination, President Johnson expanded upon programs established by his predecessor from civil rights to space exploration, but the next few years were brutal for him. Health crises took their toll, including a weak heart and surgeries to remove a kidney stone and his gallbladder. And with some 70,000 Americans killed or wounded in Vietnam and public sentiment turning against the war, Johnson announced in March 1968 that he would not serve another term as president. He retired to his Texas ranch where he died at age 64 on January 22, 1973. He and his wife, Lady Bird, who died in 2007, are buried in the Johnson Family Cemetery in Stonewall, Texas. Richard Nixon won the election to replace Johnson, with Maryland Governor Spiro T. Agnew as his vice president. The Republican takeover in 1969 wasn't a smooth transition. Agnew's views on policy matters rankled Nixon, and charges surfaced that the vice president had issues of financial chicanery and tax evasion. As Nixon was gearing up to run for reelection in 1972, he considered replacing Agnew with John Connally, now treasury secretary, but Nixon stuck with his veep, and they beat their Democratic challengers. In 1973, Agnew accepted a plea bargain to avoid jail time and, on October 9, resigned from office. On December 6, Nixon appointed his new vice president: the House minority leader and congressman from Michigan, Gerald Ford, who had served on the Warren Commission.

The Vietnam War continued until 1975, but the '70s were also rife with domestic turbulence. On June 18, 1972, five men were arrested for breaking into the Democratic National Committee headquarters at the Watergate Office Building in Washington, D.C. For the next several months, the mind-boggling investigation into the men's ties to the Nixon administration unfolded, culminating in televised hearings before the U.S. Senate. The public learned that President Nixon had approved plans to pay for and cover up the burglars' activities, and the House of Representatives began an impeachment process against Nixon for obstruction of justice, abuse of power, and contempt of Congress. The scandal resulted in the indictments of 69 individuals, with 48 convictions, including top administration officials. Among those who received prison sentences were ex–FBI agent G. Gordon Liddy and former CIA officer E. Howard Hunt, who had recruited some of the burglars from secret anti–Castro operations he had conducted. Before the impeachment came up for a vote from the full House, and because it was believed there were enough votes in the Senate to

convict, Nixon resigned from office on August 9, 1974. Congress dropped the proceedings, and Vice President Gerald Ford was sworn in as president. In a controversial move weeks later, Ford pardoned Nixon. Our government is built upon enduring
friendships, with the players protecting and rewarding each other.

In addition to President Kennedy's slaying in November 1963 and that of civil
rights activist Medgar Evers the previous June, the 1960s brought two other political assassinations in America. The Rev. Martin Luther King, Jr., was 39 when he was
shot to death on the balcony of the Lorraine Motel in Memphis, Tennessee, on April
4, 1968. A Baptist minister, King was a founder of the Southern Christian Leadership
Conference and led nonviolent protests against segregation in Georgia and Alabama.
King attained a B.A. degree from Morehouse College, a B.D. from Crozer Theolog-
ical Seminary, and a Ph.D. from Boston University. He helped organize the 1963
March on Washington and the next year received the Nobel Peace Prize. His continued efforts to end racial inequality, separated housing, and poverty, as well as his protests against the Vietnam War, made him a target of FBI Director J. Edgar Hoover,
who went after him with the kind of alacrity the top G-man never mustered against
mafiosi.

King had been the victim of a previous assassination attempt on September 20,
1958, by a 42-year-old black woman named Izola Curry. Convinced that King was
spying on her, Curry went to a Harlem bookstore where the minister was signing
his first book. She waited in line until she got close to King, then shouted, "Why do
you annoy me?" and plunged a seven-inch-long metal letter opener into his sternum. As she was arrested, a loaded pistol was found in her bra. King was rushed to
the hospital, and surgeons later told him the blade was so close to his aorta that if he
had sneezed or if anyone at the bookstore had pulled out the weapon, he would have
bled to death. After a five-week convalescence, he got back to business. Curry was
ruled schizophrenic and committed to a mental institution for most of the rest of her
life.

King's alleged shooter was an ex-con named James Earl Ray, who had served
time at Leavenworth Federal Penitentiary and Missouri State Penitentiary for
assorted burglaries and robberies. He escaped from the latter prison and traveled
throughout the states, Canada, and Mexico, using false IDs and driving a 1966 Ford
Mustang he had purchased. The month before King's shooting, Ray had gotten elec-
tive rhinoplasty, and one might well query how someone unemployed could afford
the surgical procedure, not to mention the car and extensive travel. Ray hated blacks
and, in 1968, supported former Alabama governor George Wallace's campaign for
president. Wallace was a famous segregationist. After King's murder, Ray fled to Canada, then to the United Kingdom, with plans to go to the white separatist nation
of Zimbabwe in Africa. He was caught in London with two phony IDs and extra-
dited to the United States. In the run-up to his trial for King's murder, he confessed
to avoid the death penalty and was given a 99-year sentence. Later, he recanted,
to no avail. In 1977, Ray and six other inmates of Tennessee's Brushy Mountain

Penitentiary escaped for three days but were returned to prison and given longer sentences.

There have been questions about whether Ray's involvement was part of a government conspiracy. Ballistic tests on his gun proved an inconclusive link to King's murder. I spent some time advising his final counsel, Dr. William Pepper, on the medical evidence. Pepper, a New York City attorney with an active interest in exposing governmental duplicity, believed that Ray was framed by factions within the FBI, CIA, Memphis police, and organized crime. To commemorate the 25th anniversary of King's death, Pepper represented Ray in a 1993 mock trial that aired on HBO. The 10-day unscripted procedure was taped in Memphis before an actual judge, with real lawyers and experts, then edited for broadcast. Ray testified from prison via satellite, stating that a mysterious gunman named "Raoul" manipulated him to take the blame. An out-of-town jury acquitted Ray. Although the event bore no legal weight, Ray expressed gratitude and hope that it would reopen his case. Pepper claimed that King's true assassin was a racist named Loyd Jowers who owned a restaurant near the motel.

Ray died at a hospital in Nashville on April 23, 1998, at the age of 70. Bill Pepper asked me to attend the autopsy, so I participated in the procedure with the Tennessee State medical examiner, Bruce Levy. My finding was that the death was not suspicious; Ray simply died of kidney disease and liver failure, exacerbated by hepatitis C. He would have been a good candidate for a liver transplant, which would have increased his lifespan, but the prison wouldn't allow a furlough for an operation. Up until his last breath, Ray wanted to withdraw his guilty plea and face trial for King's murder. After Ray's death, Pepper represented the King family in a wrongful death action against Jowers and unnamed co-conspirators. Jowers denied shooting King, blaming a police officer and stating that Ray was merely a scapegoat. A jury found Jowers legally liable, and the Kings were awarded the nominal sum of $100, which was all they had asked for. Jowers' story changed over the years, and in 2000, he died of a heart attack, at the age of 73.

On June 5, 1968, President Kennedy's younger brother, Robert F. Kennedy, was gunned down at the Ambassador Hotel in Los Angeles. At the time, Bobby was New York's junior senator and running for president of the United States on the Democratic ticket. Bobby had just won a major primary election in California. He was in a tight race against Minnesota senator Eugene McCarthy and Vice President Hubert Humphrey. Earlier in Bobby's career, including when he was his brother's U.S. attorney general, he was more conservative, but after JFK's death, Bobby saw that the country was slanting leftward. JFK's issue of civil rights was even more important to Bobby, and he became opposed to the war in Vietnam. In what would be his last interview—two hours before he was shot—Bobby announced to NBC News' Sander Vanocur his intention to withdraw troops from South Vietnam if elected to the presidency: "We've had more Americans killed there in the last several weeks than any time during the war.... Six months ago, we were talking about bombing Hanoi, and we're concerned about that because we're going to kill civilians. Now we're killing large numbers of them as we bomb Saigon," he said, adding, "I just think that we just have to change our policies."

Savoring his victory and more determined than ever to capture his party's nomination, the 42-year-old Bobby took the Embassy Ballroom stage to thank his jubilant supporters, with his wife, Ethel, pregnant with the couple's 11th child, at his side. He ended his speech with "My thanks to all of you. And now it's on to Chicago and let's win there!" The crowd erupted with wild cheers of "We want Bobby!" Leaving the ballroom, Kennedy and his entourage went through the crowded kitchen pantry when a 24-year-old Palestinian Christian named Sirhan Bishara Sirhan stepped into his path. Sirhan had been born in Jordan but had emigrated to the United States with his parents and brothers when he was 12. He worked in the L.A. area as a stablehand at a racetrack. He raised his Iver-Johnson Cadet pistol and began firing until the weapon was wrestled from his hand. Five people were hit by bullets and survived. The senator was also shot and died in the hospital 26 hours later.

The following year, a trial was held for Sirhan, whose legal team presented a diminished capacity defense. Two months later, he was convicted and given the death penalty—a sentence that was later commuted to life in prison. Over the years, Sirhan Sirhan has been turned down for parole 15 times. Many people believe the case is and should remain closed. I strongly disagree.

The Los Angeles Police Department provided no security for Bobby that night, and, in fact, there was hostility toward him. In the immediate aftermath of the shooting, an audio recording captured a hotel switchboard operator calling the LAPD communications desk. The operator explained that police needed to come because there was some sort of an emergency. The officer asked for details, but the operator didn't have any. She mentioned: "We have Mr. Kennedy here tonight," to which the officer sneered, "Big deal." Sirhan's gun held eight bullets, all of which were expended in the melee. Bobby was shot by three .22 caliber bullets: one fatal head shot that shattered in his brain and two that went into his armpit and/or chest in an upward trajectory. A fourth shot went through his jacket. No footage or available photographs exist of the actual shooting inside the pantry, but dozens of witnesses told the same story: Bobby was shot as he walked toward Sirhan. Sirhan was between one and five feet to Bobby's left front. But the bullet that entered Bobby's brain was fired from about one inch behind his right ear. All of the other shots were also fired from behind RFK, at a distance of no more than six inches.

Los Angeles coroner Thomas Noguchi, whom I was with when we heard the news about JFK's slaying, performed the postmortem examination on Bobby. Aware of my work on the president's case and knowing this one would garner a lot of attention, he asked me to consult, along with a team of other experts. Days later I joined him in L.A. so we could review the forensic evidence and reenact the crime. Tom explained he performed the autopsy by starting at the senator's toes and moving upward, which is atypical from normal procedure. He did so to avoid being influenced by the head injury alone. He was under great pressure and felt it would help him take the time he needed to do a competent job.

Tom demonstrated to me that the two armpit shots were not round-shaped, because the bullets hit Bobby's body as it was falling. As he examined the corpse on the morgue table, Tom manipulated the arm 15 degrees forward to represent where it was when each bullet hit it. That proved the senator was turning slightly clockwise as he went down. The first shot was likely the fatal head shot, fired with a trajectory that was back to front, right to left, and upward. The arm movement might have been a reflexive attempt to protect himself but to no avail, of course. We discussed the need to evaluate the stippling, or gunpowder residue that forms a lasting pattern in the places a victim is shot and can determine the closeness of a gun when fired. I also suggested he consult with neurosurgeons familiar with head wounds. Noguchi's morgue assistants helped him with a reconstruction, using pig ears attached to a dummy's head. He covered the head with cloth to absorb gunpowder. Then, with a similar gun to the murder weapon, test firings were conducted to measure the tattooing found at the edge of RFK's right ear. At various distances, bullets were fired into the right mastoid, the bony protuberance behind the ear. The best replication came when the muzzle was three inches from the mastoid and an inch from the outer ear when the bullet was fired. That made for an exact duplicate of the actual death-shot powder tattoo. Tom also did infrared photography and X-rays of the bits of hair taken from around the wound. This determined the powder spread and confirmed the pig ear test.

Chronicling these findings with detailed notes, photographs, charts, and X-rays would ensure that the mistakes made at President Kennedy's autopsy and death investigation would not be repeated here. This would not be "another Dallas," we both pledged. Of course, no one from the federal government was present to commandeer the senator's body and fly it to a military facility. Under Tom's watchful eye, this procedure was thorough and a dazzling display of forensic science. Based on Tom's findings, there had to be a second shooter in that room.

Sirhan was not in position to have fired those four shots at Bobby, but someone else was. Thane Eugene "Gene" Cesar worked as a plumber in a classified section at defense contractor Lockheed and had previously been employed by Hughes Aircraft, which had documented ties to the CIA. At the Ambassador that night, he was moonlighting as a freelance security guard. As Cesar ushered Bobby through the pantry, he was behind Bobby's right side and touching the back of his right arm. A famous photo shows Bobby's lying on the floor in a pool of blood, with a man's tie next to him. That tie belonged to Cesar; Bobby grabbed it as he fell to the ground. Cesar was a supporter of segregationist George Wallace in the 1968 presidential race and made no bones about hating the Kennedys. He admitted drawing his pistol when Sirhan began shooting, but he claimed he put it away once he saw that Sirhan had been subdued. Much later, the LAPD would question Cesar, who claimed he carried a .38 gun that night but had also owned a .22 that he sold to a friend before the assassination.

That was proven false when the pal produced a receipt for the gun's sale, dated three months after Bobby's death. Ballistic testing could not be compared to bullets that struck the senator, however, because the friend said the gun had been stolen. Cesar was never charged with any crime in the case and went to his grave in September 2019 at the age of 77, denying any responsibility for Bobby's murder.

When Tom testified before the grand jury, he mentioned the "three-inch" distance between Bobby's right ear and the firearm. The district attorney said, "You mean three feet?" No, Tom said, inches. "If you made a mistake, you can still change it," suggested the attorney. "I'm not going to change it," replied the determined coroner. He laughed about it when he told me, but we both knew it wasn't a good sign. Tom also testified at Sirhan's trial, but the scope of his commentary was severely limited. When he tried to explain the trajectory and position of the headshot that killed RFK, the judge stopped him cold. Around this same time, law enforcement attempted to smear Tom's reputation, and he was fired from the coroner's office. But he was soon rehired after retaining a prominent lawyer who threatened to go public with the Kennedy case's dirty laundry. To this day, Tom disagrees with the official government view that Sirhan Sirhan fired the fatal shot that killed Robert F. Kennedy.

Over the years I have made countless trips to Los Angeles, often at the invitation of news media programs that covered the case before the Ambassador Hotel was razed in 2005. Many times, I've walked the course that Bobby took that fateful night, and I interviewed assistant maitre d' Karl Uecker, who was holding Bobby's right wrist as they navigated the pantry. Uecker was slightly ahead of and to the right of Bobby and directly ahead of Cesar. Uecker observed Sirhan standing to Bobby's left front and thought he must be a busboy. When Sirhan began firing, Uecker pushed the gun up and away from Bobby. As Uecker and others restrained Sirhan, he glimpsed Cesar with his gun drawn, but Uecker was not questioned about this at the grand jury proceedings or at Sirhan's trial.

In 1975, Uecker wrote this statement of his observations and actions that night: "There was a distance of at least one-and-one-half feet between the muzzle of Sirhan's gun and Senator Kennedy's head. The revolver was directly in front of my nose. After Sirhan's second shot, I pushed the hand that held the revolver down, and pushed him onto the steam table. There is no way that the shots described in the autopsy could have come from Sirhan's gun. When I told this to the authorities, they told me that I was wrong. But I repeat now what I told them then: Sirhan never got close enough for a point-blank shot." This comports with what Uecker privately told me.

Cesar was not called to testify before the grand jury or at Sirhan's trial. Also not called as a trial witness was Donald Schulman, an employee of KNX-TV, the CBS affiliate, who told police he saw Cesar fire his gun while standing behind Bobby.

LAPD ballistics experts collected bullet fragments from the people who were hit and the ceiling tiles and door panels. They concluded all the damage was done from Sirhan's eight bullets. But the FBI entered the case and conducted its own bullet count, finding as many as 13 bullets were shot. Later, sophisticated acoustics testing confirmed 13 distinct shots could be heard. Thirteen bullets means five more than Sirhan's gun could hold, and we know he never reloaded his weapon. The proof is solid that there was more than one shooter, which means there was a conspiracy.

In the fall of 1968, I was surprised to receive a phone call at home from Sirhan's mother, Mary, whom I had never met or spoken with before. She saw some interviews I had given stating that her son could not have killed Bobby and begged me to sign on as his attorney, but I had to decline. Although I am an attorney, I wasn't prepared to drop my main career as a medical examiner to devote the time necessary to serve as Sirhan's counsel. Sigrid had given birth to our fourth child in June 1968, and with our eldest only six years old, she needed me to stay in Pittsburgh and not be in Los Angeles for months on end, no matter how tantalizing the offer.

Sirhan had confessed to police, but the trial judge did not accept that or allow him to plead guilty and be executed, as he had requested. His murder trial began on February 12, 1969, with prosecutors showing exhibits of Sirhan's handwritten journal that seemed to indicate proof of premeditation. There were multiple pages of what appeared to be automatic writing, phrases repeated again and again, such as "RFK must be assassinated," "RFK must die," "Pay to the order of…," "Who killed Kennedy? I don't know, I don't know, I don't know," "Today I must plan to come home in a new Mustang," and "Practice practice practice practice mind control mind control mind control mind control." Neither side argued that this very odd, repetitive handwriting was not Sirhan's or that someone copied his penmanship to make him look bad. The prosecution simply viewed the passages as proof of willful intent, and the defense saw them as the sad writings of someone mentally ill. Talk about missing the boat! Not one of the lawyers looked at those statements and wondered, "What the hell is this about? What is the state of mind of someone who would write these sentences?"

This subject was broached in Robert Blair Kaiser's compelling book *R.F.K. Must Die!* (the hardback edition was by Penguin-Putnam, 1970, with the subsequent paperback by Grove). A journalist who was assisting Sirhan's defense team and spent almost 200 hours interviewing the defendant, Kaiser realized the journal pages were a bombshell view into Sirhan's psyche. Sirhan's defense counsel attempted to convince the jury that the defendant killed Bobby impulsively and had a mental deficiency. They were different lawyers than the ones who had attempted that with Jack Ruby, but the results were equally futile. Unlike Ruby, however, Sirhan was allowed to take the stand in his own defense and nailed his own coffin shut with statements touting his guilt and premeditation.

Bobby's autopsy report was not shared with Sirhan's lawyers until they had already committed to a mental incapacity defense for him. When such a stunt happens, it's called "sandbagging," as it tries to win a legal argument via an unfair and unethical advantage. Not only is that frowned upon at the moment it happens, but it's also often cited when an appellate court is asked to overturn a conviction. Among we experts who followed the case from afar and heard about this ambush, it seemed certain to be a game-changer. But Sirhan's defense team seemed not to care. There was no outcry for the judge to declare a mistrial. How naïve we were to assume that the natural inclination of any lawyer would be to make the best choice for a client. Also, 2,400 pieces of evidence, including critical ceiling tiles and door panels that would have shown bullet holes, were destroyed three weeks before trial. The reason given was because the state of California didn't want to pay the storage costs! And photos that might have shown the shooting were confiscated and destroyed. But Sirhan's attorneys never went ballistic and screamed to the public that they had been railroaded. Had that been me in their shoes, I'd still be screaming.

Sirhan was convicted and sentenced to execution, but California later overturned the death penalty, and he was given a life sentence. He remains in prison to this day, claiming that he remembers nothing from the night that RFK was shot. Every five years, Sirhan appears before the parole board, but a requirement for leniency is that he renounce his crime. Due to his memory loss, he's unable to do so. His brother, Adel, appears on Sirhan's behalf, but deputy district attorneys always succeed in making the case to keep the convicted killer locked up. And that's how things went until August 2021 when there was a seismic change.

Experts familiar with brainwashing techniques have looked at Sirhan's journals and behavior over the years and feel there's a good chance he was hypno-programmed into shooting his gun that night. Some believe he only fired blanks to distract from the real assassin or assassins of Kennedy and the shootings of the other people who survived. The book *The Manchurian Candidate* by Richard Condon (McGraw-Hill, 1959), and the 1962 film version of the same name and its 2004 remake, are political thrillers about hypno-programmed innocents who become unwitting assassins with no memory of their acts. The chilling story reflected the zeitgeist of the times with dramatic, yet plausible, scenarios.

Two superb reporters decided to try to learn whether someone got into Sirhan's mind and, if so, who and how? Their book, *The Assassination of Robert Kennedy*, is one of the most important tomes you will read about this case. William W. Turner was an FBI agent from 1951 until 1961, when he resigned to become a journalist and author. He worked as a legal investigator for Jim Garrison during the probe into the president's death and has written other books about political assassinations, the FBI, the CIA, and Cuba until his death in 2015. Turner's partner was Jonn G. Christian, a former ABC newsman, who died in 2001. I never met Christian but knew Turner for years and can affirm his doggedness and skill as an investigator. The Turner and Christian book was highly anticipated when it was released by Random House in 1978. It was expected to be the publishing giant's book of the year and was the personal favorite of a top editor. A healthy run of 20,000 hardback books was printed and arrived in stores and libraries nationwide. Turner made an appearance on the *Merv Griffin Show* to promote the book, and more shows were scheduled. Then, instantly, the media tour was mysteriously canceled, and Random House whispered it was dumping the book. No paperback rights would be sold, the hardback became listed as "out of stock," and a massive incineration followed. Assassination scholars quickly bought up whatever hardbacks they could find, including my coauthor Dawna Kaufmann, who knew both authors; the book is one of her prized possessions. After years of dormancy, it was re-released in 2006 by Basic Books.

As I mentioned earlier, there is indisputable evidence that the CIA experimented with mind control techniques in the 1950 and '60s. Project Artichoke and MK-Ultra were designed to create a hypno-programmed assassin who would not be able to remember a thing afterward. The man who ran that CIA program was William Joseph Bryan, Jr., a former U.S. military psychiatrist who had an office in Los Angeles. Among Turner and Christian's revelations is that Sirhan might have been mentally manipulated by Bryan, who touted himself as a "leading expert in the world" at hypno-programming and bragged that he could hypnotize anyone in less than five minutes. He also often boasted about being called into criminal cases by law enforcement agencies, including the LAPD.

Bryan brought hypnosis into the legal realm when he used it to induce Albert DeSalvo to admit to multiple counts of murder. DeSalvo, better known as the "Boston Strangler," was believed to have molested and killed 13 women in their Massachusetts homes between 1962 and 1964. DeSalvo confessed and was sentenced to life in prison, where he was stabbed to death in 1973. DNA testing, not available when the crimes were committed, has caused modern investigators to look skeptically at DeSalvo's involvement, asserting that the murders were more likely done by multiple killers and that he was a false confessor in most, but not all, of the cases. Nonetheless, among the passages in Sirhan's journals were these handwritten words: "God help me ... please help me. Salvo Di Di Salvo Die S. Salvo." Did the reference reflect what Bryan might have told him in a hypno-programming session? According to video clips, Bryan lectured about his techniques "to brainwash a person to do just about anything," and some observers would say he became less than discreet, wrote Turner and Christian. Before Bryan died in a Las Vegas hotel room in 1987, he bragged to two prostitutes that he was the person who hypnotized Sirhan. The authors wrote that Bryan opened the American Institute of Hypnosis, a storefront clinic in Hollywood to treat sexual disorders, among other maladies. In 1969, in a response to a complaint that he had sexually molested four female patients who had been hypnotized, the state board of medical examiners found him guilty of unprofessional conduct. Given five years' probation, he was forced to have an adult female present whenever he treated female patients.

Turner and Christian reported two other interesting possible connections with Bryan: One was that he was a guest preacher at "fire-and-brimstone" churches in the L.A. area and a member of the ultra-conservative Old Roman Catholic Church, which separated from the Vatican in the 1860s. Another adherent of that very small sect was David Ferrie, who was also a trained hypnotist and was investigated by Garrison for involvement with President Kennedy's death. The second potential link was told to an associate of the authors by the doctor's former secretary. She claimed Bryan received an emergency call from Laurel, Maryland, minutes after Alabama governor and presidential candidate George Wallace was nearly assassinated on May 15, 1972. The shooting took place in Laurel, where Arthur Bremer was arrested and later convicted and imprisoned. The previous year, after Bremer was arrested for carrying a concealed weapon, a psychiatrist evaluated him as mentally ill, and the 21-year-old was put under a psychologist's care.

Bremer's diary indicated that he had planned to do something "bold and dramatic, and on May 2, he wrote that he intended to "assassinate by pistol either Richard Nixon or George Wallace." When Nixon's security proved to be too efficient, he turned to the racist firebrand who was campaigning for the Democratic nomination against the Republican candidate, Nixon. Bremer tracked the governor across the nation, following him by car, plane, ferry, and bus, and he read books about Sirhan Sirhan. When he finally got his chance, Bremer approached Wallace and shot off all the bullets from his .38 revolver. He pumped four bullets into Wallace, hitting his chest, abdomen, and spinal cord. Three other bystanders were wounded but survived. Wallace would spend the rest of his life in a wheelchair. Although his hopes for the presidency ended, he returned to serving as Alabama's governor, a role he had taken throughout the years. Wallace died in 1998 of septic shock and respiratory problems related to his gunshot injuries. Bremer was released on parole in 2007 and is on supervised probation until 2025.

Brainwashing? Real-life Manchurian candidates? Alleged assassins who keep detailed handwritten journals and seem to have expense accounts? CIA involvement and multi-platform government conspiracies? Well, if these ideas don't raise your curiosity—or, better yet, your hackles—you should get your pulse checked. A congressional panel would dig into these issues in the mid–1970s, but by now people have long forgotten the results. The subject is very worthwhile for a new generation to explore.

Since 2012, James Earl Ray's attorney, Bill Pepper, had been trying to get a new trial for Sirhan Sirhan. If he was successful, I pledged to help present the long-overdue medical evidence that was denied in Sirhan's first trial. The case of Robert Kennedy's murder begs to be reopened. There's a lot we can—and must—learn about what happened to the senator, as well as what happened to his alleged assassin.

A crucial ally for finding the truth is Robert F. Kennedy, Jr., the late senator's son, now an environmental attorney. After studying the autopsy report and evidence in the case—including visiting Sirhan in prison in 2017—Bobby Jr. came to understand that the accused assassin was not his father's killer. He referred to Sirhan's trial as just a "penalty hearing," stating, "It's unfortunate that the case never went to a full trial because that would have compelled the press and prosecutors to focus on the glaring discrepancies in the narrative."

Bobby Jr. added, "My father was the chief law enforcement officer in this country. I think it would have disturbed him if somebody were put in jail for a crime they didn't commit." He argued that the case should be reopened, and his sister, former

Maryland lieutenant governor Kathleen Kennedy Townsend, stated, "Bobby makes a compelling case."

Bobby Jr. is also troubled by the probe into his uncle's assassination, citing his father's view of the Warren Commission Report as "a shoddy piece of craftsmanship." The senator, his son declared, and was "fairly convinced" that Oswald had not acted alone in the assassination of President Kennedy.

In December 2020, George Gascón was sworn in as Los Angeles' new district attorney. One of his first decrees was that prosecutors' duties will end at convictions, thus barring them from attending parole hearings. So when Sirhan Sirhan appeared before the parole board for the 16th time on August 27, 2021, there was nobody in authority to protest his release from prison. Pepper had turned over the defense case to attorney Angela Berry, who read a letter of support for the release from Bobby Jr., and called Douglas Kennedy, Bobby's journalist son, to also back the release. Douglas spoke of interviewing Sirhan and finding him "remorseful" and worthy of "compassion and love."

After 53 years behind bars, the now-77-year-old inmate had his first real chance of seeing blue skies again as a free man. The board will take 90 days to review the decision to release, which is where things stand as this writing. The final step will be made by California governor Gavin Newsom to block or allow Sirhan's parole. The option of a new trial is no longer a consideration.

But there's a wild card involving Bobby's widow Ethel, 93, and six of their children—Joe, Courtney, Kerry, Chris, Max and Rory—who signed a letter to the parole board citing their extreme disagreement over Sirhan's proposed release. This time, Kathleen, who had previously backed Bobby Jr., refused to take sides, and her brothers Michael and David are deceased. Kerry even appeared on Ashleigh Banfield's NewsNation program to say she would "fight this with everything I've got."

We'll have to see what happens, but I tend to think Newsom, who survived a recall attempt and is expected to run for another term, will likely not challenge the Kennedy dissenters. From what I've seen and read, these Kennedy family members are reacting from pure emotion and not analyzing or understanding the forensic aspects of the case. Even though many of the children have law degrees and jobs in public service, they only echo what prosecutors said during Sirhan's discreditable trial.

During Bobby's campaign for president, his former sister-in-law Jackie had been romantically involved with Greek shipping magnate Aristotle Onassis, but, out of concern that public disclosure of the relationship could cost Bobby votes, she kept the affair out of the news. Following Bobby's assassination, that secrecy was no longer necessary. Jackie accepted a marriage proposal from Onassis and looked forward to beginning a new life for herself and her children in Europe. As she told a friend, "I despise America and I don't want my children to live here anymore. If they're killing Kennedys, my kids are number one targets."

Jackie was 39 and Onassis was 62 when they wed on October 20, 1968, in a ceremony on his private Grecian island of Skorpios. During the school year, Jackie would live in Manhattan with her children, but over summers and on breaks, the three would travel with Onassis. It wasn't a joyful marriage, and by 1975, divorce was on the table. Onassis' death from the neuromuscular disease myasthenia gravis negated that process. Jackie received a $25 million payoff from his estate. As she told a friend: "Aristotle Onassis rescued me at a time when my life was engulfed in shadows. He meant a lot to me. He brought me into a world where one could find happiness and love." Jackie and her kids returned to New York City, where she began a career as a book editor at Viking Press and later Doubleday. She had a lengthy relationship with a diamond merchant, Maurice Tempelsman, who was separated from his wife. Jackie died of non–Hodgkin's lymphoma, an aggressive cancer, on May 19, 1994, at the age of 64.

There would be four subsequent attempts at presidential assassinations. In 1975, Gerald Ford survived two separate attacks by women with handguns in California. Lynette "Squeaky" Fromme, an acolyte of imprisoned killer Charles Manson, pointed a gun that was grabbed by a Secret Service agent before she could fire a round. And Sara Jane Moore, an alleged FBI informant, fired two shots that missed the president. Both women received life sentences but have since been paroled.

On March 31, 1981—just 69 days into Ronald W. Reagan's first term as president—a ne'er-do-well named John Hinckley, Jr., who oddly hoped to impress actress Jodie Foster, fired a .22-caliber revolver outside a Washington hotel. The 70-year-old president, his press secretary James Brady, a police officer, and a Secret Service agent were all struck by bullets before Hinckley was wrestled to the ground. Reagan was rushed to the hospital in critical condition but recovered to serve out his term in office and win reelection. Hinckley was found not guilty by reason of insanity and received institutional psychiatric care until 2016 when he was granted conditional release. In June 2022, he will qualify for unconditional release.

The last serious attempt at slaying a U.S. leader occurred in 2005, while President George W. Bush was giving a speech in the Republic of Georgia. A disgruntled local named Vladimir Arutyunian lobbed a hand grenade at Bush, but the explosive device failed to detonate because it was wrapped too tightly inside a handkerchief. Arutyunian escaped but was captured two months later, put on trial, convicted, and sentenced to life behind bars.

The Ramsey Clark Panel

I've often wondered whether Jackie Kennedy was truly involved in the decisions made in her name or was just so despairing or disgusted by everything that she didn't care what happened. An example is the way her name was invoked as the reason President Kennedy's body was hijacked from Dallas and brought, not only to Washington, D.C., for autopsy, but to the National Naval Medical Center in Bethesda. Although it's true that her husband had been a Navy man when he was younger, the Army facility—Walter Reed Hospital—was better equipped for conducting such a procedure. That's where the Armed Forces Institute of Pathology was located, where skilled forensic pathologists were aplenty and had experience in assessing gunshot wounds. While I wouldn't have expected Jackie to know that—particularly, in her frame of mind in the immediate aftermath of the shooting—the president's personal physician Rear Admiral George G. Burkley would have. Burkley was a prime mover in every major decision after JFK's death, but who was giving him directions?

Another example of how Jackie might have been used to carry forward someone else's bidding happened in 1965 when an official determination was made that all the physical evidence in the Kennedy assassination was her property. In October 1966, Jackie announced she was donating these materials as a gift to the National Archives. There were some pre-conditions, however. The materials would not be available for inspection by the general public until after the president's children had died. There was one exception: A recognized expert in the field of pathology could apply to examine the evidence after five years as long as his or her intentions involved a "serious historical purpose." Between the time of the assassination and the National Archives gaining control of the evidence, the autopsy materials had been in the possession of Dr. Burkley.

I found this outrageous. First, evidence in a homicide investigation, especially autopsy reports and photographs, is never given to the family of the victim. My days are filled with dealing with families of murder victims, and I assure you that the very last thing someone would request are photos of their deceased loved one and the clothing they were wearing when slain. Showing a widow gruesome crime scene or autopsy photos, much less clothing with blood and bullet holes, would be wholly inappropriate. Those items belong in a secure location in the event a criminal case develops where they might be considered valuable evidence. Even in the 1960s, before DNA testing was in the vernacular, there would be excellent reasons to retain physical evidence in a murder case. As pertains to JFK's evidence, while a prosecution wasn't in the offing, the items must be retained in the Archives for history's sake.

President Johnson had been inaugurated into his own first full term in January 1965, and his attorney general was Nicholas Katzenbach, an east coast Ivy Leaguer and Army hero who had spent two years in a POW camp during World War II. Katzenbach was one of the first people to advise Johnson to establish a panel of experts to study the Kennedy assassination, which initiated the Warren Commission. In October 1966, Katzenbach accepted a new assignment as undersecretary of state, remaining in that role until he left in 1969 for a job with a private sector law firm. Forever an intellectual and staunch Democrat, he died in 2012. Katzenbach's deputy attorney general was William "Ramsey" Clark, a Dallas native whose father, Tom, was once the U.S. attorney general, as well as a justice on the U.S. Supreme Court until 1967. Ramsey was promoted to Katzenbach's top spot where he served until Johnson's term ended in 1969. Clark later became a law professor and prominent anti-war activist until his death at age 93 on April 9, 2021.

Johnson was always a savvy politician who understood what Americans were thinking. He could see that the Vietnam War was sullying his legacy as a great civil rights president, and the incessant criticism over the Warren Commission's work was not going away. A discussion about how to handle that began with Katzenbach and his deputy, Clark. When Katzenbach left his job for the State Department, Clark was sworn in as attorney general. Did that come to him with the promise he'd tackle the Warren detractors? I think that's likely, especially since there were similar rumors that Clark was only offered the job if his father resigned from the Supreme Court, allowing Johnson to appoint Thurgood Marshall, the first African American justice. When you come up in the trenches of politics and know every player along the way, as Johnson did, you can accomplish a lot.

In the first weeks of 1968, Bethesda autopsy doctor J. Thornton Boswell wrote Clark a letter in recognition of the controversy over the Warren Commission Report. Boswell and his co-autopsist, James J. Humes, advocated that "an impartial board of experts, including pathologists and radiologists, should examine the material available." On February 26–27, 1968, the Ramsey Clark Panel, a four-person group of experts, went into the National Archives in Washington, D.C., to inspect the JFK evidence. The names of the four men were released, but their work was top secret, with the press told a report would be written and made public. The expressed mission was to determine whether the evidence at the National Archives supported the Warren Commission's conclusion that Lee Harvey Oswald acted alone. The members of the panel were Dr. Russell H. Morgan, a professor of radiology and radiological science at Baltimore's Johns Hopkins University; Dr. William H. Carnes, a professor of pathology at the University of Utah; Dr. Alan R. Moritz, a professor of pathology at Cleveland's Case Western Reserve University; and Dr. Russell S. Fisher, a professor of forensic pathology at the University of Maryland at Baltimore. Since a key part of the evidence was the president's autopsy X-rays, I was pleased to know a radiologist was on the team. I was baffled by the inclusion of the two pathologists, since, as I explained earlier, pathologists deal with living tissue, unlike *forensic pathologists*, who deal with the dead. But seeing Dr. Fisher's name gave me confidence in the panel. He was my mentor. I had trained under Fisher from 1961 to 1962 at the Medical Examiner's office in Baltimore and had great admiration for his integrity and intellect. If anyone knew how to interpret evidence in a homicide, it was Russell Fisher.

A timeworn tradition of anyone with a modicum of press knowledge is that if you wish to release something controversial, choose a moment when the public is distracted by something greater. That way, less attention will be paid to what you're releasing, and you'll still be able to say you fully disclosed your content. That was the trick employed with the release of the Ramsey Clark Panel Report on Friday, January 17, 1969—three days before the inauguration of America's new president, Richard M. Nixon and his vice president, Maryland Governor Spiro Agnew. America's 37th president was sworn into office by U.S. Supreme Court Justice Earl Warren. Nixon once explained to his aide, H.R. Haldeman, that he had chosen the dim-witted Agnew as assassination insurance, stating: "No one in his right mind would kill me."

So, what was the conclusion of the Clark Panel? Its report stated:

> Examination of the clothing and of the photographs and X-rays taken at the autopsy reveal that President Kennedy was struck by two bullets fired from above and behind him, one of which traversed the base of the neck on the right side without striking bone and the other of which entered the skull from behind and exploded its right side. The photographs and X-rays discussed herein support the above-quoted portion of the original autopsy and the above-quoted medical conclusions of the Warren Commission Report.

The report added:

> One bullet struck the back of the decedent's head well above the occipital protuberance (base of the skull). Based upon the observation that he was leaning forward with his head turned obliquely to the left when this bullet struck, the photographs and X-rays indicate that it came from a site above and slightly to the right. This bullet fragmented after entering the cranium, one major piece of it passing forward and laterally to produce an explosive fracture of the right side of the skull as it emerged from the head. The other bullet struck the decedent's back at the right side of the base of the neck between the shoulder and spine and emerged from the front of his neck near the midline.

This was the magic bullet that the Warren Commission maintained struck Governor Connally, seriously injuring him. The Clark Report said that if this bullet had taken any path other than the one through the wound through Kennedy's neck, it "would almost surely have been intercepted by bone, and X-ray films show no bone damage." One gunman, three shots from behind and above, and the single-bullet theory to account for seven wounds to President Kennedy and Governor Connally.

Clark wouldn't comment about the content of the report or the delay in releasing it. But he said that he had consulted with Jackie Kennedy Onassis and Massachusetts

Senator Edward M. Kennedy, the only surviving Kennedy brother, before the material was shown to the panel. Burke Marshall, a former assistant attorney general who represented the Kennedys in the matter, said the widow and senator "both asked me to say that they will have no comment to make on the report or its release."

The Clark Panel did make one interesting observation: The bullet that struck President Kennedy in the head was not at the base of the head, as the Warren Commission had reported, but actually four inches higher. The Clark group based its finding on the X-rays they examined. The disparity led many to claim that the autopsy photographs and X-rays had been manipulated or altered to hide other wounds. Why the Clark Panel challenged the autopsy findings was never satisfactorily explained by its members. All the more reason, I felt, that we needed to know what their examination of the brain determined. Curiously, though, that information was not offered. And we would later discover that one of the members of the Warren Commission, Gerald Ford, purposefully mischaracterized some of the other evidence in an attempt to fool the public.

The Ramsey Clark Panel Report was merely a rubber-stamp of the Warren Commission. Nothing to see here, folks! Lee Harvey Oswald acted alone! Ignore the man behind the curtain! But, as in *The Wizard of Oz*, there really was a man behind the curtain, and he was about to spring out and spiral this case into a new direction that would explain the odd timing of the Clark Panel's disclosure. And also like in *The Wizard of Oz*, I would come to learn that the Clark Panel's work was both cowardly and brainless.

Jim Garrison

Ramsey Clark was sworn in as the new U.S. attorney general on March 2, 1967, just one day after an arrest was made in New Orleans for conspiracy to assassinate President Kennedy. The arrestee would be the only person ever charged in the case. The prosecutor bringing the charge was New Orleans' District Attorney Earling Carothers "Jim" Garrison, a charismatic 46-year-old former FBI agent. A Tulane University Law School graduate, in office as district attorney since 1961, he campaigned to reduce crime in the city's French Quarter. Many vice busts were made, often with news crews invited along by Garrison to capture the proceedings. However, there were few convictions, mostly because the tourism industry thrived from prostitution, gambling, and other so-called victimless crimes. It would be like some politician wanting to clean up Las Vegas. People go to those towns for their bawdy temptations, and as long as visitors are spending money, law enforcement is inclined to look the other way at most infractions. But the arrest Garrison made in the Kennedy case would put him on the national map and open him up to both severe criticism and near beatification.

The person arrested was a wealthy New Orleans businessman named Clay Lavergne Shaw. There was a coterie of interesting characters surrounding Shaw, and through the rumor mill, I had heard dribs and drabs about all the supposed co-conspirators until I got a phone call at my office in the fall of 1968 that filled me in on the whole shebang. The caller was Garrison, whom I had never met but who captivated me for three hours that day. It would be the first of many conversations we'd have. Garrison had heard about my displeasure over the lack of professional access to the president's autopsy materials and told me he had a plan that could help both of us attain our goals. He explained that his investigators had begun hearing tips from people who claimed knowledge about JFK's assassination and its connections to people who lived in New Orleans. I knew that Lee Harvey Oswald had ties there through his uncle, illegal bookmaker Dutz Murret, and that Oswald had passed out leaflets there in support of Cuba during the summer of 1963. But that was the tip of the iceberg, according to Garrison, who promised he had details that were purposely left out of the Warren Commission Report.

Shaw was a 55-year-old, dapper, chain-smoking bon vivant, who was 6' 4" and had thick gray-white hair. During World War II, he served as deputy chief of staff to an army general in Europe, learning the organizational skills that helped when he returned stateside. Having impeccable taste, he helped restore countless old buildings in the French Quarter, the city's historic business section. Most folks knew that Shaw was a homosexual, but he did such good for his community, no one cared. He had glamorous parties attended by the social set and handsome young men, and counted playwright Tennessee Williams as a friend. For almost 18 years, Shaw had been the managing director of the International Trade Mart, supervising its $15 million renovation into a showplace to increase commerce for the Port of New Orleans. Shaw once estimated he gave 500 speeches in his duties, and he was regularly seen on television and at fundraisers. Shaw's and Garrison's paths would occasionally cross at fancy restaurants or city functions, but they didn't know each other. Shaw told a reporter that he had voted for Garrison.

The Cuban consulate had offices in the Trade Mart, the building outside of which Oswald had been giving out those pro–Castro leaflets. Garrison told me he had news footage that showed Oswald holding the flyers, with Shaw nearby. Later, I saw the footage and wasn't convinced. The person purported to be Shaw was far away and indistinct, and, even if it were him, what did that prove? Shaw could have just been walking up the street to go into the building. It wasn't like the two men were seen talking or doing anything dodgy. Garrison thought that was a major connection between them, but I didn't recognize then that it was a sign of trouble.

As we spoke on the phone, Garrison said he heard that I thought the Warren Commission Report was a "work of fiction that should be on a shelf next to *The Adventures of Huckleberry Finn*," as I liked to say. He felt that way too, calling it a "whitewash" and "fraud." He also knew that I had seen the Zapruder film and believed my views on the medical evidence could assist him in making the case for more than one shooter and, therefore, a conspiracy in the president's murder. Garrison didn't believe Oswald shot anyone that day—not the president and not Officer J.D. Tippit. As Garrison described it, Oswald was a tool of the intelligence community, then a patsy, and then a victim. The people who assassinated JFK were still out there, and it was time to bring them to justice. It was easy to get caught up in his zeal.

During the spring and summer of 1967, Garrison had convened a preliminary hearing with three judges who agreed that there was enough evidence to hold Shaw for trial, mostly on the testimony of an insurance salesman named Perry Raymond Russo. In September 1963, Russo claimed to have been at the New Orleans apartment of David Ferrie when he overheard Ferrie, Shaw, and "Leon Oswald" discussing a plot to kill Kennedy. Russo never came forward with the information during the Warren Commission's investigation and, according to the district attorney, only felt safe to make the admission after Ferrie died. Garrison said he accepted Russo's story as fact after the young man took and passed a battery of tests his office had administered, including a polygraph, hypnosis, and sodium pentothal, an injectable barbiturate used as a truth serum. In December 1966, Shaw had come into Garrison's office for questioning, without a subpoena or attorney present, but when asked to take a polygraph test, he refused. Shaw left and lawyered up. He was arrested on March 1, 1967, but it would take almost two years for the case to get to trial.

Garrison told me that a Big Easy lawyer named Dean Andrews stated that Oswald had visited his law office a few times in the summer of 1963 seeking advice on a military discharge and immigration forms for his Russian wife. Andrews billed him a nominal amount, but Oswald never paid. After Oswald was arrested in Dallas, Andrews received a call from someone named "Clay Bertrand," who hired him to go to Texas and represent the accused assassin. Bertrand said he would cover the legal fees. Andrews would later back away from all of the claims about Bertrand, stating at Shaw's trial that he only spoke out for publicity. But, at the time, Garrison told me he trusted this witness implicitly. Garrison explained that Shaw had ties to the CIA and that it was common for intelligence operatives to use aliases. Shaw used both Clay Bertrand and Clem Bertrand as pseudonyms, he said.

The CIA was the main player behind JFK's death, Garrison said, but that didn't necessarily mean anyone who was officially employed and sanctioned by our government. The plot was more likely the dirty work of rogue forces, probably those who Kennedy fired after the Bay of Pigs disaster. The directorate in Washington had to know what their people did, Garrison claimed, and may or may not have agreed. But the CIA was forced to help cover up the caper lest their whole house of cards be toppled. Jim felt there was involvement with some members of the FBI, although in a lesser capacity, as well as among Dallas cops and city leaders. He said they were abetted by members of organized crime, including New Orleans' own Carlos Marcello, who had ties to Jack Ruby. The parties that wanted Kennedy dead hated his peace offerings toward Castro, Khrushchev, the North Vietnamese, or any communist who needed to be squashed, went Garrison's thinking. They also resented his platforms on civil rights and the Nuclear Test Ban Treaty. America was moving too fast for these people, and they wanted to slow things down. The CIA operatives who instigated the plan were assisted by Texas oil tycoons, mercenaries and gun runners, Minutemen and other far-right racists, and paramilitary hit teams who had worked together on other sniper deaths. Garrison believed there were seven to 10 assassins in Dealey Plaza that day, divided up between the Texas School Book Depository and the Dal-Tex building, and behind the wooden fence on the grassy knoll. There were riflemen who used telescopic sights and some exploding bullets, and cleanup pros who collected the spent shell casings and helped the shooters assemble and break down their rifles and make quick getaways.

Shaw's arrest was just the start, Garrison vowed. Garrison held the key to unlock the conspiracy and would expose the entire network, no matter how high up it went. And he wouldn't stop, even if it meant working for the next 30 years to get every last one behind bars. He expressed total confidence that he had the who, how, and why of the case nailed tight and that no one should bet against him. At the same time, he stated that, as a district attorney, he would rather see a guilty defendant be set free than a malicious prosecution of an innocent person. But that wasn't the case with

Shaw, he assured me. He emphasized that he would be willing to turn over his entire investigative file to the government if there was the slightest chance the feds would properly prosecute the right people. Garrison's knowledge of the case was encyclopedic, but I had to ask how he learned all of this. He wove together a narrative involving Oswald and others whose names I had heard before, but coming from someone who knew the denizens of his Crescent City, the story took on added relevance. I kept thinking that if he were this spellbinding to me on the phone, he would certainly be effective in front of a jury in his hometown—provided, that is, that everything he was telling me was accurate and could be backed up by responsible witnesses and real evidence.

Garrison began telling me about David William Ferrie, who suffered from alopecia areata, a rare immune system disorder that causes hair loss for anyone afflicted. In his case, the hair loss was almost total from head to toe. He tried to mask it by wearing a reddish wig and drawing on eyebrows, which only made him look clownish. Ferrie was an educated, seminary-trained Catholic who considered joining the priesthood and still had lace and satin vestments hanging in his closet. He had a curiosity about psychology and hypnosis, and had been conducting amateur cancer research with a local doctor. At one point, he had as many as 2,000 white mice in cages in his residence. After the doctor was murdered in what is still an unsolved case, Ferrie got rid of the mice, although the bad smell from them still lingered.

Ferrie earned his living as a pilot. Garrison said he supposedly flew mob boss Marcello back from Guatemala in 1961, after then–Attorney General Robert Kennedy had him dumped in the jungle there. Garrison's investigators were following leads that Ferrie and Oswald knew each other from when the former was a Civil Air Patrol trainer, and the former a teenaged squadron member, although Ferrie had told the FBI that he had never met Oswald at any point. Of course, Ferrie could have been asked about this, had he been called to give testimony to the Warren Commission. What a pity that august panel didn't think to invite him.

Ferrie was found nude and dead on his sofa bed on February 22, 1967, at the age of 48. The Orleans Parish coroner, Nicholas Chetta, determined the manner of death to be natural. The cause was a massive cerebral hemorrhage due to a congenital intracranial berry aneurysm that had ruptured at the base of his brain. A toxicology screen returned two days later showed nothing unusual. The coroner found no evidence of murder or violence, but Garrison felt the timing of the death, just days before Shaw's arrest and Clark's swearing in, was too convenient. Some of Garrison's office staffers had been in touch with Ferrie and told him he'd be called as a witness in the Shaw case, if not arrested as a co-conspirator. Ferrie left two unsigned, undated typed letters, which Garrison described to me as suicide notes.

Garrison suspected the pressure got to Ferrie, who took his own life. The district attorney said he had gone into Ferrie's apartment after the body had been removed and pocketed a bottle of Proloid, a prescription medication that he claimed the coroner's technicians had failed to collect. The bottle had pills missing, and Garrison wondered if the medication was used by Ferrie to kill himself. I volunteered to review the autopsy report and, grateful, he said he'd mail it to me. In a subsequent phone call, I reported back that the autopsy, performed by Dr. Ronald Welsh, was expertly done, and I agreed with the conclusion that it was a natural death. I explained that an aneurysm can frequently rupture, spilling blood into the brain. Think of it as an inner tube with a weak spot, I said. Ferrie had complained of headaches for a while, a completely consistent scenario for his condition. Ferrie had other contributing causes of trouble: hypertensive cardiovascular disease and pulmonary edema (swelling) and congestion.

Moreover, because there were two notes found, and the deceased was relatively young, the coroner asked for toxicology screening above and beyond what was typically done. The lab ran the full gamut for organic and inorganic substances, which include opioids, benzodiazepines, amphetamines, barbiturates, and marijuana, as well as alcohol. The results came back negative. Only a small amount of caffeine was detected, which comported with the cup of coffee that a reporter, the last person with Ferrie prior to his death, had said he ingested.

Garrison said there were seven pills still in the bottle of Proloid he had taken, and that he had learned Ferrie didn't even have a prescription for the medication. Garrison expected I would agree that the coroner's techs had screwed up by not collecting it but, again, I had to set him straight. Proloid was a hormone to stimulate the thyroid gland to counteract a low metabolism, and it takes time to work once introduced into a person's system. I had never heard of one case in which it was used as a suicide drug. In fact, as I explained, the only way it would make sense for Ferrie to use Proloid to kill himself would be if he stuffed the actual bottle into his throat to block his windpipe—and that didn't happen. Also, most people using drugs for a suicidal overdose generally don't leave a few pills in the bottle. They want to be sure to die, so they take all of the medication. These were the likely reasons the techs didn't bother collecting that bottle, and I reminded Garrison that his own action of taking something from a death scene was improper. Had there been something to his theory of a "Proloid suicide," he had interrupted the chain of custody. As for the lack of anyone's name on the prescription medicine, I had no idea. Maybe the pills were left over from the experiments he conducted on the white mice that had been in his apartment. I said that partly facetiously. The last people to have seen Ferrie reported that his breath was labored and he moaned in pain with each step. He had also been unable to keep food in his stomach for long. It seemed to me that his system was shutting down. He might have lived, had he gone to a hospital.

Then there was the matter of the two alleged suicide notes, which were found in separate locations amid piles of papers and books in the cluttered apartment. The first was presumably addressed to Alvin Roland Beauboeuf who, along with a friend, accompanied Ferrie on a road trip from New Orleans to Houston on the day of the assassination. Beauboeuf was rumored to be Ferrie's lover but had been keeping company with a woman he would later marry. Ferrie's letter stated:

> Dear Al: When you read this, I will be quite dead and no answer will be possible. I wonder how you are going to justify things. Tell me you treated me as you did because I was the one who always got you in trouble. The police arrest. The strip car charge. The deal at Kohn School. Flying Barragona in the Beech. Well, I guess that helps ease your conscience, even if it is not the truth. All I can say is that I offered you love, and the best I could. All I got in return in the end was a kick in the teeth. Thus, I die alone and unloved. You would not even straighten out Carol about me, though this started when you were going steady. I wonder what your last days and hours are going to be like. As you sowed, so shall you reap.

Could that have been a suicide note? Absolutely. But it also could have been the words of a jilted boyfriend who was acknowledging his own poor health. Since there is no date on it, we can't be sure. Ferrie's will bequeathed everything he owned to Beauboeuf, who has never publicly interpreted the note's meaning. The other note is even less clear. It's also undated and not directed to any particular person. It reads [typos intact]:

> To leave this life is, for me, a sweet prospect. I find nothing in it that is desirable, and on the other hand everything that is loathsome. Daily we are propagandized more and more about a rising crime rate. But how do we know it is true? We don't, for we Americans have little or no access to the truth. Today I went to the police headquarters to see these "public records" of this rising crime rate and nearly wound up in jail for my trouble. I was searched, interrogated, verbally abused, had my record checked, and finally threatened. Needless to say, I did not see the "public records." Still more irking is to hear a superintendent of police, who rose through the ranks (thus proving that zero equals super zero) stating that the solution to the crime problem was tightened and more stringent laws. A somewhat messianic district attorney concurred. Together these men prove themselves utterly unfit for office, just as they proved that an electorate cannot be depended on to pick the right man. The problems of crime rest deep in society. The problems exist in the existence of divorce and the absence of regulations.
>
> No parents would send him child to an amateur for dental work, nor a quack for an appendectomy. Yet what atrocious negligence is permitting other amateurs to raise children. Mere kids are allowed to marry because they have the "urge." How stupid can you get? Every expert tells in detail how children must be cared for physically, emotionally and intellectually. Yet society lets girls and boys, not yet capable of lover begat children who, love-starved, turn to crime for some sort of identification. However, I don't think we will often see a district attorney or a police chief with brains to realize this. We pay so much attention to the law. I have not figured out the reason. I have watched judges like [possibly J. Bernard] Cocke at work. The various police and district attorneys and the like get to bend the judge's ear long before the trial. These judges of today deny defendants due process of the law. They permit the court to try the case in chambers, to have district attorneys form their opinions and decisions long before the defense gets a chance. Further, these same judges (and I am afraid it pertains to nearly all of them) then comment, by word, glance, gesture or remark, on the evidence in front of a jury. If the defendant wins, these judges take it as a personal insult.
>
> When I was a boy my father preached that in the "American way of life" you are innocent till proven guilty. No greater lie has been told. The man charged before the court has flat got to prove his innocence. Go witness a criminal trial and watch. The state is supposed to prove guilt beyond a reasonable doubt. If you read decisions of the various courts of appeal and the Supreme Court you discover that truth and falsehood, right and wrong have no place in court. All the state needs is "evidence to support a conviction." If this is justice, then justice be damned.

This sounds more like a journal entry or letter to the editor than a missive to anyone. Was Garrison the district attorney railed at by Ferrie? When I asked Garrison about it, he presumed so but couldn't be sure. The coroner wisely discounted both letters when classifying Ferrie's death as natural.

Garrison also told me about "the most important witness" he would be calling at trial. According to a signed and notarized statement to Dallas sheriff's deputies hours after the assassination and in a later interview with a reporter, local resident Julia Ann Mercer said she was driving down Elm Street about 10:50 a.m., less than two hours before the shooting. The 23-year-old was in the slow lane, just past the grassy knoll area to her right. She had to stop her car because a green Ford pickup with a Texas license plate was obstructing her lane, with its hood up and its right tires on the sidewalk. She couldn't maneuver around it because there was traffic to her left. That gave her about three minutes to see the truck's driver, a 40-ish heavy-set, white male with light brown hair and wearing a green jacket. He was slouched over the steering wheel, but, at one point, his eyes connected with hers.

Mercer stated that a younger white man with dark brown hair and a tan complexion exited the passenger side and went to the back of the truck. This man was around 5'9" and weighed about 165 pounds, wearing a gray jacket with brown pants and a plaid shirt. He wore a wool stocking hat with a tassel on it. From the bed of the pickup, the younger man lifted what appeared to be a brown rifle case, a bit less than four feet long and with a handle. The man took the case and walked up the grassy knoll, stumbling once when the case caught on some foliage. Traffic then cleared, and Mercer was able to drive off. She added that three policemen stood by a nearby motorcycle, talking and apparently oblivious to the disabled pickup truck and its inhabitants. Mercer told police that she could identify both men in the truck if she were to see them again.

The next morning Mercer repeated her statement to an FBI agent. During her interview, he showed her photos to see if any matched the men in the truck. When shown Oswald's photo, she said she couldn't make a conclusive identification, but that he was of the same general build as the man with the brown case. But when shown a photo of another man and asked if he could be the driver, she made a positive identification. The agent flipped the photo over, and she saw the words "Jack Ruby" on it, which meant nothing to her at the time. On Sunday morning, when she watched the news coverage after Ruby shot Oswald, she recognized Ruby as the man in the photo and behind the wheel of the truck. Recall, too, that Marguerite Oswald told essentially the same story. On November 23, an FBI agent showed her a photo of Ruby and asked if she had ever seen him before. She had not. The next day, after Ruby had killed her son but before Marguerite knew the killer's identity, she saw Ruby's photo in the newspaper and recognized him as being the man in the photo shown to her by the FBI agent. Her Secret Service babysitter then told her Ruby's name.

On January 15, 1968, Garrison met with Mercer and showed her the reports she had signed. He was stunned to hear her say that they were blatantly inaccurate. Both reports stated that she couldn't identify either of the men and left out that she had chosen Ruby as the truck driver in her FBI interview. Also, both statements added that she had said the truck had an oval logo on the door that read "Air Conditioning," which was wrong. She had not commented about a logo or any writing on the truck. Worst of all, the signature on the reports was not her handwriting, and she proved it by writing her signature for Garrison. The district attorney chronicled all of her corrections for the record. He told me that Mercer was the ideal kind of witness he liked to put before a jury because she was understated and intelligent.

Obviously, Mercer's account had great relevance because it put a rifleman on the grassy knoll and showed that the feds were aware of a Ruby connection prior to his shooting Oswald. There were witnesses who saw Ruby in Houston that day, so a proper vetting of Mercer and those witnesses was something that should have been done by the Warren Commissioners.

Perhaps most daunting, the forged reports also illustrated collusion between sheriffs and federal agents to falsify evidence and discredit witnesses when necessary. Think about it: Representatives from both agencies, along with possibly other governmental bodies, sat together and analyzed the problem that Mercer's comments created for them, then determined the best way to neutralize her remarks. Whatever conspiracy Shaw might tangentially be tied to, or hoped for by Garrison, this was proof of an uber-conspiracy that extended straight into our national overlords. Mercer had given subsequent interviews to FBI agents in the days following the assassination, and the agents had the audacity to use the date of November 28 on one of those supplemental reports as when she had been shown the Ruby photo. That was another lie, designed to hide the fact that she had made that identification on the day prior to when Ruby made news for killing Oswald. Oh, and as if you can't guess, Mercer was never asked to testify before the Warren Commission. Why should it bother getting her sworn word on record when it had reports *about* her from the Dallas sheriffs and the FBI?

Garrison had a contentious relationship with Clark over the release of Kennedy assassination files. And, as he told me on the phone, he believed Clark was lying about Ferrie. Clark and·I had both caught the March 12, 1967, edition of *Face the Nation*, where Clark was asked why certain Ferrie documents had been classified by the FBI and the Justice Department. Clark shrugged and said the items were just being reviewed by the General Services Administration. But Garrison told me that FBI Director J. Edgar Hoover had personally requested the material be stamped secret. If Ferrie wasn't part of the conspiracy, Garrison asked, why seal his files?

Another key player in Garrison's hometown conspiracy was a Ferrie colleague named Guy Banister, a former FBI agent turned private eye. Both Ferrie and Banister were rabid anti-communists who, in late 1961, were involved with a munitions raid where weapons and grenades were taken to supply anti–Castro fighters. In February 1962, Ferrie had been fired as a pilot for Eastern Airlines on morals charges, having twice been arrested in the company of young men. Although the dismissal stuck, Banister had helped Ferrie as a character witness, and Ferrie returned the favor by assisting Banister with research on various cases. Both were reported to have worked on behalf of local mobster Marcello. Banister died in June 1964 without having been asked to give testimony to the Warren Commission.

As I mentioned earlier, the Banister detective agency was located on the ground floor of the Newman Building at 531 Lafayette Street. Around the corner and upstairs, but in the same building, was 544 Camp Street, the address that was stamped on Oswald's leaflets for the Fair Play for Cuba Committee. Garrison said Banister and Ferrie had recruited Oswald for pay to make the Cubans look bad. But according to Garrison's sleuths, both anti and pro–Castro Cubans were in and out of the offices, along with other shady types. Ferrie was there all the time, he told me.

On the day of the assassination, Garrison said, Banister and one of his investigators, Jack S. Martin, went to a bar to watch the news coverage. Both men were big drinkers, but Banister was a mean drunk. As they walked back to the office, Banister got mad and pistol-whipped Martin so bad that he ended up at the hospital. Martin struck back by telling people that his boss and Ferrie had something to do with the assassination. Ferrie, Martin claimed, was the one who taught Oswald how to use a rifle and scope, and was in Dallas that day to fly the assassin out of town. As we know now, that claim is in dispute, but at the time it was an idea that Garrison was willing to entertain. The FBI caught wind of Martin's commentary and interviewed him on November 25. He told them that Ferrie had hypnotized Oswald into committing the murder. Instead of acting on the lead, the agent decided the information was ridiculous and closed his files on Martin and Ferrie. But when Garrison heard about the interview, he had a meeting with Martin, who confirmed what he had told the FBI.

Delphine Roberts, who was Banister's secretary and mistress, backed up much of this, telling a reporter that she saw Oswald in Banister's office, and it was her boss' idea for Oswald to hand out the Fair Play for Cuba leaflets. She added that Banister still had deep connections with the local FBI and the CIA. Bill Turner, the former FBI agent who helped Garrison's investigation before becoming an author, said that Banister set up a CIA cover called the Anti-Communism League of the Caribbean whose tentacles extended into Latin and Central America.

Clark had said that Shaw had been investigated by the FBI in November and December 1963 and cleared. But Garrison felt Shaw was the ringmaster who presided over the New Orleans circus, and he was furious that Shaw's name wasn't even mentioned once in the 26 volumes produced by the Warren Commission. Besides, as he told me, if Shaw wasn't a suspect, why did the feds investigate him? When Garrison asked that of Clark, the attorney general reversed course and said Shaw hadn't been investigated after all.

Garrison's theories had wide public support and he was never reticent about going on TV to promote them on programs he felt he could trust. The most notable booking was on January 31, 1968, when he appeared on NBC's *The Tonight Show*

Starring Johnny Carson. In Carson's 30 years of helming that five-nights-a-week program, Garrison's appearance was the only one I can recall that only had a single guest for the full hour. As usual, the show was taped before a live studio audience and opened with Carson's topical monologue. But after the first commercial break, the lighthearted fare was over, and Carson showed America the kind of intellectual ken that was behind the twinkle in his eyes. Carson's research was solid and his questions uncompromising as he put Garrison through his paces. Carson asked Garrison if he was willing to say that when Shaw is finally put on trial the prosecution will secure a conviction "without a shadow of a doubt." Garrison replied: "I cannot make a statement which would reflect on Mr. Shaw. Since the day we charged him and arrested him, I have not made a statement that inferred that he's guilty and I cannot infer that now. But I'm trying to tell you that there is no question, as a result of our investigation, that an element of the Central Intelligence Agency of our country killed John Kennedy and that the present administration is concealing the facts."

Garrison held up enlarged photos of men known to the assassination theorists community as the "Three Tramps," which you'll read more about later. Garrison stated that the men were undercover intelligence operatives who had been arrested but released. He also emphasized that the Warren Commissioners didn't bother reviewing the 18 color and 12 black-and-white photos that were taken at JFK's autopsy, as any investigators seeking the truth would have done. The studio audience lapped up the interview, applauding both Garrison's blustery takedown of the CIA and Warren Commission, and Carson's refusal to accept everything that the district attorney was saying without seeing some proof. Garrison carefully avoided avenues that might have prejudiced Shaw's case and pledged all the evidence would be presented when the defendant got his day in court. It would take almost exactly one more year for that to happen. Due to copyright issues with the *Tonight Show* video, you'll only find a brief clip of the two men sparring on YouTube, but the entire audio feed is there.

Shaw's attorneys tried multiple times to get his trial moved to another jurisdiction outside of New Orleans. When those attempts failed, the defendant decided it was in his best interest to delay the proceedings as long as possible, hoping that Garrison would either drop the charges against him or that there would be a less emotional jury pool. Garrison didn't back down, so the conspiracy trial of Shaw began on January 29, 1969, in the Orleans Parish Criminal Court. Garrison subpoenaed the federal government to allow me to review JFK's autopsy materials.

On January 17, I had my first face-to-face meeting with Garrison. He was about 6' 6" with a booming voice and easy laugh. Later, our mutual friend Dr. Frank Minyard, who would go on to be New Orleans' 10-term coroner, would tell me that Garrison was one of his closest friends but had quirks, like never learning to drive. Garrison was smart and devoted to the law but often acted like a rumpled, absent-minded scientist. His wife, with whom he had five children, would complain to Minyard that they had no money, and Minyard would go to Garrison's office and get him to endorse a bunch of paychecks that had been stuffed into a drawer, uncashed.

Garrison asked me to meet him at the U.S. District Court in Washington, D.C., to give testimony about President Kennedy's medical evidence that was still under lock and key. Without that—and a forensic pathologist to interpret the autopsy report, photos, and X-rays—it would be harder for Garrison to prove his case against Shaw. Although the trial would occur in Louisiana, a federal jurist would decide whether he'd force the government to shake loose its secrets. I would be the only medical witness to testify. On the stand I explained to Judge Charles Halleck, Jr., how autopsy evidence was a necessary part of any homicide investigation and is, in most cases, public record anyway. I stated that Garrison had wanted me to explain the information to his jury and that the denial of it would unfairly hamstring his prosecution. By the end of the day, Judge Halleck agreed and immediately ordered that all the medical and physical evidence in the Kennedy assassination be made available for my review. As Garrison and I left the courtroom, we were elated that the judge had the brains and guts to unclog the logjam that had plagued this case for so long. Following the court's decision, however, attorneys for the federal government made it clear that they were not going to allow us to examine their evidence and that they would tie the case up in appeals for many years. Without access to those materials, I had to withdraw my offer to testify for Garrison at Shaw's trial, which could not be delayed any longer. It would not have been ethical for me to talk about something I hadn't inspected and was necessary for drawing an informed opinion. Garrison understood, but we were both very disappointed.

At every step of the investigation, Garrison found the U.S. government blocking his way. He once told me that the feds offered him a judgeship if he would drop his probe, then when he kept moving forward, he was threatened with an IRS investigation. His office was bugged, and his telephones were tapped. Double agents were hired onto his staff, and master files disappeared. Clark even stated publicly that he might prosecute Garrison, although he wouldn't elaborate about what charge he would file. The news media made the New Orleans prosecutor out to be some kind of publicity seeker yet never pointed out that during the entire investigation and prosecution, Garrison had refused to talk to the press about the evidence in the case. As he told me later, he had run into powerful forces in this country. Because he was challenging their ideas and positions, they would do anything to discredit his case or destroy him. Still, he persevered with absolute confidence that he was doing the right thing.

Shaw's trial lasted 35 days, with attorney/author Mark Lane sitting next to prosecutor Garrison and whispering points of strategy. As with the preliminary hearing, Perry Russo was the star witness, testifying that he overheard Shaw, Ferrie, and "Leon" Oswald discuss a plot to kill Kennedy, weeks before his assassination. Shaw took the stand in his own defense, stating he didn't know Ferrie or Oswald and had no connection to the CIA. (Years down the road, this would be proven false, as you'll learn.) Shaw swore that he had never used the alias of Clay or Clem Bertrand and chuckled that it was ludicrous to imagine someone who looked like him, with so prominent a public profile, getting away with using a phony identity. He spoke of the one time he met President Kennedy in Washington, D.C., and that he was impressed by him and especially his stand on social issues. The president, Shaw stated, had "youth, imagination, style, and elan." Addressing Russo's claim to having seen him with Ferrie, Shaw explained the young man probably mistook him for Banister who somewhat resembled him. Shaw insisted that if the jury convicted him on such shoddy evidence, he'd gladly go to jail because it would be the safest place to be in a world gone mad.

The 12 members of the jury were allowed to view the Zapruder film so that Garrison could argue about a second shooter. It had been screened for me in 1966, as I mentioned, but it would still take until 1975 before the public would see it. Jurors deliberated for less than an hour before unanimously agreeing that Garrison had not proven his case. Lane would claim he interviewed some of the panelists who thought Garrison was right about there being a conspiracy but just failed to make a sufficient link to Shaw. The businessman walked out of the courtroom a free man, and soon after Garrison charged him with perjury for lying on the stand. That case was dismissed. Shaw also sued Garrison's office for damages suffered from the financial burdens he endured during the trial. That case was also dismissed. Shaw died of lung cancer in 1974.

The deaths of Banister and Ferrie crippled Garrison's case, and I'll always wonder if my testimony might have helped, but it probably wouldn't have. For all of Garrison's intentions to blame the assassination on the CIA, anti–Castro Cubans, and Marcello and other organized crime figures, not one of them was mentioned during the trial. Another person Garrison chose not to call as a witness was Mercer. For reasons only known to Garrison, Mercer went from being the most crucial eyewitness to someone he only considered "peripheral" to Shaw's prosecution.

Garrison remained in office until 1973, when he was charged with accepting bribes from mobsters who controlled the illicit pinball industry in New Orleans. The jury found the charges bogus, and Garrison was acquitted. Still, he was defeated in his reelection bid by prosecutor Harry Connick, Sr., the father of jazz performer/actor Harry Connick, Jr. A few years later, Garrison won a special election for a judgeship on the Louisiana Court of Appeals, a position he retained for the rest of his life. In 1987, Garrison had a cameo role playing himself in the movie *The Big Easy*, which was shot in New Orleans. And in 1990, Garrison and I had a nice reunion on the set of the Oliver Stone film *JFK*, which was based on the trial of Shaw and for which I consulted about the medical evidence. Garrison had a small role in the film, too, portraying U.S. Supreme Court Chief Justice Earl Warren. The irony of the former district attorney appearing as the architect of the Warren Commission gave us both a hearty laugh. The movie, which came out the next year, was a gigantic hit that helped influence a new generation of critics of the government's story about JFK's death. More on that later.

Garrison died of cancer and heart disease on October 21, 1992, at the age of 70. He expired at home, in the city he loved, which didn't always return the favor. He was one-of-a-kind—provocative, inquisitive, and certain he was on the side of the angels. I never put him on the hot seat and asked why he just didn't drop the charges against Shaw when he could see the writing on the wall. And why he depended so greatly on eyewitness accounts when any prosecutor would consider them the flimsiest witnesses of all. Garrison's judgment was flawed, and he definitely got steamrolled by forces within our government, but I respected his intentions. I just expected more from someone who had often boasted that his office hadn't lost a major case in five years. In his book, *On the Trail of the Assassins: My Investigation and Prosecution of the Murder of President Kennedy* (Warner, 1988), Garrison wrote he lost the case against Shaw because he ran out of time. The book has been reissued several times, via various publishing entities, so read it and see if you agree.

Garrison told me that on January 25, 1969—Clark's final day in office as the country's attorney general—Clark wrote a memo to the Justice Department ordering them not to share President Kennedy's autopsy evidence with Garrison. Although the Shaw acquittal ended the district attorney's interest in seeing that information, Clark's actions only fueled mine. It would take more than three years before I'd get my hands on the material.

My Visit to
the National Archives

Between 1969 and 1971, very little news surfaced about the death of JFK. A few tabloid magazine articles proclaimed a conspiracy but didn't spark much attention in the mainstream press. As the summer of 1971 approached, I was acutely aware that the five-year moratorium about the Kennedy evidence was about to expire on October 29. Jacqueline Kennedy's gift to the National Archives provided that, after that date, the executor of the agreement could give permission to a qualified expert to review the assassination material. I contacted the executor, Burke Marshall, a former deputy attorney general at the Justice Department under Bobby Kennedy and, in 1971, a professor at Yale Law School.

At the time, I was president of both the American Academy of Forensic Sciences and the American College of Legal Medicine, as well as the coroner of Pennsylvania's Allegheny County. I also held four faculty positions at the University of Pittsburgh and Duquesne University in Pittsburgh. Various individuals from these and other organizations sent letters to Marshall asking that I be granted permission to review the evidence. My quest to gain access was given nothing short of a deliberate runaround. For months, Marshall ignored letters and did not return phone calls. One day, when I somehow actually reached him on the phone, he told me I needed to get permission from the National Archives—but officials there said that was untrue and that admission was Marshall's sole decision. I immediately began trying to get in contact with him again, but my repeated calls and letters were snubbed.

In late November 1971, there was finally some momentum. I had become friends with an assassination researcher named David S. Lifton who, when Kennedy was shot, had been a 24-year-old graduate student of engineering at the University of California at Los Angeles. Like so many people who followed the case, Lifton was mesmerized by it and would soon give up his advanced education to pursue writing a book. That effort, *Best Evidence: Disguise and Deception in the Assassination of John F. Kennedy*, came out in hardcover in 1980 (Macmillan), became a bestseller, and is still in print today as a paperback. Lifton's extraordinary work included obtaining the first-ever interviews of many of the young naval personnel who were present at JFK's autopsy and transcripts of Air Force One communications. Lifton's book was the first to have published X-rays and drawings representing Kennedy's body at autopsy, and later editions of the book included the first published autopsy photographs. But his overall theme was, to me, unproven conjecture that the president's head wound was altered somewhere between Dallas and Bethesda by an unidentified person or persons who sought to change the trajectory of the bullets to pin Lee Harvey Oswald as the sole shooter. The concept would have made a thrilling fictional movie but fell short as a piece of nonfiction.

Lifton knew about my desire to inspect the materials at the National Archives, and we would strategize ways to break through the barriers. Lifton contacted Fred Graham, then one of the best legal correspondents at the *New York Times*, and told him of my quandary. Soon I received a phone call in my office from Graham. We discussed the material at the archives and my qualifications, and I recited all the attempts I had made to get permission from Marshall, the gatekeeper. Graham replied: "Let me see what I can do." It's amazing how a simple call from a *New York Times* reporter will get an otherwise indifferent or uncooperative person to become friendly and helpful. No more than a few days later, a letter arrived at my office from Marshall, saying he was going on Christmas vacation, but when he returned, he would contact me. It was obvious that Graham had spoken to him.

The pressure must have shaken *something* loose. I was soon informed by Graham that he had just interviewed an independent, nongovernmental physician who had been invited into the archives to inspect the assassination materials. Graham's article on this ran in the *Times* on January 9, 1972, and was interesting for a couple of reasons. First, although I would have liked to have been the first independent physician to review the goods, at least somebody had been allowed that privilege. But second, when I learned who the chosen doctor was, I reacted quite viscerally. Think of Edvard Munch's 1893 expressionist artwork *The Scream*, and you'll get the idea.

John Kingsley Lattimer was the doctor who got the go-ahead, said to have come at the behest of the Kennedy family. Lattimer was an Army surgeon during World War II and, in 1972, chaired the Department of Urology at New York's Columbia University. He was an authority on pediatric urology and wrote extensively about renal tuberculosis. His patients included Charles Lindbergh, Greta Garbo, Katharine Hepburn, Itzhak Perlman, and top-ranking Nazi war criminals during the Nuremberg Trials. He was also reportedly the personal physician of FBI Director J. Edgar Hoover. Now, I'm not impugning the careers of urologists, but they spend their time dealing with patients who are having problems with urine flow and prostate glands. Their field of endeavor concerns matters below the belt. Lattimer was *not* a forensic pathologist. For all I know, he may have attended autopsies in his professional life, but that is not how he earned his living. I stressed that point to Graham after I read his front-page article, adding that sending in a urologist to assess a head wound would be akin to going to a podiatrist for a heart bypass. The Kennedy family might not appreciate that distinction, but it's one that should have been notable to their attorney, Marshall. In any American criminal trial, back then and now, prosecution and defense expert witnesses must gain approval from the trial judge ahead of such testimony. No sane judge would accept the qualifications from a urologist as an expert witness regarding forensic pathology, and any lawyer who brought in someone so ill-suited would be laughed out of court. Graham understood and said he would recontact Marshall and re-pitch my expertise and services that, as before, I offered free of charge.

Lattimer spent January 8 in the archives, then took it upon himself to conduct ballistic tests with a Mannlicher-Carcano rifle and ammunition similar to what Oswald supposedly used. It wasn't that Lattimer had a professional background in this area either, but he was a lifelong hunter, a collector of old weapons, and a re-enactor of famous battle scenes from the American Revolution. The good doctor wanted to see if he could duplicate the quick shots that the Warren Commission said that Oswald fired. After he completed his work on the Kennedy case, Lattimer concurred with the Warren panel! As he stated in the *New York Times* article, the materials in the archives "eliminate any doubt completely" about the validity of the Commission's conclusion that Lee Harvey Oswald fired all the shots that struck the president. But, as it turned out, the urologist had actually been "on the job" as a sub rosa Kennedy investigator for years before he was admitted into the archives. After Lattimer's death, his daughter Evan told a reporter that, when she and her two brothers were adolescents in the 1960s, Lattimer would "put us at the correct distance and angle" to fire a rifle at a cadaver from the barn roof, to demonstrate his "Oswald acted alone" theory. He'd tell the kids, "Well, there's your target, see how you do."

Lattimer died at the age of 92 in 2007, leaving his family to auction off or divide up the 3,000 rare artifacts he collected and displayed in his Englewood, New Jersey, home. Among the relics were Ethan Allen's sword, General Custer's bearskin coat, the bloodstained collar that Abraham Lincoln wore when he was shot, Charles Lindbergh's goggles, W.C. Fields' cigar, Garbo's driver's license, Adolf Hitler's drawings, Hermann Göring's underwear, and, allegedly, Napoleon Bonaparte's severed penis—an impressive assemblage of valuable souvenirs, for sure. But he also had objects from the Kennedy assassination, such as a brick from the Texas School Book Depository, Oswald's letters to his mother and his Marine Corps target-practice score book, and a swatch of leather from Kennedy's limousine. With the exception of the brick, I have to question why the rest of those items were in *anyone*'s private collection and not locked away in the National Archives where they belong.

I don't know if Lattimer was paid by the government or the Kennedy family for his services—or if he worked for free—but he managed to monetize his experience. Until he was well into his late 80s, he gave demonstrations on how Oswald could have fired those three shots in such rapid succession and made appearances for his 1980 book *Kennedy and Lincoln: Medical & Ballistic Comparisons of Their Assassinations* (Harcourt Brace Jovanovich). Perhaps even more egregious were attempted sales of Kennedy assassination memorabilia that were part of Lattimer's personal collection.

A leading document authenticator named John Reznikoff operates a respected website called the University Archives of Westport, Connecticut, which sells artifacts, letters, and relics of historic importance. In 2013, the site offered for sale 104 first-gen-photographs from the JFK files at the National Archives, a portion of which Lattimer used in writing his book. The site described the photos as the "largest and most complete grouping" known to exist. Included in the $2,900 price tag was a copy of Lattimer's book. It is unknown if this sold, but the lot is no longer listed on the site. Among the current items for sale from Lattimer's personal collection are three bloodstained fragments of leather from President Kennedy's limousine—each priced at $3,000—and a handwritten envelope sent by Oswald to his brother from Minsk, listed for $3,500. In November 2014, the highly regarded Nate D. Sanders Memorabilia Auction House put up for bid Lattimer's book and photographic reproductions of forensic exhibits of materials from President Kennedy's autopsy, all credited to Lattimer's collection. The minimum bid was listed as $2,000, but the auction closed without a single offer.

Did somebody grant Lattimer permission to take or duplicate exhibit items from the National Archives? How was he able to keep the collectibles that ended up as part of his estate? Was that part of the deal from the beginning when he was allowed to inspect this historic material? Beyond some nonspecific mention of the Kennedy family having extended the invitation to him, it has never been made clear who opened the door and put out the red carpet for Lattimer. And given his obeisance to the Warren Commission report and, by extension, the government's handling of the investigation, it's not off the mark to imagine the discussion emanating from J. Edgar Hoover, perhaps during a prostate exam, with the urologist's gloved finger probing the FBI director's most intimate cranny.

I will add that when I was finally was able to view the Kennedy collection at the National Archives, I was not allowed to photograph or take any souvenirs home with me—not that I would have ever considered doing so. But had I pocketed even the most minute portion of this esteemed collection, I would have been caught and prosecuted with the glee our government exhibits when perceived enemies of the state are put on trial and locked away. This book would have been written from a prison cell somewhere and would have consisted of far fewer chapters.

As for my pursuit to inspect the material at the archives, the rest of January and all of February 1972 came and went without a word from Marshall. I sent a couple more letters stating my request but received no response. In March, reporter Graham again called me and asked if my permission had been granted. I explained to him what had transpired and told him that Marshall was still not being responsive. Obviously puzzled by this information, he said he would certainly contact the lawyer again. Less than a week after I spoke with Graham, Marshall called, saying that, if I would meet with him at his New Haven office, we could work out the details of my visiting the National Archives. I believe he honestly thought I would not fly to Connecticut and that I would drop my request. If so, he was mistaken. After more procrastination on his part and nudging by me, we met and he finally granted me permission. My efforts and perseverance had paid off.

Since researcher Lifton had made the introduction with Graham, he flew from Los Angeles to Pittsburgh, stayed in my home and met my family, and accompanied me to the National Archives in Washington, D.C. Permission was granted for only me to enter the Kennedy section, so Lifton stayed outside, waiting for me to describe what I observed. Graham was also present, waiting with Lifton.

I spent Thursday and Friday, August 24–25, 1972, at the Archives, having brought a tape measure and ruler, magnifying glass, hand-held audio cassette recorder, batteries and blank tapes, and a notepad and pen. I was escorted into a rather large private room by the curator, Marion Johnson, who supervised the Kennedy assassination materials. He handed me a list of all the items I would be allowed to review. There was also an X-ray viewing machine in the room and a projector nearby, so I could screen the Zapruder and other films. As I would request various pieces of evidence on the list, Johnson, who was courteous and helpful, would bring them in from the storage room. The clothes worn by President Kennedy and Governor Connally were all neatly folded and separated by tissue paper. As I held Kennedy's dark gray, custom-made suit coat in my hands, I was tempted to try it on—but I didn't.

As I inspected the outfits that the president and governor wore, I was dismayed to find they had been dry-cleaned and pressed. You don't do that to items in a homicide investigation. In fact, someone who commits that infraction could conceivably be charged with tampering with evidence or obstruction of justice. Holding up JFK's jacket, I examined the bullet hole through the back. It was exactly 5¾" down from the collar. That's where the autopsy doctors stated the wound to Kennedy's back was. In fact, they went so far as to draw a diagram of the president's back, placing the bullet wounds about 5¾" down from the base of the neck. Six months later, when the Warren Commission told Dr. James J. Humes that a bullet wound 5¾" from the base of the neck did not fit its single-bullet principle, Dr. Humes volunteered that he and the other pathologists were wrong. Instead, Humes moved the bullet wound up four inches so it would match the trajectory of a bullet coming from the sixth-floor window. In other words, Humes was saying that his recollection of the bullet wound six months after the autopsy constituted better evidence than the diagram he and his colleagues made on the night of the autopsy. I found this to be ridiculous. The change, I would learn, came in a handwritten request by Warren Commissioner Gerald Ford.

Everything at the archives was listed by exhibit number, as it had been reviewed by the Warren Commission. It took me eight hours for each of the two days to go through everything. I examined Exhibit number 399—the magic bullet. It was housed in a small cardboard box with cotton bedding. I opened the box and found a missile that was in near-pristine condition. It was barely flawed. The only true deformity I could see was a slight indentation at the base of the slug, which would have been caused by the explosion of the firing mechanism. For this bullet to have done what the Warren Commission claimed it did and be in such near-perfect shape, it must indeed be magic! The Warren panel said this bullet went through two people, fractured two bones, and left bullet fragments in four places—Kennedy's chest and Connally's chest, wrist, and thigh. Despite all this, the bullet I was looking at had lost only 1.5 percent of its original weight. This kind of bullet weighs 161 grains before it is fired. However, the bullet I held in my hand weighed just under 158.6 grains. According to doctors at Parkland Memorial Hospital, fragments from this bullet weighing more than two grains were removed from Connally's right wrist in surgery, and another piece remained in Connally's leg. This point alone destroys the single-bullet theory.

Also among the evidence were details of a test that the federal government had performed at the Edgewood Army Arsenal in Maryland to see if its theory proved true. Using the same kind of ammunition and a Mannlicher-Carcano rifle, experts fired bullets into cotton wadding, the rib of a goat carcass, and a human cadaver wrist bone to simulate Connally's rib and wrist fractures. What were the test results? All the slugs fired into the listed items showed significant deformity. Even the slugs fired into cotton wadding had more deformities than the magic bullet. Keep in mind this was the government's own experiment, and it proved its theory wrong. I had known this was the case just from reading about it, but to see it proven with the

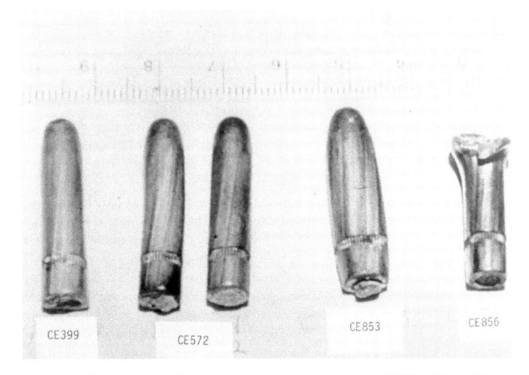

CE-399, the "stretcher bullet," was nearly pristine after going through JFK and Connally, but when the feds used a Mannlicher-Carcano rifle to fire similar ammo through cotton wadding, a goat carcass, and a human cadaver, those bullets didn't fare as well (Wecht Collection).

actual bullets—well, it was a memorable event for me. This was another argument for why the president's and governor's clothing items should not have been dry-cleaned and pressed. In 1972, a forensics laboratory might have discovered metal shavings on the items that could have linked back to the bullets. And with the state-of-the-art technology as exists today, precision tests could be done that might be very worthwhile.

Months after the assassination, Jacqueline Kennedy's suit, blouse, stockings, shoes, and gloves were dispatched to the archives by her mother, Janet Auchincloss, although not included in the box was the pink pillbox hat. Jackie's Secret Service agent, Clint Hill, recalled handing the hat to Mary Barelli Gallagher, the First Lady's personal secretary, who accompanied her to Dallas. In 1969, Gallagher wrote a book, *My Life with Jacqueline Kennedy*, but didn't disclose what happened with the hat and steadfastly refused to discuss it when asked by reporters.

Jackie's clothing was unavailable for my inspection, although they were kept—without having been dry-cleaned and pressed—at the archives in an acid-free box. I suppose the argument was that since the First Lady did not suffer physical wounds, her wardrobe wasn't germane. I would dispute that, as metal shavings could well have traveled to her outfit. As much as I'd recommend a scientific study of those items be made, it won't happen in my lifetime, thanks to a 100-year-long seal her daughter, Caroline Kennedy Schlossberg, slapped on the articles in 2003.

As I reviewed the presidential autopsy photographs and X-rays, as well as the home movies that were shot on that day, I was aware of how few people had ever seen these items. The Warren Commissioners published their report and 26 volumes without bothering to examine them, and the images had not been made public in any fashion. Even the Parkland doctors wouldn't have seen this material.

In reviewing these black-and-white and color photos, I noticed a little flap of loose tissue visible just above the hairline on the back of President Kennedy's head. Startlingly enough, no one had previously reported this piece of tissue, and it was not mentioned in the autopsy report. Because I was dealing only with the images and not the actual body, I could not determine what this defect might be. Given the questions that had been raised regarding the authenticity of the autopsy reports and photographs, the significance of this discovery could be far-reaching. The loose flap of JFK's scalp very easily could have been an exit wound, which would prove that there was a second gunman shooting from the front. But even if it were a bullet's entrance wound, it would destroy the Warren Commission Report's conclusion that only three bullets were fired. Considering the tight controls the military and Secret Service had on the pathologists doing the autopsy, it was possible the doctors simply overlooked an additional wound. Another explanation was, of course, a cover-up. Without re-examining the body or the brain, it would be impossible to ever find out what exactly this flap of tissue was.

Since it is doubtful that President Kennedy's body would ever be exhumed, I looked down the list searching for the next best thing to examine: the brain. But

I could not find the brain listed. When I asked to see the brain, curator Johnson informed me it was not there. When I asked where it was and when the last inventory was done, Johnson replied: "I don't know where it is. It was not here when I took over, and the inventory was done in 1966."

Extraordinary! The federal government had lost the brain of President Kennedy. It was gone. Disappeared. No trace of it anywhere. I immediately suspected foul play but also thought that some other agency, such as the Department of Justice, could have it secretly stored away. Perhaps the most astounding part was that, despite the brain's six-year absence, no one had reported it missing. As I went down the list, other items were missing, including some microscopic tissue slides and various key photographs of the wounds in Kennedy's chest, and Connally's Stetson hat and the gold peso cuff link that had *not* gotten blasted off the governor's shirt at the crime scene. There was no written acknowledgment of the absence of any of these items. Many individuals, including Lattimer shortly before me and the Ramsey Clark panelists who examined the evidence in 1968, obviously had discovered that the brain and other materials were missing—*but none of them made their findings public.*

I thought about my former mentor, Dr. Russell S. Fisher, the professor of forensic pathology at the University of Maryland at Baltimore, under whom I trained at the medical examiner's office, and fellow trainee Dr. Richard Lindenberg, who served with the German military in World War II and would go on to become a neuropathologist. During our training, we would dissect and study human brains, and Fisher was a tough taskmaster when it came to assessing the quality of our labor. Yet, Fisher sat on the Clark Panel and didn't notice or care that the president's brain was absent? I can't even fathom what kind of reaction he would have shown his students if they had presented such a cavalier attitude toward a missing brain—of a victim who died of a gunshot wound to the head, no less! A failing grade would be the very *least* humiliation such a student would suffer from Fisher. And Fisher brought Lindenberg in as a consultant, even though there was no brain for a neuropathologist to evaluate.

You'll recall that, in a previous chapter, I described the Clark group's work as reminiscent of *The Wizard of Oz*, in that it was cowardly and brainless. This is why I said that. This perfectly illustrated how people of the highest order had permitted themselves to be compromised by the federal government's influence and pressures.

As I looked over the scalp photographs one more time, something else appeared to be out of order. Where the doctors at Parkland Memorial Hospital had earlier said they saw a large hole—at the top back of Kennedy's skull—there was now hair. Where was the gaping hole from which JFK's cerebellum matter dripped onto the floor, as they witnessed? And that wasn't all. Because it was the top of the head, the hair in that spot should have been long. But in the Kennedy scalp photograph, it was very short hair—less than an inch long. It was the kind of hair found at the base of the scalp. Was it possible that the scalp had been rearranged to cover up the wound that the Parkland emergency surgeons say they saw? Only those who were present at the autopsy when the photographs were taken can tell us for sure, but this certainly raises a question as to whether the body had been tampered with.

I picked up the rifle that the government claims Oswald used to kill the president. I can't explain the feeling I had as I held the rifle up to my shoulder and looked down the end of the barrel of the most infamous rifle in American history, wondering if it had been wrongfully accused. With one more review of all the photographs, X-rays, and films, my two-day mission was complete. It was an experience I will never forget.

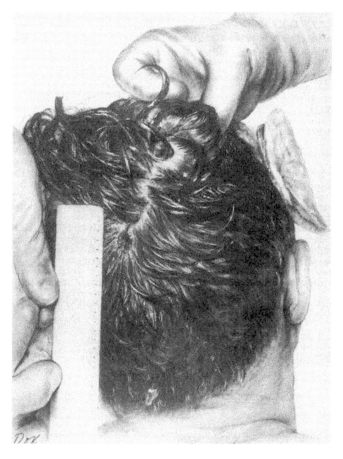

Parkland doctors described JFK's skull as having a large defect in the right occipital area that exposed cerebellum, yet Bethesda doctors did not describe that injury. How is that possible? (Wecht Collection).

Friday evening, as I departed the National Archives, Graham was waiting to ask me a few questions. I appreciated the role he had played in helping me gain access to the evidence, so I had no hesitation about sitting down and talking with him for a few hours. When he asked me what I saw that interested me the most, I responded that the most newsworthy finding was what I did not see. Later that evening, I boarded a plane at Washington's National Airport and headed home to Pittsburgh. Other than my family, Graham, and Lifton, no one else was aware I had even been to the National Archives.

That Sunday, as on every weekend, I went to the store to buy fresh bagels and the *New York Times*. There it was, splashed all over the front page of the world's largest and most influential newspaper: "Mystery Cloaks Fate of Brain of Kennedy." The lengthy article detailed how I, Cyril Wecht, "a noted forensic pathologist," had discovered that the president's brain, supposedly preserved in a container of formalin, was gone. According to the article, on April 26, 1965, JFK's personal physician, Rear Admiral George Burkley—four days after receiving a letter from then–Senator Robert

Kennedy—itemized all the Kennedy assassination materials, and the brain and other items were listed on his inventory. However, when all the materials were inventoried again for the logging in of Mrs. Kennedy's "private gift" to the National Archives on October 29, 1966, these items, including the brain, were not among those listed.

I told Graham that questions about President Kennedy's head wounds might never be answered as long as these objects were not available for thorough examination. In the years that followed, I requested of numerous federal agencies, including the Department of Justice, the FBI, and National Naval Medical Center in Bethesda, that the location of these items be determined. However, officials at each agency said that they could not comment on the case or that they did not know the whereabouts of the missing items. To further complicate matters, Burke Marshall told the *Times* that neither the brain nor the slides were part of the autopsy materials given to him by the Kennedy family and that he had never possessed them. In 1966, then–Attorney General Ramsey Clark ordered that all the items relevant to the assassination should go to Mrs. Kennedy, who then gave everything to the National Archives.

The records of the Warren Commission show only that the brain was "removed and preserved for further study." After the autopsy, records show that the Secret Service and FBI delivered various medical items to Dr. Burkley. After Burkley made his inventory on April 26, he turned the items over to President Kennedy's personal secretary, Evelyn Lincoln, who was working on the Kennedy memorabilia at the National Archives. Lincoln acknowledges receiving the items, saying they came in a padlocked chest. However, she says she never opened the box and turned it all over to Angie Novello, a personal secretary to Bobby Kennedy who by then had been elected to the U.S. Senate from New York. After reviewing the items, Bobby then put Marshall in charge of the materials, and they were returned to the National Archives.

Curator Marion Johnson was quoted in the *Times* article as saying the brain was among the items he gave to Lincoln but that it was not returned when the evidence came back in 1966. On the evening I sat and talked with Graham, I believed the brain was still around somewhere. "Who would have taken the responsibility to destroy the brain?" he quoted me as saying.

In the *Times* article, I described the pristine condition of the Commission Exhibit 399 bullet and explained why it could not be the magic missile that the government claims it is. I pointed out that a bullet that goes through two men, breaking bones and leaving fragments in four places, would surely have lost more than 1.5 percent of its original weight and would have been severely deformed. I also informed Graham about the little flap of loose tissue I found on the back of President Kennedy's head. Despite the *Times* article, there was little or no public outrage. People simply must no longer care, I thought. But as the years went on, I learned how wrong I was.

Tracking JFK's Brain

In an attempt to determine when President Kennedy's brain vanished and who might be responsible, I have assembled the following timeline of events, including some which occurred after my visit to the National Archives. My sources include the reports of the President's Commission on the Assassination of President John F. Kennedy (also known as the Warren Commission) and the House Select Committee on Assassinations (established in 1976); documents obtained under the Freedom of Information Act from the U.S. Secret Service, the National Archives, the General Services Administration, the Armed Forces Institute of Pathology, and the Department of the Army; and the *New York Times*.

1963

November 22: At the conclusion of President Kennedy's autopsy, Captain John H. Stover, Jr., commanding officer of the U.S. Naval Medical School, handed all the film taken by medical photographers during the examination to U.S. Secret Service agent Roy Kellerman. Kellerman was also given the X-ray film by Commander John H. Ebersole, the chief of radiology. Sections of other organs were placed in glass jars in the pathology department safe. The brain was set in formalin and placed in a stainless-steel bucket in the closet of Admiral George Galloway, commanding officer of the National Naval Medical Center in Bethesda.

November 23: Kellerman delivered the film and X-rays to Robert I. Bouck, special agent in charge of the Protective Research Division of the Secret Service.

November 24: The autopsists met in Galloway's office to review and sign their report. Sections of organs were reportedly taken for microscopic analysis. That night, U.S. Navy pathologist James J. Humes hand-delivered the report to Admiral George G. Burkley, JFK's personal physician at the White House.

November 27: On the orders of Bouck, Agent James K. Fox and Robert L. Knudsen, Mrs. Kennedy's personal photographer, took the autopsy film to the Naval Processing Center in Anacostia, Maryland, for processing by Lieutenant Vince Madonia. Fox later returned the prints and negatives to Bouck.

A few days later: Under instructions from Bouck, Fox had additional black-and-white prints made in the Secret Service lab at the Executive Office Building.

December 2: The three autopsists, observed only by a U.S. Navy photographer, met at the hospital to examine the formalin-fixed brain, which was described, in part, as weighing 1,500 grams (an upper limit for a normal intact brain) with a parasagittal laceration of right cerebral hemisphere, extending from the frontal to the occipital lobes and exposing the thalamus; its corpus callosum was lacerated, with the convolutions of the brain flat and the sulci narrow. This was interpreted as a "fixation artifact" because the change was not observed at the time of autopsy.

They noted "no metallic fragments" but found "numerous small bones fragments … in the container where the brain was fixed." Humes made sections of the hemorrhage on the left side of the brain and of the laceration of the right side but decided not to make "coronal" or cross-sections "in order to preserve the specimen."

Color and black-and-white photos were taken of the specimen at this time.

December 6: Burkley picked up and signed a receipt for all the autopsy materials, including the brain, which he said the family wanted to inter with the body. Burkley then personally transferred everything to a locked Secret Service file cabinet at the White House. This material supposedly remained in this location, under Burkley's authority, until its transfer to the National Archives in 1965.

December 9: Under instructions from Bouck, Fox had enlargements of the color photos made and returned the enlargements and positives to Bouck, who placed them in a locked safe in the Executive Office Building, the combination for which only Bouck and his administrative assistant, Edith Duncan, knew.

The autopsy photos and X-rays were not included among the materials given to the Warren Commission on this day.

1965

April 22: Senator Robert F. Kennedy wrote to Burkley, authorizing him to release all autopsy materials to JFK's former personal secretary, Evelyn Lincoln, who was now working with his effects at the National Archives.

April 26: After meeting to take an inventory of all the material, Burkley, Bouck, Secret Service Inspector Thomas J. Kelley, and two other agents hand-delivered a locked chest and a two-page inventory to Lincoln, "for purposes of secure storage and pursuant to an arrangement with RFK under which material may not be opened without his consent." No key was included. Listed under #9 on the inventory were the following items:

> One 9 by 6½" plastic box containing paraffin blocks of tissue sections
> Another such box, also containing 35 slides
> A third box containing 84 slides
> A 7 by 8" stainless-steel container containing "gross material"
> Three wooden boxes containing 58 slides of blood smears taken at various
>   times during JFK's life

The complete autopsy protocol, signed by Humes, plus seven copies

A letter of transmittal of autopsy report, plus one copy

A November 29 office memo from Fox to Bouck concerning the processing of
film in the presence of Madonia, plus two copies

A November 29 memo from Madonia to Fox concerning the receipt of film
films and prints, plus one copy

A "certificate of destruction of preliminary draft notes" on the autopsy protocol
signed by Humes, plus one copy

A November 22 memo from Ebersole to Kellerman concerning X-rays, plus two
copies

A copy of a November 22 memo from FBI agents Francis X. O'Neill, Jr., and
James W. Sibert to Stover concerning "receipt of missile"

A copy of a December 5 letter from Bouck to Stover concerning "graphic film
holders"

A November 22 memo from Stover to Kellerman concerning the receipt of
photographic material

A few days later, RFK called Lincoln to tell her that his secretary, Angela Novello,
would be coming to move the footlocker that day. Novello arrived with Herman
Kahn, assistant archivist for presidential libraries. Lincoln gave them the trunk and
two keys; it was unknown when she received the keys, as they had not been given
to her when she accepted the chest. Lincoln later told investigators that it was her
belief that Novello and Kahn were simply moving the materials to another part of
the archives where RFK was storing other materials. She added that she was certain
Novello signed a receipt for them but was uncertain where it would be today.

1966

October: U.S. Attorney General Ramsey Clark contacted RFK about acquiring
the autopsy photos and X-rays, but RFK was unsympathetic. An argument between
Clark and Burke Marshall, the representative of the executors of JFK's estate, ensued,
the result of which was an agreement on a "deed of gift" to the General Services
Administration (GSA). Reportedly, no other autopsy materials were discussed.

October 29: Marshall outlined the agreement formally transferring JFK's
personal clothing as well as autopsy X-rays and photographs to the GSA in a letter to
GSA administrator Lawson B. Knott, Jr. No mention of any other autopsy materials
was made. In his letter, Marshall noted that "the family desires to prevent the
undignified or sensational use of these materials ... or any other use which would
tend in any way to dishonor the memory of the late President or cause unnecessary
grief or suffering to the members of his family and those closely associated with him."
The following restrictions were attached:

1. That none of the clothing shall be placed on public display and that access shall be permitted only to government officials or "any serious scholar or investigator of matters relating to the death of the late President…."

2. That none of the X-rays and photos shall be placed on public display, and that access shall be permitted only to government officials until five years from the date of the memo, at which time "any recognized expert in the field of pathology or related areas of science or technology" may examine them "for serious purposes relevant to the investigation."

October 31: Marshall formally transferred the locked footlocker to the GSA. Just prior to this transfer, Assistant to the Deputy Archivist Trudy H. Peterson later told investigators, the footlocker was brought to the archives, suggesting that Novello may have previously removed it from the building rather than just moving it to another part of the building. Peterson added that Assistant Archivist Kahn, now dead, may have been the only employee present for the transfer and that no record of delivery was available.

Novello provided the key to open the footlocker. After it was opened, she and Marshall left. Various officials of the GSA and the Department of Justice then inspected the contents, which they discovered include only inventory items 1 through 8, plus three manila envelopes containing copies of JFK's military service records.

November 1: Humes and U.S. Navy pathologist J. Thornton Boswell were summoned to the archives to help categorize the autopsy materials and were shown the photos for the first time.

1967

March 14: JFK's coffin was secretly reinterred at Arlington National Cemetery under tight security. Later asked by investigators whether someone could have slipped additional material into the grave at this time, John Metzler, the cemetery superintendent from 1951 to 1972, said that at the time of the original burial, the coffin was placed in a tar-sealed vault, and that during reinterment there was no way anyone could have gotten anything inside.

October 3: The Secret Service forwarded the original autopsy protocol to the archives, raising the question of what the inventory was referring to.

1968

January 26: Boswell wrote to Clark, asking that "an impartial board of experts" be appointed to "examine the available material."

February 26–27: Clark fended off New Orleans District Attorney Jim

Garrison's lawsuit forcing the disclosure of these materials by naming a panel of four private physicians led by Maryland medical examiner Russell Fisher to examine them.

Summer: After the assassination of RFK, Lincoln later told investigators, she called former JFK aide Kenneth O'Donnell to make sure the family was aware of the autopsy materials. According to Lincoln, O'Donnell then called Senator Edward Kennedy, later phoning her back to tell her everything was under control.

1969

January: Clark released the panel's report. Although raising questions about the location and size of the back wound, it essentially corroborated the autopsy findings and neglected to mention the missing autopsy materials.

February 7: After hearing my testimony as to the need to examine the autopsy materials, Federal Judge Charles Halleck ruled that the government must make them available for my review. The government promptly appealed this decision, effectively tying the materials up long enough to outlast the trial.

February 12: GSA General Counsel Harry Van Cleve called a meeting of Secret Service agents and archivists to address the matter of the missing items. In a report filed the next day, Secret Service Assistant Director Kelley wrote:

> Mr. Van Cleve is concerned that writers like [Harold] Weisberg or Mark Lane, when they learned that such an inventory existed, would demand to see the inventory and items covered by it. He indicated that he saw no legal reason how the existence of this inventory could be kept from writers of this kind, and that when they learned of the inventory and then learned that some of the items ... were not in the possession of the Archives, that this would lead to all sorts of speculation and accusation that the government was not being perfectly frank and open in handling this matter, and that was further proof of the various conspiracy theories which these writers are alleging....

February 13: Kelley visited Burkley at home in Chevy Chase, Maryland. Burkley said he was surprised to learn that all the materials were not there and called Lincoln in Kelley's presence. She told him that she never opened or disturbed the trunk, but that "sometime after the receipt," everything was turned over to Novello, now secretary to Angier Biddle Duke, the U.S. ambassador to Denmark. Burkley also mentioned a "Henry Giordano," whom he identifies as a "former White House driver" and "employee of the Kennedy family" who now worked as a doorkeeper at the U.S. Senate.

Kelley called Van Cleve later and advised him that "we should not contact Giordano." In his report, he wrote that Van Cleve "agreed with this and stated he felt that the inquiry would have to remain as it now stands, that perhaps we were borrowing trouble in exploring it any further...."

1971

Summer: I began trying to gain access to the autopsy materials.

October 29: The Kennedy family's restrictions to access of the autopsy materials ended.

1972

January 8: Dr. John K. Lattimer, head of the urology department at Columbia University College of Physicians and Surgeons, became the first person not under government auspices to examine the available autopsy materials. He told the *New York Times* that they "eliminate any doubt completely" about the validity of the Warren Commission's conclusions, but he neglected to mention the missing autopsy materials.

March: I was finally granted access to the materials at the archives.

August 23–24: I reviewed every piece of physical evidence available at the National Archives and discovered that the brain and microscopic tissue slides were not there. Afterward, I gave an interview to Fred Graham of the *New York Times*.

August 27: All of the above information pertaining to the missing autopsy materials was made public for the first time in a front-page *New York Times* story. In it, I was quoted as asking, "Who would have taken the responsibility to destroy the brain?" National Archivist Marion Johnson related the above history, adding that the inventory of the missing items was being kept secret at the behest of the Kennedy family on the ground that a mention to some of them would be "objectionable." Marshall was quoted as saying it was "offensive for there to be all this probing … it is a terrible thing to do to that family."

1975

January: President Gerald Ford appointed the Commission on CIA Activities Within the U.S. (the Rockefeller Commission). Amid the ensuing public criticism of the Commission's choice of medical panelists, a group of doctors and I presented a petition calling for full disclosure of all the scientific evidence.

June: In its report, the Rockefeller Commission neglected to mention the missing autopsy materials.

1978

September 7: I testified before the House Select Committee on Assassinations (HSCA) as a member of its nine-person forensic pathology panel. Asked by Staff Counsel Andrew Purdy to what extent access to the brain would enable a determination of whether JFK was hit by a shot from the front, I testified that "the brain would be extremely important to help us determine whether more than one missile had penetrated" it.

Later, asked by Pennsylvania Congressman Robert Edgar what I would do to locate the brain, I testified: "I would get the best trained investigators ... and with an attorney for proper legal guidance.... I would go back to day one.... I would get the people who were in charge of the Archives. I would depose them under oath." Further asked what I would do if these efforts did not produce the brain, I pointed out that, if nothing else, "at that point it would be a matter of record. We would know what had happened to that ... evidence, and we would know who was responsible for it and that would be the end of it." I added that if and when an examination was done, it "would be performed in the most private, discreet circumstances by a competent neuropathologist or forensic pathologist."

1979

March 29: The HSCA released its final report. In the section dealing with the missing autopsy materials, the committee recounted its efforts to locate them by contacting all of the above-mentioned individuals, as well as several others. According to the report, Novello "had no recollection of handling a footlocker, or of handling any of the autopsy materials." Marshall was reported to have said that although he did not know what became of the items, "it was his speculative opinion that Robert Kennedy obtained and disposed of these materials himself, without informing anyone else" because he was "concerned that these materials would be placed on public display in future years in an institution such as the Smithsonian." Marshall was also reported to have added that he was "certain that obtaining or locating these materials is no longer possible."

In the report's conclusion, the HSCA wrote that, although it had "not been able to uncover any direct evidence of the fate of the missing materials, circumstantial evidence tends to show that Robert Kennedy either destroyed these materials or otherwise rendered them inaccessible." This opinion has never been officially corroborated by the FBI, the Secret Service, the National Archives, Admiral Burkley, the Kennedy family, or anyone else who would have firsthand knowledge of the items' whereabouts.

The final specific reference to the president's brain was on December 6, 1963, when Admiral Burkley signed a receipt for the brain and autopsy material, stating that the Kennedy family wanted the items interred with the body. But by that time, JFK had already been buried. On April 26, 1965, the list of inventory items turned over to RFK included a nonspecific entry of "gross material" in a 7-by-8" stainless-steel box. Was that the brain? What else could it be? There is nothing else that would even remotely qualify. *Of course*, it was the president's brain!

An inadvertent answer may have been offered by historian and author Anthony Bergen who runs an excellent website on the U.S. presidents. Bergen reminds us that JFK's original bronze coffin from Vernon Oneal Funeral Home in Dallas was not used for the burial, since it was bloodstained. When the Washington, D.C., team from Gawler's Funeral Home finished preparing the body, they put it in a mahogany coffin, which was buried at Arlington Cemetery. The original casket was stored in a local D.C. warehouse until Oneal asked for it. He had submitted a bill for $3,995 to the federal government, then knocked off $500 when told the amount was excessive. But Oneal really wanted the casket returned. He had offers as high as $100,000 from souvenir hunters and felt the item was his property since it hadn't been paid for. The Kennedys, apparently fearing that the casket would be made a spectacle, insisted that Oneal be paid, so he received a check, and the coffin became the property of the General Services Administration.

After the U.S. House of Representatives passed a bill in September 1965 that turned over JFK assassination materials to the National Archives, the original casket was transferred there. But a curious turn of events occurred. The mayor of Dallas at the time of the assassination, Earle Cabell, was now a U.S. congressman, and he sent a letter to the nation's new attorney general, Nicholas Katzenbach, stating that the casket had no purpose but to pander to "the morbidly curious." The Kennedy family had used another casket for the burial, Cabell reasoned, so the old one was "surplus" and expendable. He urged that it be destroyed. Cabell's brother, as you may recall, was Charles Cabell, a deputy director of the CIA under Allen Dulles until both lost their jobs in the agency's purge by President Kennedy following the Bay of Pigs calamity. Katzenbach was only too willing to comply with Cabell's request.

Bergen's research states that on February 18, 1966, members of the U.S. Air Force picked up the casket and brought it to Andrews Air Force Base. A team from the 93rd Air Terminal Squadron loaded the coffin onto a C-130 four-engine military transport aircraft for a burial in the Atlantic Ocean. To ensure that the casket did not float ashore, it was drilled with more than 40 holes, filled with three 80-pound sandbags, then placed into a sealed wooden crate. The plane then flew 100 miles eastward to a remote part of the ocean that was approximately 9,000 feet deep. The plane's tail hatch was opened, and then the coffin crate was pushed out at a height of about 500 feet. Parachutes had been attached to lessen the impact, and when the item hit the water, it sank quickly. The C-130 circled for about 20 minutes to make sure it didn't resurface.

Why was this elaborate rigmarole undertaken when the coffin could have been simply and privately incinerated? Were President Kennedy's brain and autopsy materials part of that burial at sea? Bergen doesn't mention it, and no such information is publicly available elsewhere.

Some Kennedy scholars have an alternate suggestion. JFK's burial casket was exhumed and moved to its permanent location at Arlington National Cemetery on March 15, 1967, during a very early morning ceremony attended only by Jackie

Kennedy, RFK, LBJ, and a few others. If the family wished to inter the items with the president, this would have been an opportunity for that to happen. But the cemetery supervisor denied that anyone opened the sealed coffin, so I'm skeptical about this theory. Other assassination buffs have questioned whether the president's brain and autopsy items might be residing in a private safe in the mansion of some Kennedy family member. The hope is that once the current generation of Kennedys dies off, the brain will then be reintroduced to the world, and a qualified forensic pathologist will be able to examine it. I feel this is both unlikely and a ghoulish idea. But for the life of me, I don't understand why a Kennedy family member or authorized representative doesn't speak up and settle the matter. It's infuriating that I, and others, must keep this subject alive with speculation when a spokesperson could simply say, "The brain and the other items were buried, period. It was our choice to make and we made it." I would be the first person to applaud that reaction. But the absence of any knowledgeable statement keeps the gossip mills rolling.

In the late 1970s, I was chairman of the Allegheny County Democratic Committee. The committee held an annual fundraising dinner where a nationally known political figure would be invited to speak. One year I invited Senator Ted Kennedy. I picked him up at the Pittsburgh airport, sat next to him in a private limousine on the way to his hotel, stayed beside him for three hours during the event, and rode back with him to the airport that evening. During all those hours alone with me, he was friendly and comfortable but never once discussed his brothers' assassinations. And he certainly never said anything to me about the missing brain. Ted had to have been aware of my criticisms of both murders and my public derision over the mishandling of JFK's brain, and he could have simply said, "Please don't talk about the missing brain, we buried it; it's unpleasant for his children and my family." But he remained mum on the subject. The inference I drew was that he was not at all unhappy or discomfited by my frequent, publicly expressed critical comments concerning both JFK's and RFK's assassinations. I'd like to think the senator was pleased that I was doing the work that he couldn't do himself.

Dan Rather

Jim Garrison's prosecution may have been flawed, but it contributed greatly to the American public's insistence to know what happened to its slain president. There were floods of interest everywhere, with the mainstream media doing its best to control the waters on behalf of the government. You'd think that an open press would be keen to explore the obvious lies and inconsistencies in the Kennedy case, but there seemed to be monstrous collusion to hide the details on television, radio, and the printed page. The European and world press didn't have that reaction, and because of my prominent position as a Warren Commission critic, I was offered various book deals to spill the beans, as I saw them. As flattering as that was, for the first several years, I resisted the opportunities, partly because my career as a forensic pathologist and courtroom witness was so active, but also because I felt any such book would be missing a final chapter that tied up the case with a neat ribbon.

Every November, there would be an outbreak of attention to commemorate the assassination, and many times I would make appearances on news documentaries. My first major invitation came in 1967, from Dan Rather of CBS-TV. As you may recall, Rather was one of the first Dallas reporters to describe the assassination to *CBS Evening News* anchor Walter Cronkite, and Rather's access and contacts in Texas made him a valuable asset. His natural ambition didn't hurt either, and, in 1964, he was brought to Washington, D.C., and named the network's national White House correspondent. More acclaim for the newsman followed, with Rather being assigned to both London and Vietnam before reclaiming the White House beat during the Nixon administration. During that period of the mid–60s, most every broadcast of the *CBS Evening News* contained an important report from Rather.

For the 1967 assassination program, I was filmed ahead of time and told by Rather that the interview would appear in the documentary. For his camera, I methodically explained my criticism of the Warren Commission Report and its single-bullet hypothesis. I also staged a demonstration with a mock limousine and four "passengers," showing the trajectory of the bullets, how there had to have been more than three shots, and where a second shooter might have been hiding. I left the studio very pleased that I had made a compelling argument for a conspiracy. By doing such an exclusive and elaborate interview with CBS News, I would be effectively barred from appearing on other network shows. So you can imagine my surprise when I watched the broadcast with my family and saw just a line or two of my views and no re-creation of the shooting. The next day I called Rather, who profusely apologized and explained that he had filmed too many interviews for the program, and his bosses had to edit mercilessly to comport with the network's time restraints. I was miffed because the overall program supported the government's position, but I assumed Rather was being genuine with me. Besides, there wasn't anything I could do about it. On September 30, 1970, Rather traveled with President Nixon to Belgrade, Yugoslavia, for a historic meeting with that country's leader, Josip Tito. I was there at the same time for an international conference on forensic science. The next day, as I was walking through the town square, I ran into Rather, and we had an amiable chat. I told him that I was attempting to secure a visit to the National Archives to review the JFK assassination materials, and he said if that happened, I should talk about it with him on CBS.

In 1972, after my visit to the archives was headline news, Rather called and extended another invitation to take part in an assassination round-up. He recalled the demonstration I did in 1967 and asked if I'd do it again, assuring me that this time he would make sure it was included in the broadcast. By this time, Rather was increasing his presence at CBS with appearances on *60 Minutes,* and he convinced me that his new stature would extend to editorial control of the segment. So, I agreed, and we filmed the exclusive interview, discussing the president's missing brain and other information I derived from my research at the archives. This time, when the program aired, I had a full house of family and friends eager to see me decimate the single-bullet silliness on coast-to-coast television. And, once again, my demonstration ended up on the cutting-room floor, and there was only a passing mention of my work at the archives. All that remained of me was a bare whisper of dissent, surrounded by loud voices from talking heads who promoted the government's official party line. Apparently, a clown car pulled up to the CBS studios, and out came every half-baked Warren defender who spoke about the integrity of the Commission's work and hinted that it was just not "patriotic" to keep questioning a matter that had been settled. Let President Kennedy and this investigation rest in peace, they demanded! Of course, the other participants were not challenged in any way by Rather or anyone else with his network.

I realized that Rather invited me on this program and the previous one to give the illusion that CBS had no bias. There wasn't much I could do about it—except to send off a blistering letter to Rather. I wrote that he was unethical, dishonest, and a shame to his profession. I can't recall, and don't care, if he responded. We never spoke again.

Rather should have been canned the minute he was caught mischaracterizing the Zapruder film in the hours after the assassination, when he stated to national viewers that the president's fatal head shot caused his head to "move violently forward" instead of backward. Whether that was a mistake on his part, or purposeful, I don't know. Later, I saw Rather interviewed about the assassination, and he added a detail I had not heard before. He stated that he was positioned just beyond the grassy knoll, a block past the triple underpass, waiting for the motorcade to arrive. He didn't know about the assassination and hadn't heard the bullets but was puzzled when the presidential limo suddenly zoomed past him. It made me curious as to who informed him that the president had been shot, because his was the first phone call with the scoop to Cronkite, who was live on CBS News.

In 2005, Rather was encouraged to resign as the *CBS Evening News* lead anchor after a scandal over purported phony memos about President George W. Bush's Air National Guard service during the Vietnam War. His departure was, in my view, 42 years too late. In 2015, a docudrama starring Robert Redford as Rather was made about the incident. Its title is *Truth*. You can find it on Netflix.

Since December 2016, away from broadcast news and relegated to sending out messages via social media, Rather expressed his disappointment about the election of Donald Trump as president. Scolding that "the press has a very important role to play" in keeping the erratic Republican accountable for his often-bizarre behavior, Rather has prompted newshounds to "do deep-digging investigative reporting, ask tough questions, particularly ask tough follow-up questions, and not be intimidated." Too bad he didn't follow that advice himself when it mattered.

Although Rather didn't care to tell his audience about JFK's missing brain, in time many other media outlets welcomed me and others on their programs to discuss the matter and its implications. The blizzard of lies from our government's snow job was melting with each shovelful of facts. It wasn't just the Kennedy case and other political assassinations that caused Americans to grow angry at our leaders; there was a myriad of governmental missteps that piled on citizens' distrust. From Nixon's Watergate downfall to the public lack of confidence in J. Edgar Hoover, to demands to end the Vietnam War, to revelations about CIA dirty deeds, skepticism was becoming a growth industry.

More Commissions
and Committees

In 1969, America traded Chief Justice of the U.S. Supreme Court Earl Warren for a similarly named gentleman, Warren Earl Burger, as our next high-court leader. Warren, who had been ready to resign his post before forced by LBJ to stay and work on the Commission named after him, was no doubt pleased to finally be set free. Burger served until his resignation in 1986 and was replaced by Associate Justice William Rehnquist. Warren died in 1974, at age 83, and Burger in 1995, at 87; both are buried at Arlington National Cemetery.

With Gerald Ford's ascendency as America's president, we had another example of a Warren Commission member whose career seemed blessed. From 1949 to 1973, Ford served as a Republican member of the U.S. Congress from Grand Rapids, Michigan. As House minority leader and an ally of Richard Nixon, Ford was a natural choice for vice president when Spiro Agnew resigned. While waiting for the vice president's official residence in Washington, D.C., to be remodeled, Ford was informed of the "smoking gun" audiotape that showed Nixon's failed attempt to blame Watergate on the CIA. For Ford's first four months as president, he had no vice president, but eventually the job went to New York Governor Nelson A. Rockefeller. Months later, Ford ended the Vietnam War. He remains the only U.S. president to have assumed the office without having been previously elected president or vice president. Ford's unpopular pardoning of Nixon, along with rampant economic inflation, contributed to his loss to Democratic Georgia Governor Jimmy Carter in the 1976 presidential election.

Ford considered another run in 1980 but was advised by fellow Republicans that the nomination would go to Ronald Reagan. Ford, the last surviving member of the Warren Commission, died at the age of 93, on December 26, 2006. His wife, Betty, died five years later, also at 93.

In 2008, a 500-page declassified FBI file on Ford was released, and it detailed the politician's mutually beneficial relationship with J. Edgar Hoover and the Bureau. In 1942, Ford had applied to become an FBI agent and passed a background test. The only blemish was that, at Yale, Ford had been an "isolationist" and active organizer of the America First Committee, which was against U.S. involvement in World War II. Ford soon withdrew his application for undisclosed reasons. Once

Ford became a member of the Warren Commission, he volunteered to work closely with Hoover's Deputy Director Deke DeLoach, the Bureau's liaison with the panel. DeLoach had had a listening device implanted in the room where the hearings were conducted, ostensibly for security reasons. But when he wanted to know what else was happening behind the scenes, Ford was his fly on the wall. DeLoach wrote that Ford was committed to keeping the Bureau apprised but had requested assurance that his disclosures would be kept off the record.

According to the file, a December 1963 memo from the then-congressman ratted on two unnamed Commissioners who rejected the Bureau's claim that the bullets that hit Kennedy all came from the book depository's sixth-floor window. And three unnamed Commissioners were confused about the government's trajectory theory of the shots. It was not stated whether the initial two doubters were part of these three skeptics. With only seven members, such dissension could spell trouble. But Ford promised DeLoach that there would be "no problem," although there was no elaboration about what he meant by that statement. The Commission's internal debates were apparently so serious that the group missed its expected deadline of July 1964 to issue its report, ahead of when the presidential campaigns would be gearing up. Instead, the report that indicated Lee Harvey Oswald was the sole assassin was not released until September. In another memo, DeLoach wrote that he discussed press leaks with Ford, insisting that the Bureau was not responsible for stories planted in *Newsweek* and the *Washington Post*. Both men agreed that they didn't like either publication, which had the same owners. Ford requested that the Bureau give him a copy of a confidential report, and DeLoach had it delivered in a special locked briefcase that Ford took with him on a family vacation.

After the conclusion of the Commission's work, Ford's cordiality with the Bureau continued. In 1965, he asked FBI technicians to check out his home for secretly installed listening devices, but none were found. On another occasion, he asked that background checks be performed on a household maid, as well as on a man with a Swedish accent who was running for office in Grand Rapids but had not answered certain personal questions to Ford's satisfaction. The FBI file also showed flattering correspondence between Ford and Hoover, including notes of sympathy from the latter when Ford's parents died and of appreciation when Ford praised the Bureau on the House floor. Hoover also sent Ford a signed copy of a book he wrote and an autographed publicity photograph. After a party at DeLoach's home, attended by Hoover as well as Jerry and Betty Ford, the director wrote a gushing note, stating his pride in a congressman so "alert and vigorous" and offering him a tour of FBI headquarters. Not covered in the declassified file was whether Hoover or the Bureau had influence over Ford's misrepresentation of President Kennedy's bullet wound, which shifted it four inches higher—from JFK's back to his neck—to conform to the single shooter idea.

In the early stages of the Warren Commission, Hoover testified that Oswald acted alone, and there was no conspiracy. When Ford asked him to confirm that

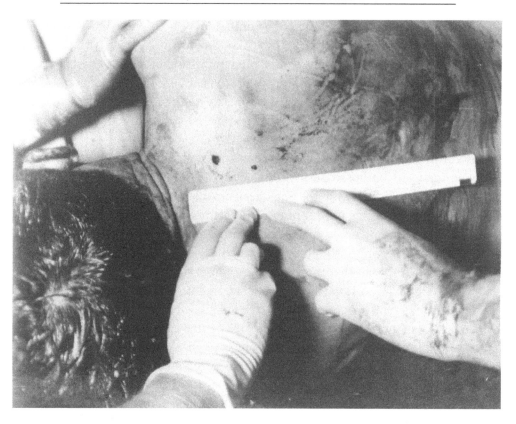

A declassified FBI file indicated that, while a member of the Warren Commission, Congressman Gerald Ford redefined the bullet wound to JFK's back as occurring four inches higher to comport with the "one lone shooter" scenario. Rewarded for his perfidy, Ford went on to serve as Richard Nixon's vice president, and, when Nixon resigned in 1974, Ford became the nation's 38th president (Wecht Collection).

Oswald was never an FBI informant, Hoover lied, "That is correct. I couldn't make it more emphatic." He added that, as director, he and his top associates would know and approve of anyone working as a Bureau informant. Hoover never again testified under oath in the matter. He died on May 2, 1972, at the age of 77 and is buried in Washington, D.C.'s Congressional Cemetery.

After the flurry of media attention over my disclosure about the president's missing brain, I was booked as a public speaker at assassination conferences beginning in the fall of 1972 and continuing through today. From October through early December, I am scheduled solidly, sometimes to deliver the keynote address and other times as part of a panel, or both. It's a part of my career that I enjoy, and it's always satisfying to deliver these speeches to full houses and receptive audiences. The fashions and hairstyles may change but the elan and great questions persist from Kennedy buffs who are always up-to-date with case news and views.

In 1970, I had become the chief coroner for Allegheny County, and eventually one of the doctors who worked for me was Robert P. Smith, whose background in engineering was valuable in reconstructing crime scenes and, in the JFK case, calculating the movement of the limousine, the people, and the bullets. He studied my notes from my visit to the National Archives and about the Zapruder film. In 1974, we coauthored the article "Medical Evidence in the Assassination of President John F. Kennedy," which was published in the *Journal of Forensic Science*. Despite the fact that this was a trade publication, the article was picked up and promoted in the media and caught attention in Washington, D.C. President Ford had the unfortunate timing of being in office during a period where Americans felt great unease toward their country's leadership. Not only was the smoke from so many political assassinations still thick in the air but also books and articles abounded that cast blame squarely on the government. I certainly did my part to inform the public that their cynicism was reasonable with the article I coauthored for the journal.

It wasn't just the assassinations that caused concern. News reports on the extraordinary means by which the FBI and CIA spied on and punished its citizens were commonplace. The names of CIA employee E. Howard Hunt and admitted spy and anti–Castro operative Frank Sturgis became known as more than just Watergate burglars with ties to the Nixon White House. Now, serious journalists were investigating whether the two men with confessed ties to the CIA's covert actions throughout South America and the Caribbean also had involvement in President Kennedy's murder. As previously mentioned, in response to all the criticism, on January 4, 1975, President Ford signed an Executive Order, appointing a nine-man Commission on CIA Activities Within the U.S., better known as the "Rockefeller Commission," since it was chaired by Vice President Nelson Rockefeller.

The Commission's executive director was David W. Belin, who had been an assistant counsel for the Warren Commission and had recently written a book asserting that Lee Harvey Oswald was JFK's lone assassin. Why anyone would think that Belin would be an unbiased party tips that the Rockefeller Commission was doomed from the get-go. In 1999, Belin slipped and fell in Rochester, Minnesota, suffering a head injury that put him in a coma for days before he died. During the 12 days he was unconscious, family members whispered Kennedy assassination conspiracy theories in his ear, in an attempt to rouse him. Other commissioners were John T. Connor, LBJ's former U.S. secretary of commerce, with ties to both the military and the pharmaceutical industry; C. Douglas Dillon, a Republican and Eisenhower's U.S. ambassador to France and undersecretary of state, as well as the U.S. secretary of the treasury under Kennedy and Johnson; Erwin N. Griswold, a Republican and former dean of Harvard Law School, and U.S. solicitor general under Johnson and Nixon; Lane Kirkland, a Democrat and president of the AFL-CIO, the country's leading labor union; Lyman L. Lemnitzer, a U.S. Army general who served as chairman of the Joint Chiefs of Staff and later as supreme allied commander of NATO. He had engaged in several military operations against Castro and Cuba, including the Bay of Pigs, and had testified to the U.S. Senate about the radical political beliefs that got General Edwin Walker bounced from the military; Ronald W. Reagan, a Democrat-turned-Republican in 1962, former Hollywood actor and

Screen Actors Guild president; from 1967 to 1975, and the governor of California who would later run unsuccessfully for U.S. president in 1976 before winning in 1980 and serving two terms; and Edgar F. Shannon, Jr., former president of the University of Virginia who increased the recruitment of black students and faculty, and also opposed Nixon's invasion of Cambodia.

The Rockefeller Commission issued its final, 2,900-page report on June 10, 1975, with most of it assessing any possible involvement in the assassination by Hunt and Sturgis. Both men gave testimony and swore that they, respectively, were in Washington, D.C., and Miami, Florida, on November 22, 1963—and family members verified their whereabouts. There were reports that Hunt was the acting CIA station chief in Mexico City when Oswald visited in September and not just earlier as he had claimed. Still, the Commission found "no credible evidence" to contradict Hunt's and Sturgis' accounts and denied that Hunt worked in Mexico City in September 1963.

Further, the Commission countered a claim by some assassination critics that Hunt and Sturgis looked like two of the three clean-shaven tramps found in a boxcar in the railroad yard near Dealey Plaza immediately after the assassination. The men claimed they had been in a homeless shelter where they had gotten fresh clothes, then went to the freight car to hang out. No weapons were found on the trio who asserted they hadn't known about the assassination until Dallas police officers told them. As the drifters were walked to the sheriff's office for questioning, they were photographed by observers. Seven black-and-white photos exist, but the imagery is imperfect. Dallas cops apparently questioned the men, let them go, then conveniently lost all pertinent information, such as photos or fingerprints. The absence of verifiable identification led to conjecture about whether the men had a more nefarious purpose there that day. If there was a shooter on the grassy knoll, it was a reasonable thought that he had associates who could break down and hide his rifle while he made his escape. Moreover, there were accounts of unauthorized federal agents in the vicinity who could have eased access for an assassin and provided team members with credentials to ensure that only selected personnel were present. For experts familiar with intelligence capers, having operatives in place to assist a main player was good training.

FBI photographic expert Lyndal L. Shaneyfeld told the Rockefeller Commission that any resemblance between the tramps and Hunt and Sturgis was faulty, causing the panel to determine that any notion the CIA had planted the three men was unproven fantasy. In 1989, the three men were identified by Dallas police as Harold Doyle, John Forester Gedney, and Gus W. Abrams, and deemed unconnected to the assassination. In the decades to follow, other men have been named as the vagrants. One was the father of actor Woody Harrelson, who first gained fame as the dim-witted bartender in the sitcom *Cheers*, then attained a remarkable resume in feature films. Charles Harrelson was a Texas hit man who died in prison in 2007 after his conviction for the 1979 fatal contract shooting of a San Antonio federal judge at the request of a drug dealer. A career criminal, Harrelson was also rumored to have been a hired gun for Santo Trafficante and Jack Ruby, and involved in attempts to kill Fidel Castro, although he was never charged with any Cuba-related offense. When he was arrested for the judge's murder, he confessed to it, as well as to the Kennedy assassination, but later recanted both claims, stating that he was high on cocaine when he made the statements. Still, many JFK buffs believed he was the tallest and youngest of the three tramps.

Before he died of cancer in 1997, a man named Chauncey Marvin Holt went to extraordinary lengths to assure the world that he was one of the Dealey Plaza derelicts. He wrote letters to the editor, gave countless interviews, wrote a posthumously published autobiography titled *Self-Portrait of a Scoundrel* (Trine Day Books, 2013), and helped his daughter become an expert on the subject, continuing to tout his story after his demise. Holt's account was certainly powerful, but was it true? Holt, who would have been 42 in November 1963, said he was the eldest of the boxcar trio. He considered his JFK assignment as just one of many in a long, checkered career as an undercover intelligence operative. He stated that he had been an accountant for organized crime boss Meyer Lansky and used his talent as an artist to help the CIA, making phony IDs for the assassination team and for other covert jobs. He boasted of having numerous identities and businesses that could facilitate whatever spooky gig he was working at a particular time, and that he was a licensed pilot. He also claimed close working relationships with key members of the Dallas Police Department and city government, as well as with Joseph Ball, an attorney who served as an assistant counsel to the Warren Commission.

Holt said he didn't know Ruby, but they had associates in common, and that his only encounter with Oswald was a favorable impression when he saw the younger man working for the Fair Play for Cuba Committee in New Orleans. Holt's primary job in Dealey Plaza, he said, was to furnish guns to his fellow tramps, whom he identified as Charles Harrelson and Richard Montoya, who was also known as "Charles Rogers" and "Frenchy." Holt claimed to have met Montoya before through anti–Castro Cubans in Miami. Holt said he and his cohorts were questioned by the Dallas sheriff's deputies, as well as FBI agents. The trio told the officers they were undercover agents with the Bureau of Alcohol, Tobacco, and Firearms, and indeed had guns on them. Chauncey had two, he said, including a small and rare .45 caliber pistol that fascinated the federal agents. He later wrote that none of these guns were used to shoot the president but were intended solely for protection for himself and his fellow tramps in case trouble should arise. When they heard the gunfire and shouts that JFK had been shot, the men hid in the boxcar, feeling they had been set up. Although Holt said he didn't know who shot the president, he's certain that Oswald and Ruby were also tools of the forces who orchestrated the event.

Is it possible that a man who appeared disheveled and homeless could wax eloquently at length, with the knowledge that comes from studying a vast amount of documentation on the subject? Or was his profundity proof that he was a valuable intelligence asset, wanting to clear his conscience before shuffling off the mortal coil? I can't say, but I wish I knew.

I was one of the 51 witnesses who gave sworn testimony to the Rockefeller Commission. It began when I received a phone call in April 1975 from the panel's senior counsel, Robert B. Olsen, who asked for my views on the case. I was then invited to appear before the Commission provided I paid my own way to and from Washington, D.C., which I did. On May 7, I spent almost five hours being questioned by Olsen, who entered Bob Smith's and my *Journal of Forensic Science* article as an exhibit. I asked if I could give my testimony to the whole Commission, but David Belin denied my request.

Olsen was interested in having me admit that I had stated in the *Journal* piece and elsewhere that the evidence pointed to the president having been struck only by two bullets that came from the rear. Specifically, I had written in the article: "If any other bullet struck the President's head, whether before, after, or simultaneously with the known shot, there is no evidence for it in the available autopsy materials." Olsen and other of my critics suggest this means that no missile was fired from the grassy knoll area. As I explained to him and to countless others over the years, that is hardly the case, and they should focus on the last five words of my quote. What could have helped make a positive determination was the brain, which was conveniently missing. Also mitigating against a solo from-the-rear shooter was the president's body movement after the fatal head blow. That "back and to the left" movement, shown so clearly in the Zapruder film, could only have come from a front shot. As usual, the opposition was trying to win an argument by only citing facts to prop up its contention, rather than assessing all of the information. Hilariously, Olsen tried to cast doubt on my expertise by getting me to confess that I had never shot a rifle at a live target. He was right about that. As frustrated as I may have been by some of our government's apologists, I never once considered using them for live target practice!

Regarding the matter of the missing brain, Olsen stated that I should acknowledge it was in the possession of the Kennedy family, which had the right to do whatever it wished with it. I disputed both parts of that. I said I didn't know who had the brain, and it should be retained in a scientific setting where it could be microscopically examined by a qualified forensic pathologist, as would happen in any typical murder case. My questioning ended with Olsen attempting to ascertain that fees from my speeches about the assassination were fattening my bank account. I replied that almost every speech I gave on the subject—whether live on TV or radio, or in print—was done without payment, and the small amount I had ever received over the years probably represented less than 1 percent of my income and actually cost me money, considering the time it meant I had to take off from my actual job as the county coroner.

The Commission had a medical advisory panel consisting of U.S. Marine Corps Lieutenant Colonel Robert R. McMeekin, a forensic pathologist from the Armed Forces Institute of Pathology (original autopsy doctor Pierre Finck's alma mater);

Dr. Richard Lindenberg, the director of neuropathology and legal medicine from Baltimore's Department of Mental Health; Dr. Werner U. Spitz, the chief medical examiner from Wayne County, Michigan; Dr. Fred J. Hodges III, radiology professor from Baltimore's Johns Hopkins School of Medicine; and Dr. Alfred G. Olivier, a supervisory research veterinarian from the Aberdeen Proving Grounds in Maryland. They wrote separate reports but concluded that the shots came from behind and above the president, no bullet came from any other direction, and Kennedy's violent whiplash movement was not proof of a shot from the front. I was not the only outside medical expert who gave testimony for the Commission. J. Edgar Hoover's favorite urologist, Dr. John Lattimer, gave testimony, repeating his assertion that the bullets came from the depository's sixth-floor window. The Commission also interviewed Dr. E. Forrest Chapman, a medical examiner from Belleville, Michigan, and member of the far right-wing American Independent Party. Chapman's interview was conducted by telephone, possibly because he wasn't willing to pay for his own travel to our nation's capital. He studied the autopsy photos and X-rays before concluding that if there were any assassins firing at the president from the grassy knoll, "they must have been poor shots because they didn't hit anything." Whether he had been shown the Zapruder film at that point is unknown because he didn't factor in JFK's head movement.

Amid the ensuing public criticism of the Commission's choice of medical panelists, a group of other doctors and I presented a petition calling for full disclosure of all the scientific evidence. We might as well have been yelling into the Grand Canyon. The next month when the report was made public, I hit the roof. The Commission determined that there was no evidence that proved Kennedy was struck by bullets from two directions. In a flagrant misrepresentation of my testimony to Robert Olsen, the authors had artfully edited my quotes to support their assertions. The next day I gave an interview to the Associated Press that blasted the Commission, saying that the panel's summary distorted my views on the case and demanded that they release the full transcript. My demand was denied on grounds of "national security." As I stated in my interview: "If that transcript shows in any way that I have withdrawn or revised my thoughts of the Warren Report, I'll eat the transcript on the steps of the White House." When I calmed down, I realized that despite their editing being utterly reprehensible and despicable, it was also a great compliment that they would consider my testimony that much of a threat. I followed up with an article titled "Why is the Rocky Commission So Single-Minded about a Lone Assassin in the Kennedy Case?" that was published in the July/August 1975 *Journal of Legal Medicine*. And I was interviewed at length for a two-part article by Washington editor Ken Rankin in the October and November 1975 issues of *Physician's Management* titled: "A Civilian M.D. in on the Kennedy Autopsy Says More Than One Gun Killed JFK." You can read my testimony at the maryferrell.org archive.

In the end, the Rockefeller Commission found that the intelligence community had been out of control and listed 30 recommendations to tighten up procedures. In its summation, the Commission failed to mention the missing autopsy materials. The March 6, 1975, broadcast of the Zapruder film on the ABC late-night television program, *Good Night America* featuring Geraldo Rivera, illustrated to the nation what I had been saying since I had first seen the footage myself years earlier: The final bullet that exploded the president's head was shot from the front right, causing JFK to jerk violently backward and toward the left. It was simple physics, and one didn't need a college degree to understand it. That television airing released the genie from the bottle, and there would be no forcing it back inside. Citizens who might have just thought of the assassination in the abstract were confronting it

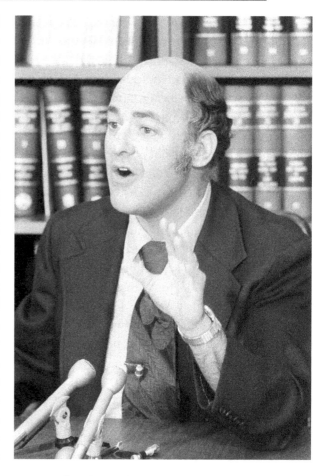

Furious that the Rockefeller Commission distorted my testimony, I held a press conference on June 12, 1975, and aired my complaints (Associated Press/Charles Bennett).

in the comfort of their living rooms, and it made them realize how the government had persistently lied to them about what happened to JFK. For the next week's follow-up show, Geraldo called me to be a guest. His invitation came as I was on a family vacation in Vail, Colorado. With their approval, I left my wife and kids on a ski slope and flew to New York City for the live program. As Geraldo ran the Zapruder footage, I narrated how the bullets his Kennedy and Connally. The show was a ratings smash.

As you'll recall, the Warren Commission was only established after LBJ and J. Edgar Hoover panicked at learning that both the U.S. House of Representatives and the U.S. Senate were embarking on their own investigations into JFK's murder. In 1975, history repeated itself as both of the legislative bodies created their own studies on the broader issue of intelligence malfeasance. The Senate established an 11-member Select Committee to Study Governmental Operations with Respect to Intelligence Activities to delve into the 58 federal agencies involved in government law enforcement or intelligence. The goal was to determine whether those agencies' covert and overt dealings were necessary and legal. The chair of that new select committee was Idaho's Democratic senator, Frank F. Church.

The Church Committee heard testimony in the summer and fall of 1975 and brought out eye-opening information on Operation Mongoose, the CIA's plan to assassinate Fidel Castro. An inextricable connection was made between these attempts and the American mobsters who provided assistance for the failed capers. Chicago crime boss Sam Giancana once described the Cosa Nostra and the CIA as being "different sides of the same coin." Days before Giancana was due to give testimony to the Church Committee, he was found shot to death in the kitchen of his Oak Park, Illinois, home. His associate, Johnny Roselli, testified three times for the committee and was asked what he knew about any conspiracy to kill President Kennedy. He was due to appear for a fourth session, with the JFK case as the main topic, when he went missing on July 28, 1976. The FBI investigated the disappearance, and on August 9, Roselli's decomposing remains were recovered from a 55-gallon metal container floating in the waters near Miami, Florida. Who wanted these two men dead, and why? Other factions of the mafia? The CIA? The FBI? Castro? There are good arguments for any scenario.

The House version was a 10-member Select Committee on Intelligence, chaired by Michigan's Democratic representative, Lucien N. Nedzi, who was also the chairman of the House Armed Services Intelligence Subcommittee. Their primary focus was on possible misdeeds by the CIA and FBI, but they also examined the National Reconnaissance Office (NRO), which was collecting space satellite-based intelligence. When news reports revealed that Nedzi had known about CIA involvement in the Watergate break-in but had not reported it to the full House, there were concerns that he was too friendly with the agency to be in charge of investigating it. He resigned from the committee, and later that year, the full House voted to create a new committee, chaired by New York's Democratic representative, Otis G. Pike. Eight members of Nedzi's panel joined the new committee, and three new members were added.

Both Select Committees completed their work in April 1976, just in time for the Gerald Ford versus Jimmy Carter presidential race. Carter made hay with the idea that, if elected, cleaning up the intelligence abuse of the past would be a top priority. To my mind, both committees sacrificed a forest's worth of trees to generate paperwork that didn't say much. There was general agreement that we could and should do better, and plenty of bloviating about how change could be implemented. The best thing was the creation of an ongoing Senate Select Committee on Intelligence. It was an admirable addition, but one governing future deeds, not past ones. The House Permanent Select Committee on Intelligence was established the next year. In case you're wondering whether I was called to testify before either of these panels, the answer is no—not that I didn't try to be included. While Capitol Hill chose not to hear what I had to say, the American public's curiosity was still burning as bright as the eternal flame on JFK's grave.

The House Select Committee on Assassinations

In October 1976, I appeared on the ABC News program *20/20* to demonstrate the irrationality of Arlen Specter's single-bullet theory and garnered a lot of positive feedback from viewers. That same year, the House of Representatives established a panel to probe whether our national intelligence agencies and policies were responsible for the murders of President John F. Kennedy and the Rev. Martin Luther King, Jr. It would be a two-year investigation costing $5.8 million, but I believe that was money well spent, although why they excluded Senator Robert F. Kennedy's murder is mystifying.

The House Select Committee on Assassinations was first helmed by Virginia Democrat Thomas N. Downing, but he retired and ceded the leadership to Texas Democrat Henry B. Gonzalez. I was delighted that Gonzalez took over because I had been impressed with his forcefulness on issues in the news and felt he had the right temperament for this job. I was especially happy that the committee's chief counsel was Richard A. Sprague, a hard-boiled prosecutor from Philadelphia. He was the chief deputy district attorney in his office, and his specialty was homicide. Finally, now the Kennedy case would be handled by someone who knew how to put together a proper investigation! Alas, my optimism waned when the two men had difficulties working together, sparring over budgets and methods. Gonzalez resigned, and Sprague soon followed after the CIA refused to cooperate with his questions about Oswald in Mexico. Sprague's expert deputy, Robert K. Tanenbaum, was the next to resign.

Despite its turbulent beginnings, the committee coalesced and was extended for another two-year term. A Democratic congressman from Ohio, Louis Stokes, was now the chair. His chief counsel and staff director was G. Robert Blakey, a former professor at both Notre Dame and Cornell University law schools, who had served as a consultant on organized crime and racketeering for Presidents Johnson and Nixon. Blakey would bring those same skills to the HSCA, obtaining and listening to vast amounts of wiretapped conversations between mobsters with grudges against JFK. I had never met Blakey before, but it became abundantly clear that he manifested palpable hostility toward me and was unwavering in his support of the Warren Commission's view of the medical evidence. Most of the other members of the panel were Democrats: L. Richardson Preyer of North Carolina, Walter E. Fauntroy of the District of Columbia, Yvonne Brathwaite Burke of California, Christopher Dodd of Connecticut, Harold Ford, Sr., of Tennessee, Floyd Fithian of Indiana, and Robert W. Edgar of Pennsylvania. The Republican members were Samuel L. Devine of Ohio, Stewart McKinney of Connecticut, Charles Thone of Nebraska, and Harold S. Sawyer of Michigan.

The HSCA's probe included assembling a nine-person forensic pathology panel, and I was a member. Rather than wait for an invitation that might not come, I requested that I be allowed to give testimony and my request was granted. The other eight members were Michael M. Baden, the panel's chairman and the chief medical examiner of New York City; John I. Coe, the chief medical examiner of Hennepin County, Minnesota; Joseph H. Davis, the chief medical examiner of Dade County, Florida; George S. Loquvam, the director of the Institute of Forensic Sciences in Oakland, California; Charles S. Petty, the chief medical examiner of Dallas County, in Dallas, Texas; Earl Rose, the former Dallas medical examiner who should have performed JFK's autopsy and was currently a professor of pathology at the University of Iowa in Iowa City, Iowa; Werner U. Spitz, the medical examiner of Detroit, Michigan; and James T. Weston, the chief medical investigator at the University of New Mexico in Albuquerque, New Mexico. We had all reviewed the autopsy report, as well as authenticated photographs and X-rays, and other pertinent data.

Blakey's influence on our medical panel was crystal clear as he tried to close down inquiries and steer the other doctors toward another whitewash conclusion. After several long sessions where we debated the medical evidence among ourselves, I found myself alone in speaking out against the single-bullet and sole-assassin theories. When the panelists tried to insinuate that the single-bullet notion was credible because JFK "could have" bent over, I laughed loudly and reminded them the Zapruder film makes clear that the president was not tying his shoelace or scratching his groin at just that right moment. They all knew that, but that's how desperate they were to justify their absurd claim. At one point, I openly challenged the other eight pathologists on the panel regarding the weight and condition of this magic bullet: "Go back to your respective cities and search through the thousands and thousands of bullets you have recovered from cadavers and show me one bullet that has done what you say this bullet has done and looks like this bullet looks." I asked my colleagues on the panel to reconstruct or repeat the bullet firing test. When Blakey nixed that, saying such a test was too expensive, I offered to pay all the costs for such an experiment. He still refused. I could not believe it. The other doctors even stated that a cadaver bone would be different than a bone in a live person. It was not like I was asking to have an Egyptian pharaoh exhumed and used in the experiment!

One of the three Bethesda autopsy doctors testified before our panel on March 11, 1978, at the National Archives. Pierre A. Finck, who was brought in from the Armed Forces Institute of Pathology after the president's procedure was already underway and had been living in Brussels, Belgium, since 1970, was a familiar face to me. The last time I had seen him was at my American Academy of Forensic Sciences' lecture where he privately expressed the utter panic at the postmortem and his reluctance to reveal the horrors he beheld. Now, under oath, he would finally talk, and I would be one of the panelists asking questions. In a cordial, conversational tone, I asked him to cite his professional experience before we delved into the autopsy information. While the years had calmed his nerves, they hadn't improved his memory—he couldn't recall which Army general instructed him not to dissect the bullet wounds in Kennedy's back and neck. He stated he was the one who ordered the full-body X-ray to confirm there was no intact bullet in the corpse, since the upper back/lower neck wound had no exit wound, and there were only metallic fragments in the head.

The brain had already been removed from the skull when he arrived, Finck explained. When asked to describe where the back of the head entrance was, he used my head as a guide and pointed to about 2.5 centimeters to the right of the midline, just above the bony occipital protuberance. All of his notes and measurements were handed over to Dr. Humes, he said, and none of the doctors were able to review the photographs or X-rays taken during the procedure before their report was written. He didn't even have the materials when he testified before the Warren Commission in 1964, because Arlen Specter said the then–U.S. Attorney General Bobby Kennedy would not make those items available. When the three doctors visited the National Archives in 1967, they learned the brain was missing, and although Finck believed they should list the autopsy as "incomplete," Humes convinced him it had accomplished its purposes to determine the number of wounds, the direction of the projectiles, and the cause of death. It wasn't ideal, but Finck found it satisfactory. He dismissed rumors that shots had come from the front and stated that even if he had seen the images before signing the report, he wouldn't have changed his mind.

As for the other two autopsy doctors, much later I learned that most, if not all, of my eight colleagues had a private interview with Drs. Humes and Boswell. I never heard whether the Bethesda duo declined to testify if I was present, but, incredibly, no one felt an ethical duty to disclose this big secret to me.

On September 7, 1978, I took my turn on the hot seat. Staff counsel Donald A. Purdy, Jr., did most of the questioning, but others contributed input as well. I cannot accuse any of the members of short-changing me when it came to my being able to discuss a myriad of issues that I felt needed attention, from the single-bullet theory to my ideas of how I would like to harness their investigation, if given the opportunity. Like the other panel members, I was given 30 minutes to make my case, and I used every second of it. The representatives and staffers were polite and seemed intrigued by my testimony. After I made the point that the president's brain was missing and unavailable for study, Purdy asked to what extent access to the brain would detect whether JFK was hit by a shot from the front. I resisted laughing out loud and merely replied that examining the brain could determine whether more than one bullet had penetrated it, as well as possible directionality of the missile or missiles. Later, I expressed to Congressman Robert Edgar that I felt the proper procedure should include deposing under oath all parties who might have had knowledge of or involvement with the chain of custody of the brain and other autopsy material. If that failed to turn up the items, at least the record would show that a sincere attempt was made. I added that if the brain were recovered, it should be examined by a well-qualified expert in forensic pathology or neuropathology.

On March 29, 1979, the HSCA released its final report. In the section dealing with the missing brain and other material, the committee recounted its efforts to locate the items, which included getting perfunctory statements from the key individuals at the National Archives and within the Kennedy offices. Nobody was put under oath. When all individuals responded that they didn't know what happened to the goods, that was the end of the subject. Kennedy family attorney Burke Marshall basically put the onus on the now-slain Bobby Kennedy as being the likely source for whatever occurred with that critical evidence.

The other eight doctors were unanimous in their conclusion that JFK was shot by two bullets, both which entered from above and behind him—corroborating the Warren Commission findings. I, of course, could not hop aboard that bandwagon. I wrote a solo dissenting opinion that the single-bullet concept was impossible and included drawings to illustrate my view. In my five-page, single-spaced letter for the record, I stated that Professor Blakey was dismissive of my suggestions to conduct tests to replicate the contention of the panel regarding the single missile that it insisted did such damage to the president and Governor Connally yet was apparently recovered in pristine condition. My letter and exhibits are online at the Mary Ferrell site.

Of course, the authors of the HSCA report got the last word. An addendum states: "The panel majority has considered all the issues raised by the panel minority of one. The conclusions of the panel majority remain unchanged in the absence of additional bona fide evidence." It was troubling that my brethren on our forensic pathology panel all echoed the Warren Commission findings. I had known some of these men for decades and respected their experience and competency, but I couldn't justify their positions on this case. A frequently asked question is if the Warren Commission missed the boat so badly, as I say it did, then why did so many of my colleagues disagree with my assessment? I believe it was a predetermined mindset on the part of the other panelists that a cover-up or conspiracy of this magnitude by the federal government was unthinkable or, at the very least, unlikely. Just as lawyers disagree over what a particular law or court ruling means, forensic pathologists frequently have differences of opinion.

I have no reason whatsoever to doubt the other doctors' sincerity. However, it should be noted that many of these same people had a long-standing involvement with the federal government, and many had received research grants and appointments to various influential governmental boards. To be overly critical of a government action might end that friendly relationship with Uncle Sam. It was around this time that I began seeing doors once opened to me as a nationally recognized forensic pathologist starting to close. Several invitations to participate as a faculty member in seminars at the Armed Forces Institute of Pathology were no longer offered to me. There is no doubt that if I had kept my mouth shut and toed the government line in the Kennedy case, I would have been appointed to many more medicolegal positions directly or indirectly controlled by the U.S. government. I also have gotten the cold shoulder from several national pathology organizations since I became an outspoken critic of the Warren Commission.

Beyond the medical testimony, there were more fruitful developments in the HSCA probe. In the 15 years since the assassination, great strides had been made in forensic science, and the panel availed itself of more sophisticated tests and experts. Sadly, this also meant that the government could use better sources to lie about the evidence, as in the case of the ballistic evidence that the committee linked to Oswald's rifle to the exclusion of any other weapon. Its way of dealing with the magic bullet was to just deny it. A team of photographic experts also weighed in to verify the accuracy of all the photos and X-rays of JFK and Oswald, and reject that there was any tampering. Handwriting experts linked Oswald's penmanship to the rifle purchase, the application form for the post office box, and the signature on his backyard photo where he held the rifle. And Oswald's fingerprints and palm print were matched to the rifle, boxes in the sniper's nest, and on the brown paper bag used to bring the weapon to work. No one ever denied that those items should be linked to Oswald, but were they part of a plan to make him the fall guy or even left there after his death to frame him? The HSCA never considered those possibilities.

Days before the HSCA was scheduled to wrap up its session, significant new evidence was unveiled by acoustics experts who had obtained an audiotape. The recording had been made from a Dallas police officer's radio microphone as the officer, who was riding his motorcycle with the presidential motorcade, talked with a dispatcher back at the police station. All radio transmissions between officers and the dispatchers are routinely recorded on a Dictabelt, the state-of-the-art method of the era. The analysis of the tape recording, several independent nongovernmental experts testified, made it clear—there were four gunshots fired at President Kennedy, three from the back and one from the right front, the area of the grassy knoll. Much later, new testing would provide different interpretations of the sounds on Dealey Plaza that day.

In its final report, the House Select Committee ruled that, with a high degree of probability, President Kennedy had indeed been the victim of a conspiracy and that there was little doubt a second gunman was involved. However, the committee added, the second gunman missed his target. The committee went on to say that certain members of the Mafia had the motive and means to kill our leader, but there was no direct evidence proving it beyond a reasonable doubt.

At last, the ball was really rolling, I thought. Now we will be seeing some serious action. The Kennedy case will be officially reopened, new evidence will be unveiled, and possibly additional suspects will be brought to justice. Here you had the Congress of the United States, the governmental body that most represents the general public, finally saying the Kennedy assassination did not happen the way we had been told. I thought that would certainly force the FBI or the Justice Department to take immediate action and find out once and for all what happened that day in Dallas. I could not have been more wrong. Not only was there no intensive, massive investigation but also essentially nothing at all happened thereafter. The response by the FBI and Justice Department was zero. Each agency said they planned to examine the evidence that the House Select Committee had uncovered. To its everlasting discredit, the committee did not press the FBI or the executive branch of government to do anything about their findings. They simply presented them as if it were an academic exercise. My frustration level by this point was at an all-time high.

The HSCA also determined that Martin Luther King, Jr.'s death was also part of a likely conspiracy but hedged about blaming the government and gave full credit to James Earl Ray as the assassin who fired the fatal rifle shot. Although the panel's investigation filled 12 volumes and included a single-volume summary, the underlying documents were put under seal for 50 years. That would eventually change and lead to the creation of the Assassination Records Review Board.

An upcoming book entitled *Medical Betrayal* by a British physiologist and lecturer named Russell Kent will shed new light on the inner workings of the HSCA. The depth of Mr. Kent's research has greatly impressed me.

Willem Oltmans and
George de Mohrenschildt

Jumping back a bit in time, in the early part of 1977, I received a phone call from a man named Willem Leonard Oltmans. I had heard about him in the Kennedy assassination circles, as he had been following the case for years, but we hadn't spoken before. He set up a meeting that would be memorable for several reasons.

Oltmans was born in the Netherlands but educated at Yale at the same time William F. Buckley, Jr., attended the university. On graduation, the latter joined the Central Intelligence Agency, and the former returned to his native land to begin a lengthy career as a globe-trotting journalist, often writing pieces that rankled the Dutch government. He emigrated to the United States in 1958 and had connections in North Vietnam, Cuba, New Guinea, South Africa, and Indonesia. Whether he was recruited by the CIA or he was its sworn enemy is up in the air, but he liked to be in the thick of whatever intrigue was roiling. Since there was no bigger journalistic story worldwide than JFK's assassination, Oltmans delved into it, befriending Marguerite Oswald and writing articles about her view that her son was the victim of a conspiracy. Later, Oltmans helped Jim Garrison with press coverage for his prosecution of Clay Shaw.

Oltmans claimed to have been told by a Dutch psychic, Gerard Croiset, that a man fitting George de Mohrenschildt's description had manipulated Lee Harvey Oswald into becoming the fall guy in the assassination. Croiset believed that the phantom string-puller, at the behest of Texas oil millionaires, arranged for the president's murder using voodoo techniques he had perfected in Haiti. Marguerite helped Oltmans track down de Mohrenschildt, the Belarus-born geologist who was Oswald's mentor after Oswald's return to the States from Russia with his bride Marina. Oltmans was 14 years younger than de Mohrenschildt, but the two men shared the same patrician roots and love of adventure. I had known about de Mohrenschildt, of course, but hadn't met or spoken to him. De Mohrenschildt told Oltmans that he had a fond friendship with Oswald but had no part in the assassination.

As the House Select Committee began preparing to hear testimony, no schedule was made public about who would be called as a witness, and when—but it seemed obvious to me that the panel would definitely want to hear from de Mohrenschildt, and I guessed that he would be an early witness. What I couldn't have known was that he was an absolute basket case about what he was going to say. He was also distressed from the 1973 death of his daughter, who had suffered from the same disease that had claimed her brother in 1960.

In September 1976, de Mohrenschildt felt he was getting death threats and decided to reach out to then–CIA director and future U.S. president George H.W. Bush. Years before, Bush had been a prep school roommate of de Mohrenschildt's cousin, although there is no evidence the two Georges had ever met. De Mohrenschildt's letter read (typos intact):

> You will excuse this hand-written letter. Maybe you will be able to bring a solution to the hopeless situation I find myself in. My wife and I find ourselves surrounded by some vigilantes; our phone bugged; and we are being followed everywhere. Either FBI is involved in this or they do not want to accept my complaints. We are driven to insanity by the situation. I have been behaving like a damn fool ever since my daughter Nadya died from [cystic fibrosis] over three years ago. I tried to write, stupidly and unsuccessfully, about Lee H Oswald and must have angered a lot of people—I do not know. But to punish an elderly man like myself and my highly nervous and sick wife is really too much. Could you do something to remove the net around us? This will be my last request for help and I will not annoy you any more. Good luck in your important job. Thank you so much.

Bush replied:

> Let me say first that I know it must have been difficult for you to seek my help in the situation outlined in your letter. I believe I can appreciate your state of mind in view of your daughter's tragic death a few years ago, and the current poor state of your wife's health. I was extremely sorry to hear of these circumstances. In your situation I can well imagine how the attentions you described in your letter affect both you and your wife. However, my staff has been unable to find any indication of interest in your activities on the part of Federal authorities in recent years. The flurry of interest that attended your testimony before the Warren Commission has long subsided. I can only speculate that you may have become "newsworthy" again in view of the renewed interest in the Kennedy assassination, and thus may be attracting the attention of people in the media. I hope this letter had been of some comfort to you, George, although I realize I am unable to answer your question completely.

The exchange caused the CIA to urge the FBI to keep an eye on de Mohrenschildt and shortly thereafter he was scheduled to give his testimony to the HSCA—but he would never keep that appointment.

Sometime in the first few weeks of 1977, I got a phone call from Oltmans who said he was at de Mohrenschildt's home in Dallas. He said de Mohrenschildt was fearful about his upcoming appearance and asked if I would fly there and convey what I knew about the HSCA. I wasn't going to turn down the opportunity to meet both of these men, so I flew there and spent a long afternoon with them at de Mohrenschildt's home, which he had designed. They told me that they had been audio recording de Mohrenschildt's story over the years and were intent on turning it into an autobiography. Oltmans was helping with the editing and looking for a publisher. De Mohrenschildt had been working as an assistant professor of foreign languages at Bishop College, a small, local liberal arts school. He and his wife Jeanne had quietly divorced in 1973 but maintained a close relationship. She wasn't present for our meeting.

When it came to relating what de Mohrenschildt might expect in front of the HSCA, I couldn't speak from personal experience because, at that time, my request to testify had not yet been granted. But from reading the Warren Commission Report, I knew that de Mohrenschildt had given two full days of testimony, which may have been more than any other witness. This HSCA grilling would be a different panel but basically the same structure. I was puzzled why he seemed unnerved about this Commission when his responses had been so assured with the Warren panel. Yes, it was years later, and many more questions had surfaced about de Mohrenschildt's connections to Oswald, but he and Jeanne had been in Haiti at the time of the president's murder. They had a solid alibi, and no one could logically accuse him of long-distance voodoo. But the upcoming event was making him uneasy. I suggested that he try to bring an attorney in the room with him, who could intercede if need be—and that he should first tell his full story to an attorney he trusted. I wanted him to talk to an outside party besides Oltmans whose duties as a journalist might not protect de Mohrenschildt's legal rights. Oltmans seemed to agree with that idea, too.

George was kicking himself over answers he gave the Warren Commission which, to him now, seemed glib and unsupportive of Oswald, whom he enjoyed intellectually. If the Warren lawyers could trick him into talking trash about his young friend, he groused, the HSCA lawyers might make him go even farther into accusing Oswald of acts of murder. When I asked de Mohrenschildt's opinion of Oswald, he replied that he was bothered by Oswald's increasingly extremist views, such as he held toward General Edwin Walker. But Oswald had only said good things about JFK, so being charged with the president's murder was difficult to comprehend. He regretted that he never had a chance to talk to Oswald about what happened on that day but said he was inclined to believe Oswald's last words to reporters: "I am a patsy." De Mohrenschildt personally believed Kennedy was shot by some anti–Castro Cubans who were still angry about the Bay of Pigs.

When I asked de Mohrenschildt if he was, or had ever been, a CIA agent he denied it but admitted that many people assumed that he was. He *had* encountered CIA operatives in his travels and was debriefed by intelligence agents when he returned to the states from certain countries. In Dallas, de Mohrenschildt and his wife socialized with J. Walton Moore, the CIA's local head of the Domestic Contact Division. It was Moore, he said, to whom they complained when they learned Oswald had been beating up Marina. But Moore insisted that Oswald was "a harmless lunatic" and encouraged them to stay in the ex–Marine's life. At one point, de Mohrenschildt suspected that Moore or his colleagues had broken into his home and photocopied files about Oswald when the de Mohrenschildts were out of town, but Moore denied it. De Mohrenschildt said one of the things he was finding hard to process was that so many people who knew him over the years would now and forever connect his name to the Kennedy assassination instead of his other accomplishments. During the period when de Mohrenschildt gave testimony to the Warren Commission, he told me that on more than one occasion he would privately eat lunch with Allen Dulles. I was stunned to hear that the former CIA director would extend an invitation for an off-the-record meeting with *any* witness, but de Mohrenschildt insisted that that the Kennedy case was not discussed and that the conversations centered solely on foreign oil exploration. De Mohrenschildt clearly walked on clouds of rarified air.

After a while, de Mohrenschildt said he needed to take a nap, which allowed me a more private meeting with Oltmans. He was worried about his friend who had always seemed of sound mind and athletic even for a 65-year-old. But now de Mohrenschildt was having a mental breakdown, with suicidal depression, paranoia, and delusions where he would hear voices and see visions. He told Jeanne that the CIA was coming to get them. It got so bad, Oltmans said, that in November 1976, Jeanne had her former husband institutionalized for weeks at Parkland Hospital where he was given a regimen of strong anti-anxiety drugs. Privately I wondered if being in that particular hospital might have increased his distress. On some days, de Mohrenschildt was enthused about writing his book, Oltmans said, but on others he panicked about what could happen if he divulged what he knew. Oltmans was still trying to ferret out the details behind de Mohrenschildt's relationship with Oswald and whether de Mohrenschildt might have had advance knowledge of the murder. I flew back to Pittsburgh wondering whether Oltmans had de Mohrenschildt's best interests in mind or if he was contributing to de Mohrenschildt's angst. I never saw or spoke to de Mohrenschildt or Oltmans again.

In early March 1977, de Mohrenschildt told Oltmans that he wanted to leave the United States, so the men flew to Europe. They packed a copy of de Mohrenschildt's completed manuscript, which was titled *I Am a Patsy!*, and Oltmans had scheduled a meeting with a Dutch publisher. Oltmans brought de Mohrenschildt to Brussels where some friends, including a KGB officer, would join them for lunch. De Mohrenschildt said he wanted to take a short walk and would be back in an hour. Instead, he left Europe and returned to the United States.

De Mohrenschildt went to visit Alexandra, his daughter from his first marriage, who had been staying with a friend in Manalapan, Florida, about an hour north of Miami. He had apparently expressed suicidal ideations to his daughter. On Tuesday, the 29th, he was interviewed by author Edward Jay Epstein, who had written the Kennedy book *Inquest*, and the author asked George pointblank if he was a paid employee of the CIA. De Mohrenschildt said no, but he had done some occasional favors for CIA agents who, in turn, helped with his overseas business interests. That same day, Gaeton Fonzi, an investigator with the HSCA who wanted to discuss de Mohrenschildt's appearance before the panel, stopped by the Manalapan home. De Mohrenschildt wasn't home, but Alexandra was. Fonzi handed her his business card, which she gave to her father when he returned. He put it in his shirt pocket, then walked upstairs, sat in a chair, and blew his brains out with a rifle. The coroner's office ruled the death a suicide, and when the HSCA probed the death, its investigators concurred with the coroner.

De Mohrenschildt could have had a fatally guilty conscience, regardless of whether he was involved in the conspiracy. He might have felt he should have done more to report to authorities Oswald's criminally dangerous frame of mind, especially after the Walker shooting when he was well aware that his young friend had attempted to murder someone. But the prevailing conjecture is on him agreeing to babysit the Oswalds for the CIA in exchange for the agency's help with de Mohrenschildt's business efforts in Haiti. While he flatly denied that when I asked him, others closer to him had a different view. Even his former son-in-law Gary Edward Taylor, who divorced Mohrenschildt's elder daughter before JFK was gunned down, was suspicious of the mysterious White Russian's possible connections to the CIA. In testimony before the Warren Commission, Taylor noted the extensive travel George and Jeanne de Mohrenschildt had made, including countries behind the Iron Curtain and those where Cuban refugees were being trained to invade Cuba. Taylor added that it had occurred to him from the beginning that "if there was any assistance or plotters in the assassination that it was, in my opinion, most probably the de Mohrenschildts."

Fonzi's own digging assured him that de Mohrenschildt was a "CIA intelligence asset" and said that CIA records proved that contention. He believed George felt he was being set up by Oltmans for the purpose of making him seem like he was a KGB agent, which would have provided a link for people to think of Oswald as a KGB operative. Fonzi also noted that around the time of the assassination, $200,000 in deposits from a Bahamian bank appeared in de Mohrenschildt's Haitian bank account, ostensibly as payment for George and a partner operating a sisal plantation that they actually never visited. Was that accurate or was it monies from the CIA for services rendered, paid through a shelter account? Fonzi never got to the bottom of that deal.

One interesting sidebar to this story involves the former host of Fox News' *The O'Reilly Factor*, Bill O'Reilly, who has long refused to see any evidence of a conspiracy behind the president's murder. As he described in his book, *Killing Kennedy: The End of Camelot*, O'Reilly spent considerable time as a professional journalist looking for proof that Oswald had associates but never found any. But what O'Reilly *did* find, according to the book, was trouble. He wrote that as a Dallas-based WFAA-TV reporter, he traveled to Florida to track down de Mohrenschildt and showed up at the home where he was staying. As he knocked on the door, he heard from inside the gunshot that took de Mohrenschildt's life. There's even an audio recording from 1977 where O'Reilly tells the details.

In 2013, former *Washington Post* journalist-turned-JFK author Jefferson Morley posted the audio on his website, JFKFacts.org. There you can hear O'Reilly make a phone call to Fonzi to verify the suicide and adding that he'll be arriving in Florida the next day—meaning, there was no way that O'Reilly personally heard the gunshot as he had always maintained. He wasn't in Florida, he wasn't at the door—he just made it up. As Morley explained: "It is what these guys all do, they inject themselves into a dramatic situation. O'Reilly was chasing this story, but he wasn't there. He made it sound like he was more on the scene than he was. It was show business."

O'Reilly's former WFAA colleague Tracy Rowlett had stronger words, calling him a "phony" and adding, "There's no other way to put it. He was not up on the porch when he heard the gunshots, he was in Dallas. He wasn't traveling at that time." But the then–Fox News host had a supporter at his publisher's office. Henry Holt spokesperson Patricia Eisemann said: "We fully stand behind Bill O'Reilly and his bestseller *Killing Kennedy* and we're very proud to count him as one of our most important authors. This one passage is immaterial to the story being told by this terrific book and we have no plans to look into this matter."

De Mohrenschildt's autobiography was never published and is available online for free. While rife with typos, it's a fascinating account of the aristocrat's views of Oswald and Marina, and the Kennedy assassination. The audiotapes in which Oltmans interviewed de Mohrenschildt are also online and available for sale.

Fonzi, who was an investigative journalist with the *Philadelphia Inquirer* and other outlets, was diligent and knowledgeable, and unafraid to change his opinions when new information surfaced. Like me, he began his exploration into JFK's death by accepting the Warren Commission Report, but we both amended our views when confronted with better evidence. In Fonzi's case, it was reading Philadelphia lawyer Vincent Salandria's critique of the single-bullet theory. Fonzi studied the facts, then interviewed his local district attorney and Warren panel lawyer Arlen Specter, who created the theory. When Specter suffered a convenient memory lapse at Fonzi's tough questioning, it was all over. Fonzi knew then that the Warren Commission Report had been a hoax and began writing about it. He was first hired as an investigator for the Church Senate Committee, and then the HSCA by Philly prosecutor Richard Sprague before he left the case. Fonzi stayed on and turned up much valuable material. When the HSCA's report was published, Fonzi was angry as it didn't include his solid links between Oswald and the CIA. He continued to write about the case and became a regular at assassination conferences. I enjoyed speaking with him on many occasions. He died in 2012 from complications of Parkinson's disease at the age of 76. Fonzi's book, *The Last Investigation: What Insiders Know About the Assassination of JFK* (Thunder's Mouth Press, 1993; republished in paperback by Skyhorse Publishing 2013), is one of the absolute must-haves for any scholar of this case as it unravels the CIA and Cuban connection that was surely the engine that drove the assassins and provided the getaway car for the cover-up. Fonzi's wife of 55 years, Marie, who has a doctoral degree in education and was the chief ally in his work, continues to pursue the truth in the JFK case.

Oltmans wasted no time solidifying his views of de Mohrenschildt. In a special closed-door Saturday session, four days after de Mohrenschildt's suicide, Oltmans appeared before the HSCA panel and pinned his dead friend to the mat. There was no longer any hesitation about de Mohrenschildt's intentions. For three hours, Oltmans swore under oath that de Mohrenschildt had implicated himself in the murder plot and had discussed the crime "from A to Z" with Oswald. Now, it was revealed, that de Mohrenschildt had given the young Marine explicit instructions of what he was expected to do to perform the assassination. De Mohrenschildt had also indicated the CIA and FBI were heavily involved with the caper. Oltmans told the panel that de Mohrenschildt's death released him from his pledge not to discuss the matter.

We'll never know how much, if any, of Oltmans' testimony was true. It's possible that he felt implicating de Mohrenschildt would be more financially beneficial should he pursue giving paid interviews around the globe or exploiting the story for profit in some form. It's also possible he was sitting on a secret that was eating him alive, and he couldn't wait to release it after de Mohrenschildt died. And it's surely possible that the facts are somewhere between both choices. Oltmans continued writing about world events and was eventually kicked out of South Africa after being deemed a spy. In a funny, karmic way, Oltmans had one last blast in the Kennedy case, portraying de Mohrenschildt in Oliver Stone's 1991 film about the assassination, *JFK*. Oltmans died of liver cancer in 2004 at the age of 79. Perhaps someday someone will make a movie about him.

Trials, Tribulations, and Triumphs

As the 1980s rolled by, it became evident that there was little interest in the JFK case by anyone with the authority to make things happen. But it was not a forgotten issue, at least to two lawyers who decided to push some buttons. Bernard Fensterwald, Jr., was a Harvard Law School graduate who had worked in the U.S. State Department in the early 1950s, defending its members against Senator Joseph McCarthy's communist witch hunt. In the 1960s Bud became an investigator for the U.S. Senate Judiciary Committee. Fensterwald and Washington, D.C., attorney James H. Lesar briefly represented James Earl Ray after he regretted the guilty plea he had entered in the death of Martin Luther King, Jr. In 1984, Fensterwald and Lesar joined forces to establish the Assassination and Archives Research Center, a nonprofit organization that chronicles and publishes an online library of documents involving American political assassinations, especially that of President Kennedy. Fensterwald died in 1991, but Lesar remains the president of the group today and is an avid litigator for Freedom of Information Act documents. Members of the AARC board of directors include a Who's Who of the most auspicious and well-respected fact gatherers and analysts from a variety of disciplines.

Other than that, every once in a while, a newspaper article would pop up about some person making an accusation in the JFK case. Polls by *Time* and other magazines showed that three of every four Americans believed there was a cover-up in the Kennedy assassination. Yet there were no renewed investigations and no real push by the all-powerful news media. But with the 25th anniversary of the murder approaching in 1988, I knew that there would be a series of media events. I pledged to accept every offer I could reasonably schedule—from TV and radio appearances to civic clubs and professional organizations—to make sure my position on the case was part of the national dialogue.

One opportunity came my way in 1986, courtesy of some British documentarians who posed the question: *What would have been the outcome if Lee Harvey Oswald had been put on trial for the death of President Kennedy?* It wasn't the first time a film project on the topic was broached. In 1964, a black-and-white drama called *The Trial of Lee Harvey Oswald* was released by self-described "schlockmeister" director/writer Larry Buchanan and starred a cast of actors few movie fans would recognize. Billed as an "exploitation film" due to its paltry budget and quickie shooting schedule, it had a tagline that said it had been "secretly filmed in Dallas." I would imagine that meant the movie makers lacked the location permits that are standard in that industry. As might be expected from a down-and-dirty project with no historic perspective, it didn't attract much of an audience. The upshot of this movie is that viewers would compose the jury, and it was up to them to decide whether or not to agree with the contention that Oswald was criminally insane when he shot JFK.

The Trial of Lee Harvey Oswald was also the title of an ABC TV movie that aired in 1977 and was produced by Charles Fries Productions. It was a more upscale film with some recognizable actors, including Ben Gazzara and Lorne Greene as lawyers and John Pleshette as Oswald. The script stuck close to the Warren Commission Report and had a gimmicky ending—just as the defendant was led back into the courtroom to learn the jury's verdict, he was fatally shot by Jack Ruby.

The 1986 production had greater ambitions. *On Trial: Lee Harvey Oswald* was an unscripted mock trial in a simulated courtroom. It was produced by London Weekend Television for the United Kingdom, with a running time of 21 hours. For its subsequent American broadcast on the Showtime cable network, it was pared down to five hours. The program featured an all–American cast, led by two superstar real-life attorneys: Gerry Spence as the defense attorney for the deceased Oswald and Vincent Bugliosi as the prosecutor for the people. The judge hearing the evidence was truly a former Texas judge. Witnesses included many actual people who would have testified if this case had ever made it to a courtroom: individuals who knew Oswald over the years, law enforcement personnel, Dealey Plaza observers, and the like. I was called as a defense witness, and, not to toot my own horn, my cross-examination by Bugliosi is widely considered the explosive highlight of the program. Presented as a real trial would have been, both sides had opening statements and closing summations, with a jury of 12 sworn-in citizens from Dallas hearing the evidence. The prosecution began its case and called witnesses, and then the defense did the same. In all, there were 21 witnesses, but Marina Oswald, as well as the Parkland and Bethesda doctors, were not among them. If Oswald had actually been tried in a proper venue, there would have been more than 100 witnesses, induced by subpoena to testify, and the procedure would have gone on for months.

The mock jury found that Oswald was guilty and had acted alone. Needless to say, there was no evidence admitted that would have pointed a serious finger of blame toward any governmental entity, so the verdict was what you might expert. For what it's worth, a phone poll that followed the Showtime version revealed that 85 percent of viewers rejected the mock jury's verdict and found Oswald not guilty.

For me, it was a free trip to London, a scholarly exercise, and that's about it. The program has been transferred to DVD and is available online. I'd mostly recommend it to see what I looked like with more hair on my head and appearing younger than I do now. The high ratings that the program earned in the United States. and around the world were noticed by famous Hollywood writer/director Oliver Stone, who would shortly announce his intention to tackle the subject with a mega-motion picture.

The mock trial also inspired Bugliosi to write his 1,648-page "Oswald acted alone" opus, *Reclaiming History: The Assassination of President John F. Kennedy*. Hibbing, Minnesota-born Bugliosi had been the Los Angeles County deputy district attorney who prosecuted and won convictions against the Charles Manson "family" for its depraved murder spree of August 1969. With Curt Gentry, he wrote the 1974 bestseller *Helter Skelter* about the case and, after his retirement, wrote several other interesting true crime and political books. He had an eidetic memory for trial details that Dawna Kaufmann enjoyed during the many discussions they had. Bugliosi, 80, died in a Los Angeles hospital on June 6, 2015, from cancer that had been ravaging him for his last few years. Dawna had spoken to him weeks before his death and said he was aware his time was ticking down. He was interred at Forest Lawn Cemetery, in Glendale, California. On June 10, I received an email from Michael B. Padden, a Minnesota lawyer and Bugliosi's longtime friend. He wrote that in their last conversation, Bugliosi had asked him to reach out to three people who might speak at his memorial, and I was on that short list. I dictated the following letter to my secretary, who quickly dispatched it to Bugliosi's wife, Gail. I understand that my letter was read at the event.

> Dear Mrs. Bugliosi, I very much regret that I am unable to attend the services that are being held to honor your beloved husband. I am in Alaska with my family and will not be returning until late next week. I would like to extend my deepest sympathies and personal condolences to you, your children, and all the members of your family on the passing of this remarkable individual.
>
> Vince was a brilliant attorney and a true gentleman. His keen intellect and scholarly analysis of every legal matter that he dealt with made him an articulate spokesman for his beliefs and a formidable opponent for his adversaries. Our first encounter in London for a TV program dealing with the JFK assassination was not a pleasant experience for either of us. However, quite ironically, it was the beginning of a warm, genuine friendship that was based upon a deep feeling of mutual respect for each other's beliefs regarding the Warren Commission Report.
>
> Vince Bugliosi epitomized the beauty of our country's adversarial justice system. He was a courageous, ardent, and eloquent advocate for the positions that he arrived at. His scholarly, erudite analysis of controversial, difficult legal matters engendered esteem and admiration from allies and opponents alike. As the great debate continues in the years ahead regarding the death of President Kennedy, I shall miss the cerebrally stimulating discussions with this extraordinary gentleman. I shall always be extremely proud of the fact that Vince Bugliosi considered me a close friend and colleague.
>
> With deepest sympathies. Sincerely, Cyril H, Wecht, M.D., J.D.

In the spring of 1987, I was introduced to Jean Hill, the famous "lady in red" who stood on Elm Street directly opposite Abraham Zapruder as President Kennedy's motorcade went by. Jean was an unhappily wed mother of two who would soon get divorced. She was in Dealey Plaza that morning to see the presidential motorcade but also because she had a crush on J.B. Marshall, one of the Dallas motorcycle cops who were escorting the motorcade. Marshall's helmet and bike would soon be covered with JFK's blood and brain matter.

Jean testified to the Warren Commission and felt intimidated by Arlen Specter's aggressive questioning of her, yet she never backed down from the main premise of her account. By the time I met her, she had stopped talking to the press because her ex-husband and assassination critics poked fun at her. She had stated that she thought she saw a "white and fuzzy" dog in Kennedy's limousine—but the quick flash she thought was an animal turned out to just be flowers. After hearing Jean's whole story, I encouraged her to continue sharing it with others, which she did.

Jean was standing at the edge of the street, closest to where the motorcade would pass. Her friend, Mary Ann Moorman, stood next to her, snapping Polaroids. As JFK's limo approached, Jean noticed that the president and First Lady seemed to be looking downward at the car seat between them. Jean wanted to make sure they looked up so Mary Ann could get a good photo, so she yelled out: "Hey, we want to take your picture!" The president looked up just as the ladies heard the first gunshot and Moorman clicked the image. Hill told me she heard three shots, then there was a pause, followed by more shots. Altogether, she heard four to six shots. As JFK slumped, Mary Ann hit the ground and tried to pull Jean down, warning that they might get hit by bullets, too. But Hill didn't heed the advice.

As Jackie began crawling onto the back of the now-speeding limo, Jean crossed the street and ran toward the grassy knoll, where she was adamant the shots came from. It wasn't a sensible thing to do, she explained to me, but her reaction was autonomic, and she wasn't the only person to run up the slope. She noticed one man in a brown hat running from the depository to the knoll and told the Commission that he looked like Jack Ruby. As she neared the picket fence, she saw two men. One was holding a rifle behind the fence, and both were preparing to flee. That's when two other men in trench coats grabbed her and forcibly took her to the Dallas County Records Building for a lengthy interrogation. Upon informing the "police agents" that she had heard four to six shots fired and had seen the men on the grassy knoll, they rebuked her and issued this stern warning: "You would be very wise to keep your mouth shut about this." Hill endured regular harassment from the FBI and other law enforcement personnel, and she believes someone tampered with her car on two occasions in an attempt to silence her. With coauthor Bill Sloan, Jean wrote a book called *The Last Dissenting Witness* (Pelican Publishing, 1992). Jean died in November 2000 but is remembered as a brave observer to history and someone who I was privileged to know.

In 1988, the FBI released a short and disappointing statement saying it had reviewed the conclusions of the House Select Committee on Assassinations, particularly the acoustical tape, but found no persuasive evidence of the conspiracy.

In happier, personal news, my wife Sigrid had attained her master's degree in

International Affairs from the Graduate School of International and Public Affairs at the University of Pittsburgh in 1985. In 1989, she graduated from the University of Pittsburgh School of Law. Her specialty was family law, and together we established the Wecht Law Firm, which our son Daniel later joined until he became a judge. Today, Sigrid manages my Wecht Pathology and Associates office.

Oliver Stone's *JFK*

W illiam "Oliver" Stone, born in 1946, is the son of a politically conservative Wall Street stockbroker, Louis, and his French-born wife, Jacqueline. Stone entered Yale University in 1964 but left after a year to join the U.S. Army as an infantryman. His tour of duty in Vietnam brought him a posting with Bravo Company, a Bronze Star for Valor, and a Purple Heart. His experiences overseas helped him home in on visual storytelling and forge a different political identity from that of his father. Stone's entrée into show business began with short films, but his prolific writing skills brought greater opportunities. His screenplay for *Midnight Express* won him an Academy Award for Best Adapted Screenplay in 1978 and was followed by scripts for *Conan the Barbarian* in 1982 and *Scarface* in 1983. It wouldn't be long before the entertainment industry realized that his vision for pop culture hits should translate into directing and producing. His template became medium to big budget features, with dramatic casts, often controversial topics, and actors with a good chance at being recognized for an Academy Award. This winning system extends through today and includes such films as *Platoon, Born on the Fourth of July, Wall Street, Talk Radio, The Doors, Heaven & Earth, Natural Born Killers, Any Given Sunday, Alexander, World Trade Center, W., Snowden*, a 10-part documentary series about American history, a four-hour documentary on Russian leader Vladimir Putin, and others.

At the 1988 Latin American Film Festival in Havana, Stone was promoting his political thriller, *Salvador*, about an American journalist who breaks the true story behind the headlines in a death squad-ridden Central America. Ellen Ray, a representative for Jim Garrison's publisher, handed him a copy of the New Orleans' district attorney's just-released book, *On the Trail of the Assassins*. Stone had no strong opinions about President Kennedy's murder and was in Vietnam during Garrison's quest for justice, but as he devoured the book, he knew it would make a great movie. The dramatist in him could not resist the story of the homespun civil servant and father of five who ached to crack history's biggest whodunit, against the backdrop of quirky New Orleans' characters and the wide assortment of challenges JFK faced at the time. Stone and the Warner Bros. studio optioned Garrison's book for material about the Clay Shaw prosecution and Garrison's home life. For an overview on other facets, an option was made for Dallas journalist Jim Marrs' book, *Crossfire: The Plot That Killed Kennedy* (Carroll & Graf Publishers, 1989, for the hardback version; reprinted in paperback by Basic Books, 1993). Stone then hired several researchers to immerse themselves in the case. Stone and his co-screenwriter, Zachary Sklar, who edited Garrison's book, also spent considerable time interviewing Garrison, his co-workers and family, and as many of the actual individuals connected to the case as were alive.

The film, directed by Stone, was shot in 72 days under the production title of "Project X" in an attempt to keep the press at bay. Actors who had brief cameos were only shown "sides," or the script pages that pertained to their scenes, and everyone involved was asked not to discuss the production with outsiders. Locations included Dallas; Fort Worth; New Orleans; the Louisiana State Penitentiary in Angola; Washington, D.C.; and Arlington National Cemetery. A full tenth of the $40 million budget was spent on reverting Dealey Plaza to what it looked like in 1963, and there were arduous negotiations with the former Texas School Book Depository officials to permit filming in the building. The city of Dallas even allowed the camera into the actual basement of Dallas City Hall where Ruby shot Oswald. Stone paid a $40,000 licensing fee for use of the Zapruder film footage and spent another $45,000 on digitally stabilizing the imagery via a new and revolutionary process. The first draft of the script was an unwieldy 190 pages, followed by subsequent drafts until they arrived at the shooting script's tight 156 pages. The finished movie's running time is 3 hours and 10 minutes, with a half-hour more material in the director's cut DVD.

The cast of *JFK* was a galaxy of stars. Kevin Costner portrayed Garrison, and Sissy Spacek played his wife, Liz. Tommy Lee Jones played Clay Shaw; Joe Pesci was David Ferrie; Ed Asner was Guy Banister; Jack Lemmon was Jack Martin; Donald Sutherland was "X," a prominent military informant who believed that Garrison was on the right track; Gary Oldman was Lee Harvey Oswald; Brian Doyle-Murray was Jack Ruby; John Candy was Dean Andrews; Walter Matthau was Senator Russell Long; Kevin Bacon played a composite of shady characters in the Big Easy; and Jay O. Sanders, Michael Rooker, Laurie Metcalf, and Wayne Knight were members of Garrison's staff. Archival footage of many of the newsmakers of the era was incorporated and, in an exhibit of spectacular stunt casting, Perry Russo, who was one of Garrison's chief sources, played an angry bar patron; Willem Oltmans, who knew George de Mohrenschildt, played him; and Garrison acted as Chief Justice of the U.S. Supreme Court Earl Warren. Jean Hill, the "lady in red" closest to the presidential limousine, was filmed for a cameo role as the stenographer who takes down her statements to authorities, who are seen questioning an actress playing Hill.

In the summer of 1991, I received a personal telephone call from Stone, asking if I would kindly review the script to ensure that the medical and autopsy details were accurate. "Certainly," I said with gusto. "Just send it to me and I'll get right back to you." I didn't realize that some high-profile Hollywood movies do not allow their scripts to be read off-site, at least until the film is released. Instead, I was invited to New Orleans, where the film, already in production, would be shooting. I would be paid and listed in the credits as a "technical advisor." Within days, I was on a plane to Louisiana.

A production assistant met me at the airport and drove me to a location that represented Garrison's office. We tiptoed onto the set, and the assistant found me a chair that was out of camera sight, but close enough to see what was going on. Stone, Costner, actors playing Garrison's aides, and Pesci were rehearsing the scene they would soon shoot. I had seen photos of Ferrie, the colorful Garrison witness who died before he could testify in the Shaw case, but seeing Pesci in costume and makeup was a reminder of how outlandish Ferrie was. It was quite a different look from the two characters that the actor had played in movies released the previous year: the bumbling burglar in the John Hughes' comedy *Home Alone*, the highest-grossing film for 1990, and the hot-tempered gangster from the Martin Scorsese drama *Goodfellas*, for which Pesci won a 1991 Oscar for Best Supporting Actor. Now, Pesci wore an overly-large reddish wig and thick, painted-on eyebrows to illustrate the real Ferrie's alopecia. Pesci's Ferrie was a bundle of jitters, in fear of his life. Costner had had an outstanding last few months, too. The 1990 film that he directed and starred in, the lush and spiritual Civil War tale *Dances with Wolves*, had just won Oscars for Best Picture and Best Director, and he had received a nomination for Best Actor. Now, dressed and made up as Garrison, Costner had the kind of quiet, masculine strength that Gary Cooper exhibited in his films of an earlier era.

As Stone called for another run-through, he noticed I was in the room and gave me a friendly nod. The scene was the one where Garrison asked Ferrie if he had ever worked for the CIA. Ferrie, manically puffing on a cigarette, confessed that the agency was calling the shots with him, Shaw, and even Oswald and the Cubans. Jack Ruby, he said, was a bag man for the mob, and ran guns for Castro. "Everyone's flipping sides all the time," he snarled. "Fun and games, man. Fun and games." When Ferrie was asked what he was doing on November 22, the actor echoed the alibi of the real Ferrie by saying "I was duck hunting!" The remark was so absurd that the actors and crew broke into guffaws, and the scene had to be restarted. But things got serious when Garrison asked who killed the president, Ferrie waved that the answer was "too big" for the lawyer to understand, adding "The shooters don't even know!" Then, borrowing Winston Churchill's line about Russia, Ferrie sobbed: "It's a mystery wrapped in a riddle, inside an enigma." Watching Pesci dissolve into tears and seeing Costner, as the audience's surrogate, realize the tentacles of his prosecution and wonder what he got himself into, I was swept away by the "movie magic" I had never seen up-close before. Stone worked with his actors to find the best ways to convey their lines and went over where the camera would be placed and how they could move to stay in the proper lighting. I felt fortunate to watch these three men engage in what they did best and would have liked to watch the actual filming—but that wouldn't happen.

Stone called for a 10-minute break to talk to some of his technical crew, while Costner made a beeline toward me. With his hand out to shake mine, he smiled and said, "Dr. Wecht, I've seen you on TV so many times and I've read a lot about you. I'm honored that you're involved with our film." I had promised my wife Sigrid that, if given the chance, I would tell Costner what a big crush she had on him, but in all honesty, I can't recall what I replied to him. When one of the world's most popular movie stars comes over with a handshake and compliments, all rational thoughts leave one's mind. Pesci didn't speak to me or anyone else, perhaps wanting to stay in character. But Stone joined us and gave me a warm greeting. He handed me a full script that had Post-It notes on the pages he wanted me to read. He told me that this was the sixth or seventh draft of the screenplay, and there would be more as the production rolled along. An assistant walked me into a comfortable production trailer and stayed outside while I perused the medical and autopsy information and made notes, then he took the script back after I had finished. It took me a couple hours to formulate my thoughts, but the time was pleasant, with plenty of food and iced tea brought in to keep me working.

After I completed my analysis, I was walked back to the set, where they had already completed filming the Ferrie/Garrison scene. Stone and Costner were discussing their next location. There were three areas that I wanted to make certain were strongly hit. The first was to emphasize that the Parkland doctors saw a gaping hole in the back of Kennedy's head and that his cerebellar tissue and blood were leaking onto the floor, despite the Bethesda autopsy photos that don't reflect that. That suggests, I said, that the fatal head blow had to come from the front and that the autopsy photos must have been tampered with. The Dallas and Parkland locations had already been shot by the time the production moved to New Orleans, but Stone said that my information would be easily added, likely with a voice-over by one of the Parkland doctors.

The second area was the "back and to the left" motion of President Kennedy's head when the bullet from the front fatally struck him. That needed to be delivered to Garrison's jury even more vociferously than the district attorney had described in his book. Stone understood perfectly what I was saying and assured me that would be clearly portrayed in the film.

The third area was a courtroom scene in which Garrison demonstrated to the jury just how inane and incomprehensible the single-bullet theory is. The script had Garrison use a chart and two assistants, one sitting in front of the other just as Kennedy and Connally were that day in Dallas, to show the angular turns and gyrations the bullet would have had to make. The chart was very similar to the one I had first displayed almost 15 years earlier on the ABC News show *20/20* and had repeated often over the years. But I thought I should demonstrate my patter live to Stone and Costner so they could add some inflections and styling to their shoot.

With the two men paying rapt attention, I put out two chairs—one in front of the other—and asked two production assistants to portray Kennedy in the rear seat and Connally in front of him. I began my pitch, stating that bullets can only travel in straight trajectories. But if, indeed, the magic bullet had been fired by a shooter on the sixth floor of the depository, its path was anything but straight. With my finger I poked "JFK's" upper back where the missile would have entered his back and exited his neck. With dramatic effect, I explained that the bullet would then have had to travel from back to front, from right to left, and at a downward 17-degree angle. That would have required the bullet to make a hard stop in midair for 1.6 seconds, before taking an acute turn to the right for 18 inches, stopping again, then turning downward at an angle of 27-degrees. In contrast to the fictional single-bullet premise, the actual trajectory of the bullet in Kennedy from the back wound to the neck exit had an upward angle of 11 degrees.

Again, I pointed my finger, this time poking "Connally's" back under the right armpit, where the bullet would have then entered the governor, tearing through four inches of rib, rupturing his lung and exiting his chest, about two inches below and to the left of his right nipple. Only then did I realize that the young assistant who was filling in for Connally was female, and I would have to touch her breast to make my point. I halted my thrilling presentation to explain that I'd never had a female in that role before in all the times I had done that demonstration. I spared the woman from being groped, even in the interest of science and art. We all shared a good laugh, and then I continued the display showing how the bullet then went through the governor's right wrist before landing in his left thigh. And I emphasized that the shattering of Connally's wrist, severing his radial nerve, would have made it impossible to continue grasping his Stetson hat that, as we know from the Zapruder film, is what he did. I also pointed out that the Zapruder film showed no pain on the governor's face at that time.

My suggestions were implemented, and, when I saw the film at its premiere in December 1991, I beamed at how the scenes were beautifully choreographed for maximum drama. Garrison's summation to the jury was an acting tour de force for Costner who had mastered Garrison's passion and languid patois. He held the jurors in the palm of his hand and brought tears to Mrs. Garrison's eyes as she watched her husband, while the camera followed the prosecutor's every purposeful move. His demonstration of the magic bullet theory, which he described as "one of the grossest lies ever forced on the American people" is phenomenal, as is his "back and to the left" speech. The last minute of the summation focused on Costner's face. He explained the duty the jury had to bring a conviction against Shaw for conspiracy to assassinate the president and paraphrased from Lincoln's Gettysburg Address: "Show this world that this is still a government of the people, by the people, and for the people. Nothing as long as you live will ever be more important." Costner then looked straight into the camera lens to utter the final sentence: "It's up to you"—a reminder to all Americans to keep seeking justice in this matter. There is no footage of the real Garrison delivering his summation, but if he had used the words Oliver Stone and Zachary Sklar wrote for the film, and had Kevin Costner's powerful delivery, perhaps the jury would have spent more than just a few minutes deliberating before they let Shaw walk out, a free man.

Since I had not read the full script, I didn't know what else would be in the film until I saw the completed version. But when my wife and I left the theater, we were struck by the movie's boldness in targeting the Central Intelligence Agency as both the planner of the assassination and the architect of its cover-up. There's a delectable scene in Washington, D.C., between Garrison and X, the spooky military bigwig who served as this movie's "Deep Throat." He encouraged the district attorney to keep digging to find the answers to three most critical questions: "Why was Kennedy killed? Who benefited? And who had the power to cover it up?"

As the end credits rolled, I spotted my name as a technical consultant— an accolade shared by these other individuals: Colonel L. Fletcher Prouty, the inspiration for "X" in the film, was a former Air Force colonel who served as chief of special operations for the Joint Chiefs of Staff during Kennedy's administration and knew about assassinations abroad. Retired U.S. Army Major John M. Newman wrote scholarly books that analyzed subjects like the impact of JFK's murder on the Vietnam War and Oswald's involvement with the CIA, and believes Kennedy was assassinated for planning to end the Cold War. John R. Stockwell, a CIA officer-turned-author, was outspoken about how the agency systematically lied to Congress about its illegal operations. U.S. marine-turned-mercenary Gerald P. Hemming, Jr., had worked with the CIA on attacks against Cuba in the early 1960s, was allegedly Oswald's case worker at the Atsugi Naval Air facility, and was involved with the intelligence community's dirtiest tricks. Roy Hargraves was another mercenary with a background similar to Hemming's. Dr. Marion Jenkins, Parkland's chief of anesthesiology who tried to resuscitate both Kennedy and Oswald, advised on how JFK's brain matter leaked out from the back of his head, showed Stone a diagram he drew of all the people in the room that day, and helped re-create the operating room as it appeared in 1963. Jean Hill and a witness named Beverly Oliver had been present on the grassy knoll during the assassination and told Stone what they experienced. Perry R. Russo revealed details about Ferrie in New Orleans, and authors David Lifton and Robert Groden, respectively, advised on the military personnel at the National Naval Medical Center at Bethesda and photographic evidence.

Stone's *JFK* is a wonderfully written and produced movie with dazzling acting and technical direction—the kind of film that is about something that should matter to everyone and deserving of all the awards the Academy of Motion Picture Arts and Sciences may bestow. At the 64th Academy Awards ceremony in 1992, it celebrated nominations in a spectrum of categories: Best Picture, Best Director, Best Adapted Screenplay, Best Supporting Actor (for Tommy Lee Jones), Best Original Score (by John Williams), and Best Sound Mixing (by Michael Minkler, Gregg Landaker, and Tod A. Maitland). But the only wins the movie achieved were for Best Cinematography (by Robert Richardson) and Best Film Editing (by Joe Hutshing and Pietro Scalia). *The Silence of the Lambs* swept the big awards that year, winning Best Picture, Best Director (by Jonathan Demme), Best Actor and Actress (Anthony

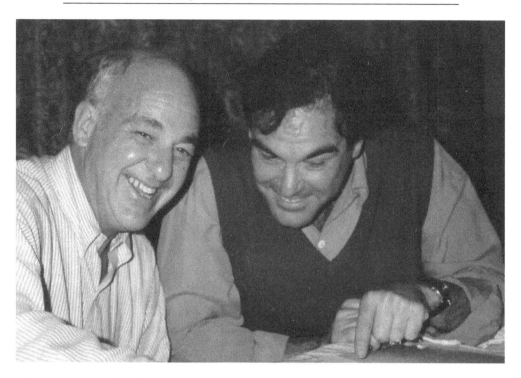

After the success of his film, *JFK*, for which I was a consultant, director Oliver Stone and I kept in touch. He has spoken at assassination conferences at my institute, and I consider him a good friend (Wecht Collection).

Hopkins and Jodie Foster), and Best Adapted Screenplay (by Ted Tally, from a book by Thomas Harris).

JFK was released on December 20, 1991, and I attended its Pittsburgh premiere. A year later, when the movie came out on video, I received a gift in the mail. It was a copy of *JFK* from Stone, and there was some scribbling on the cover: "Dear Cyril, I admire you enormously. You're a man that has ushered in the important evidence that the official medical bodies have—much to their shame—wholly ignored. My gratitude forever, Oliver Stone."

I very much enjoyed the movie but was bothered by the negative press it received. My 1993 book, *Cause of Death*—which included one chapter on President Kennedy's murder—gave short shrift to Stone's epic. This book you're reading now has allowed me the benefit of time and space to expand my views on areas I touched on before and to accommodate new thoughts based on more recent information. Over the years, I've seen the film a few more times and wish to give it a proper defense. For one thing, some people were upset that no one was specifically named as the real shooter or shooters, or if Lee Harvey Oswald was just, as he claimed, a patsy. Folks must understand that every answer in a conspiracy may not be known. This is not an hour-long television episode where all the circles get closed. Identities of shooters on the grassy knoll or elsewhere should not be stated as fact unless there is sufficient proof of culpability. Stone was duly briefed by mercenaries and intelligence operatives who were privy to inside information. Why not accept that he very responsibly stated all that he was willing to state on such a permanent record as a film? As often as I've spoken out about this case, I've never put names to other possible riflemen because the research is not solid enough to reveal any names. Perhaps in time those names will surface and be given the kind of vetting they deserve. Until then, should we avoid discussing the assassination? Of course not.

Also, people complained that the protagonist of the film should not have been Garrison, whose prosecution fell apart as witnesses died, bailed, or changed their testimony. Critics seem to have expected the New Orleans district attorney to pull the plug on his obsession to convict Shaw. But—rightly or wrongly—Garrison didn't do that, and, for Stone, it added to why he was an excellent choice to build the movie around. Stone has told me that he knew Garrison followed a lot of false leads and trusted too many people—but it wasn't the filmmaker's job to prosecute Jim for making errors. *JFK* is very much a human story, and most moviegoers appreciate seeing a battle-scarred Don Quixote who keeps tilting at windmills, even if they're only in his imagination. A character's idealism makes for better cinema than does his or her practicality. It also appealed to Stone that Garrison's seeming willingness to put the case ahead of his family life made for fertile exploration.

How about focusing on what Stone got indisputably right about Garrison? *The JFK Assassination: The Jim Garrison Tapes*, is a 1992 documentary written, directed, and hosted by Los Angeles news personality John Barbour. It opens with Barbour's voice-over stating: "On January 31, 1992, NBC conducted a telephone survey asking American citizens who they thought killed President John F. Kennedy. NBC received 30,000 calls in three hours. Fifty-one percent said the CIA did it. In 1967, only one man said the CIA did it. Jim Garrison." Barbour says Garrison told him: "These people had no qualms about dropping napalm onto women and children running around in black pajamas who were yellow and burning them to death. Do you think they had any problem eliminating a solitary five-foot-nine-inch [*sic*], blue-eyed, red-headed, Irish American?" Barbour's documentary offers a nice counterpoint to the criticisms of Garrison and has been updated with new material over the years. I strongly suggest you order a copy online.

Stone has given many interviews where he's stated that he is "not a historian." But he surely has affection for the topic, as is clear from the many biographical movies and documentaries he's made. He's educated about world events and the people who lead us into or out of wars, and he draws conclusions that are intellectually stimulating and visually provocative. In fact, I can't think of any other filmmaker who has such a successful track record at making history entertaining to the masses. His *JFK* is not a documentary. It's a drama, a mystery, a thriller. The never-static camera movements propel the action and are complimented by newsreel footage or black-and-white re-creations that make for compelling storytelling. For example, in the scene where Garrison is relating to the jury the magic bullet hoax, there is a shadowy re-creation of a man who seems to be Jack Ruby slipping the pristine bullet—Commission Exhibit 399—onto an empty stretcher at Parkland. Did that really happen? Ruby said no, but he was caught telling many lies, and three unyielding witnesses swore they saw him at the hospital around the time that bullet was deposited—witnesses who were either ignored by the Warren Commission or were otherwise discounted. We can be sure that *someone* placed that bullet there, so it's not a fantasy to suggest that person was Ruby.

Whether or not you accept everything in the film as gospel is your choice. But you can't fault Stone for not having valid sources for what he portrayed. This case, unlike any I've seen, is jam-packed with detailed information and speculation, and I give Stone credit for not featuring some of the more outlandish theories that were available to him at the time. One of the most exasperating aspects of this homicide investigation is how rigid some people in the JFK assassination community get about information that they have uncovered or written about. If you don't accept their work without question you become an enemy—even if you agree about many ideas they put forth. JFK buffs often sow seeds of their own destruction because giant egos and hurt feelings overwhelm sensible debate. And, over the years, it's been noted by many that some of the critics may have a professional stake in closing down discussions or fomenting feuds. Researchers of that ilk are best avoided, but Stone's film brought out disinformation artists to spread unconstructive discourse. The Internet has only accelerated these arguments.

Long after I visited the set in New Orleans, I learned why there was such a strict rule about protecting the secrecy of the script. Harold Weisberg, one of the early-case critics who wrote *Whitewash* and other books, had been one of Garrison's chief supporters for the first two years of the district attorney's probe into the New Orleans' conspiracy. But he turned against Garrison for reasons that remain unclear. When Weisberg learned that Stone was going to use Garrison as his chief character, he decided to do what he could to harm the project. Weisberg somehow got hold of a first draft of the script and passed it along to George Lardner, Jr., a writer for the *Washington Post*. Lardner visited the set and then wrote a column to warn readers that a terrible film was being shot. Reviewing a film based on observations from a first draft of a script is unheard of in show business, I'm told, and giving a pan to any movie before it's edited and ready for release is highly unprofessional. Weisberg also went on a CBS News program to further castigate the film. Weisberg died in 2002, so I can only wonder if another factor was his jealousy that Garrison's book, and that of researcher Jim Marrs, were chosen as Stone's sources rather than anything Weisberg wrote. With a major studio like Warner Bros. backing the production, that could have netted a nice payday for the authors who were chosen and may have seemed a betrayal for someone whose research was not optioned.

The long knives of the Warren Commission's cheerleaders extended to other major press sources. Post-release reviews were generally nasty, with many media outlets claiming that the story was trashy fiction and exaggerated. The *Chicago Sun-Times* film reviewer Roger Ebert—then the most prominent and influential film critic in the business—gave *JFK* five-out-of-five stars, calling it the "Best Film of 1991." He, and his partner Gene Siskel, who hosted a popular weekly film criticism series on TV, both gave the film their top honor of "two thumbs up!" Ebert's praise drew a dressing down from Walter Cronkite, who told him there wasn't a shred of truth in the film. But the reviewer had followed the case closely, so he wasn't impressed by anyone trying to pretend that Oswald acted alone. Ebert also wrote that in 1979— 10 years after Shaw's trial—former CIA director Richard Helms testified under oath that Shaw indeed worked part-time for the agency as an informer regarding Latin American concerns.

In an interview with Ebert, Stone expressed his annoyance over the pre-release barrage of bad publicity. "It was disturbing to have this film attacked so early," he said. "Never before in the history of movies has a film been attacked in first draft screenplay form. All the established media seem to be terrified of my movie, as if it's somehow going to destroy their lives. I'm amazed at their fear. What stake do they have in it?" He added: "I think it was the most distressing film I've had to make. I knew I'd have eyes on the back of my head while I was directing this film. It was very difficult not to be rattled by the attacks saying this film was a monstrosity. Any piece of work like this is an act of love and trust, and a leap of faith. You need to nurture something like that. To be attacked and stabbed in the back was not easy."

Perhaps Stone's most significant contribution occurred not long after the original movie came out: He addressed a U.S. Senate subcommittee over the continued secrecy of documents relating to the president's assassination and, shortly thereafter, the government began declassifying documents. That, alone, should earn our ongoing appreciation.

My Lunch with Marina

In early November 1991, I was fielding my usual requests for JFK media appearances, which were even more plentiful as we approached the release of the Oliver Stone film, *JFK*. I had spent much of the month out of town at various engagements but happened to be home after dinner when the phone rang. It wasn't unusual for me to get calls at home about the Kennedy assassination. Throughout the years, my family, especially Sigrid, has probably wished that I had never gotten involved in the JFK case. The time spent, the heartache endured, the criticism directed at me, and the late-night telephone calls from so-called tipsters were routine after so many years, but that didn't make them any less disruptive. Sigrid and my children have been the one constant source of strength, in that they have listened to me babble on and on about new evidence. But this time as Sigrid answered the ringing phone, I could tell from the way that her eyes widened that the caller had to be special. She handed the receiver to me and whispered, "It's Marina Oswald! She's calling from Dallas and wants to talk to you."

I had never before spoken to or met Marina, although I had long been fascinated by her plight and circumstances. In footage of her soon after the assassination, she could only communicate in Russian. Now, over the phone, her voice still had her native accent, but her command of English was excellent. She said she had been asked to appear on a television program but didn't feel right about doing it and wondered if I would fill in for her. I agreed, she gave me all the details, and I ended up adding that TV show to the list of appearances I would make that month. Marina appreciated my open-mindedness about her former husband, and as we spoke it became clear that she was an astute scholar of the case. She recalled everything that I had ever said with remarkable clarity and expressed that same knowledge about other peoples' comments in TV and radio interviews, books, and magazine articles. While I had her on the phone, I took the opportunity to broach the topic of Lee Harvey Oswald. "Lee was such a mystery to me," she said. "He was a lousy husband, a lousy father, a lousy person. First he told me he had no mother, that she had died. Then one day, his mother showed up. I could never figure him out. I was not and am not the enigma. Lee was the enigma."

After becoming America's second most famous widow in 1963, Marina began a relationship with Kenneth Porter, a neighbor who protected her and her daughters,

June and Rachel. She and Ken wed in 1965, had a son they named Mark, then divorced nine years later. Yet she and her ex-husband still lived under the same roof, she told me, in a small house on a large property outside Dallas. The whole family used "Porter" as their last name. Through she seldom spoke about Oswald publicly, Marina was very open with me for two reasons. First, she said, there were very few people she trusted. This caused her to hold back telling others of her insights and opinions, which was frustrating to her. Second, she wanted to help me investigate the case. She wanted answers as much as I did. I asked her as many questions as I could think of off the top of my head and later thought of many more I wish I had asked, had I been prepared for her phone call. Like me, she was looking forward to the *JFK* movie, which she hoped would change people's perceptions about her first husband. We ended the conversation with my getting her phone number and a promise that we could delve even further into the topic in a face-to-face meeting the next time I was in her neck of the woods.

That opportunity came up the next year, November 1992, when I was booked for a lecture in Dallas. I called Marina to say that my wife and I would like to take her to lunch. Marina made arrangements at a local restaurant where the three of us could have a leisurely meal. Sigrid and I showed up at the appointed time to find that Marina had secured a booth in a quiet corner. Her hair was pulled into a ponytail, and she wore no makeup. Her outfit was a simple wool sweater and a pair of slacks. Although I had only seen Oswald in photos and news footage, I was struck by how similar he resembled the woman sitting across from me. Perhaps it was the clear blue eyes, delicate features, and dark brown hair. When I mentioned that to Marina, she said that she and her husband had noticed the same thing when they first met. "He said that looking at me was like looking in a mirror," Marina chuckled, adding: "Maybe that's why he fell in love with me."

She showed us photos of her family and smiled at the pictures Sigrid had brought of our kids. June and Rachel, then attractive young women on either side of 30 years old, both spoke with typical Texas twangs, their mother said. In November 1963, June was aged 21 months and Rachel aged one month, so neither girl remembered their biological father. But Marina had saved every book and magazine article on Oswald and the Kennedy assassination, expecting that they might one day want to learn about him. But as she explained, Marina couldn't be sure what to think about him. As she had said on the phone, Oswald was never a good husband, but now she added more details. He beat her, including when she was pregnant, and would force himself on her sexually. Worse yet, he constantly insulted her and crushed her spirit. After they moved from Russia to the United States, he made fun that she couldn't speak English but didn't want her to learn the language. He criticized the way she handled their babies, not liking how she bathed or fed the girls, and would act as if he were "saving" them when he'd sweep in for a visit. He would fluctuate between playing peek-a-boo games with June and railing at Marina for not giving him male heirs. His precarious moods left her emotionally imbalanced and often in tears. Marina called it "psychological torture."

We asked if Oswald exhibited that aggressive behavior when they were in Minsk, and she said it wasn't as bad then. He seduced her with tales of how she'd love America with its sunshine, fresh food, and big cars, and he'd do funny impressions of Nikita Khrushchev and the old gray men of the Politburo. Once she and Lee wed, KGB agents surveilled their every move and read their mail. Marina knew what Russia had to offer, and it wasn't inspiring. Starting over in the United States sounded like bliss, she said. But reality soon set in. In the 18 months Marina lived in the United States prior to the assassination, she felt isolated and terrified. Oswald's mother, Marguerite, never warmed to Marina and would frequently act impatient with the girls. Ruth Paine, the newly separated friend with whom Marina lived, helped her learn English and American customs, and both women leaned on each other for support. Ruth also brought in Russian-language reading material for Marina, which gave the younger woman something to concentrate on other than the American television programs she couldn't understand. Reading biographies and novels by the great Russian authors fed Marina's intellectual needs and imagination. Marina considered leaving Oswald but, with her mother's death, there wasn't much waiting for her back in Russia. And, as miserable as Oswald was as a father, she couldn't deprive him of his children—they were her best hope for him growing into a normal adult and treating his family better. Plus, she had no money. Oswald was a dreadful provider and what little money he did give to her had to be accounted for to the penny. So, she was stuck.

I asked Marina if she thought her husband shot the president. Surely, she was of that frame of mind when she spoke to authorities and the Warren Commission early on. When one of the lawyers suggested that Oswald's motive was to become famous, she agreed because she had no other sensible explanation. But in the ensuing years, as she analyzed the case and became exposed to more skeptical thinking, she modified her position. At our lunch, she stated that she now believed Oswald was telling the truth when he said he was a "patsy." Marina asserted the U.S. government had lied to both her and her late husband. I knew that Marina, her daughters, and Marguerite had been in "protective custody" from right after the assassination until her attorney asked law enforcement to back away and let the women live freely. Now, so many years later, Marina told me, she wondered whether the FBI or CIA were still tapping her phone. She remembered how brutal Russian justice could be and was observing the same bullying and cover-ups from American authorities. On a personal level, she felt tremendous guilt over Oswald's actions, whatever they were.

The man she first met when she was 19 had always seemed peculiar. In those early days in Russia, she wondered if he were some kind of intelligence agent because he spoke Russian so fluently. She asked me if I had been in the military, and I told her briefly of my U.S. Air Force stint. Then she asked if I had been taught a foreign language while enlisted, and I replied that I had not. So why, she questioned, would a U.S. marine like Oswald learn Russian if there wasn't some nefarious purpose? When she asked that of Oswald, he'd laugh and say it was so he could defect. But she didn't understand why he'd want to do that, since his descriptions of life in the United States seemed so much better than conditions in Russia. With Oswald's abrupt decision to move back to the United States with Marina and June, the American embassy provided the paperwork without question and gave the couple money, too. Once back in the states, Oswald wasn't treated as a security risk or tossed into prison, as might have been expected. No, he and his family were welcomed back with open arms. Even to an inexperienced and young woman as Marina was, it all seemed bizarre, and I had to agree. I mentioned how I was grilled for hours by two FBI agents after my professional trip to Moscow and Leningrad, and I had certainly not tried to renounce my citizenship and pledge allegiance to Mother Russia, as Oswald had.

Marina had a lot to say about Marguerite, who had died in 1981. The two women had not kept in contact for years before the older woman's death. Marina felt that Marguerite had come unglued. Marguerite seemed to accept his death but was intent on making money from it in any way possible, from selling family keepsakes to hawking her own autographs and photos. She impressed upon Marina that Oswald was a great hero who was sent on a spy mission by the U.S. government to infiltrate Russian life, then was brought back to the states to continue his spycraft. But when Marina would ask why Oswald was seemingly eliminated by the same government he had helped out, Marguerite didn't have a clue.

Marina, Sigrid, and I tried to talk it through. Why would the U.S. government go to the expense of training someone to become a double agent and carry out a mission successfully, returning to the states with a souvenir in the form of a wife and child, be dispatched to New Orleans on a phony pro–Cuba stint, set up with a doppelganger to advance a cover, only to be disposed of so callously in Dallas? Wouldn't someone who proved his value, as Oswald ostensibly had done, be reassigned another spooky duty? Did he do something to lose the support of his intelligence handlers? What was the exact point when he went from being an ace asset to collateral damage? How many weeks or months of planning was involved, by whom, and at what point was Oswald informed?

We reasoned that if Oswald's chosen profession was more than that of a shipping clerk at a book warehouse, he had to know what he was part of. Maybe not everything, but enough to recognize that he had to keep his mouth shut and do what was needed. If that involved firing a gun, he had to do that, too. The polite thought would be that he was being forced into this and had to perform out of fear. But the more pragmatic view was that he relished the work and wouldn't have walked off if given the chance. If that meant keeping his family in a secondary position, that had to be okay with him. I asked that if Marina had married a real "James Bond," why wasn't her quality of life more exotic? She grinned at the irony of being with someone who, if the rumors were true, was this international man of intrigue and yet kept his wife and two babies in near poverty and upheaval. "I never wanted such drama," she said, shaking her head. "I wanted to be in love, enjoy our daughters. Maybe go out for dinner and a movie, nothing fancy. But he was never there, and when he *was* there, he wasn't *there*."

Marina was familiar with my spiel about the magic-bullet fraud and had viewed the Zapruder film when it aired on Geraldo Rivera's television program in 1975, so I didn't have to tiptoe around the medical evidence. She understood that one of the fatal shots came from the front and right of where the president was, which meant that there had to have been a grassy knoll shooter. And she knew the debate about whether Lee could have shot from the book depository's sixth-floor window, then run to the downstairs lunchroom so quickly and nonchalantly, as witnesses maintained. She wanted to believe that he couldn't have been involved at all, but there were things that nagged at her. When I asked what Oswald thought of President Kennedy she was clear that he loved America's young leader and had been pleased that he was elected over Richard Nixon. In August 1963, when news broadcasts announced that the president and First Lady had lost their two-day-old son to lung disease, Marina felt bad, but Oswald shed tears. She had a difficult time imagining that Oswald could cause such pain for the First Lady and Kennedy children, much less end the life of a man he admired.

Then again, there were numerous incidents where Oswald's mind-boggling exploits caused grief for Marina. Why did he use a phony name when he sent away for his mail order firearms and to rent the room on North Beckley Avenue? She was also puzzled when, in April 1963, he asked her to take a photograph of him, holding his rifle, handgun, and communist newspapers. He signed the photo to their friend, George de Mohrenschildt, and made Marina mark it with Oswald's anti-fascist taunt. Days later, when Lee was late in getting home, Marina found the fatalistic note he wrote about what she should do if he were to be arrested. When he finally showed up, his frantic wife learned that he had fired a bullet into the front window of the home of the conservative gadfly General Edwin Walker. Oswald told Marina that the shooting had been planned for months and that he was disappointed that Walker was only slightly wounded from flying glass. "It was excruciating for me to hear about such violence," she exclaimed. "What kind of man does this? People have strong opinions and if you don't agree with someone, you ignore him. You don't shoot and try to kill him."

Oswald sneered that she didn't understand politics and that Walker was despicable. If someone had been able to kill Adolf Hitler, millions of lives would have been spared. Marina just wasn't smart enough to know how the world worked, he insisted. The remembrance of that upset her. She dabbed at her watery eyes and reached for a cigarette, her go-to habit when she felt stress. I posited that the Walker hit might have been an assignment by some handler to test Oswald's mettle and see if he could be depended upon for the JFK murder. If you viewed all of the strange behavior in Oswald's past through that prism, what came into focus was: Oswald was ordered to do certain things in a certain way, for certain reasons that might have made sense to him but weren't clear to us. Oswald was definitely involved in this mess, but to what degree? And at what point did he realize he had been duped and would die? Maybe Oswald thought he was doing his best, Marina rationalized. He did leave her emergency instructions the night he fired at Walker's house. And, after her last hours with Lee, before he went to work on November 22, he left Marina all of his money and his wedding ring. Whatever mission he was on, he had realized that he might not return.

Very gingerly, I mentioned a passage in her Warren Commission testimony, where she was asked about a suicide attempt. She had responded affirmatively to the panelists, after which the subject was dropped to save her the shame of having to discuss it on record. It was true, she confided, and came at a time where she had lost all hope. She and Oswald had had an awful fight that left her crying in the bathroom. She stood on the toilet and wrapped one end of a ligature around her neck, and looked for something to affix the other end to so she could hang herself. Oswald barged in, pulled her to the floor, and smacked her across the face. He extended no sympathy to her. If she were going to get through this, she'd have to find the strength within herself. She worried that her children would one day learn about this act of desperation but was resigned to the fact that she could have no secrets. It happened, she dealt with it, and she went on to the next crisis.

I asked Marina if she had heard the story that, a month prior to the assassination and days before the president's motorcade was to travel through Chicago, a phone call came in to the FBI's office in Washington, D.C. The caller was said to be an informant named Lee who warned that JFK would be fired upon at a turn in the expressway by a team of assassins with high-powered rifles. Chicago's Secret Service agents quickly rounded up some suspicious Cubans, and the motorcade was canceled. Although there is no record of the caller's last name, some people—including Marguerite Oswald—believed it was Oswald, trying to avert a disaster. Marina had heard about it and also about Thomas Edward Vallee, the man with reported mental issues who Windy City cops said had numerous weapons and anti-JFK clippings in his home. Vallee, like Oswald, was a former marine who had been assigned to a CIA spy base in Japan, and had ties to anti–Castro radicals. At the time we discussed this, we didn't know how this whole episode would be covered up in the official records, as would later be revealed. And Marina wasn't shy about stating that Jack Ruby's murder of her husband was no accident. Someone in the government feared what Oswald might say, so Ruby, through his mob contacts, was told to eliminate him.

As Marina offered her views on these issues, I was in awe of how she could so astutely separate fact from conjecture, giving each appropriate weight. When I later discussed this with Sigrid, we joked that perhaps authorities had made a mistake in recruiting Oswald for complex assignments when Marina might have made a better candidate. Behind Marina's bravery, and despite having moved on with her new life, she harbored a troubled heart as Sigrid learned when she asked the pointed question, "Do you still love Lee?" Marina mulled it over, then shrugged: "I don't know. I don't understand how he could betray me and his daughters like that. Did we mean nothing to him? He owes us explanations we will never get."

Marina's daughters were shielded for years from learning their birth father's story. The Dallas area schools—along with most of the other schools in America—taught students that "lone nut" Oswald murdered a cop and assassinated the president on one of the nation's darkest days. Marina kept the Oswald memorabilia tucked out of sight but, eventually, June, Rachel, and their half-brother Mark caught on to their Oswald connection. Even though the sisters used the Porter last name, many people knew who they were from their first names and respective ages, particularly as they still lived so close to where JFK and their father died. Each autumn would bring a barrage of phone calls, with family members overhearing Marina turn down offers to do TV interviews. She had a bigger goal, one that would last all year long: to keep her kids safe and raise them well. Marina knows there will always be people who judge her and her family unfairly, and may even believe she was part of the conspiracy to kill Kennedy. There have been death threats from time to time, and the Porters have had to walk a fine line between being cautious yet not paralyzed by paranoia. "People can be cruel, but Junie and Rachel did nothing wrong. They are smart and kind, as are Mark and Ken. We contribute to society and just want to blend into our community," she said.

In 1991, Marina became a U.S. citizen, and, at our luncheon, she spoke of an upcoming trip with the family to her homeland. For decades, Marina's and June's passports, family photos, and personal effects were part of the Kennedy assassination files in the National Archives. It took some effort to get the items returned to the women. Before retiring, Marina worked as a store clerk, and Ken was a carpenter, but both now live on Social Security. She and her daughters have made very few media appearances and continue to eschew publicity. The Porter children have all thrived and enjoy fulfilling careers and their own families. Despite the kooks who have made their lives miserable, there are many more strangers who have wished them well. Dawna Kaufmann grew up thinking of June and Rachel every November—just as she thought of the Kennedy children—hoping they were having better luck than what befell them in 1963. Sigrid and I both have often discussed the fond memories we shared with Marina that day.

In 2013, Marina sold Oswald's wedding ring that he had left behind on the morning of the assassination. An auction house arranged for the sale of the gold band, which Oswald had bought in Minsk and had engraved with a tiny hammer and sickle. An unnamed buyer paid $108,000 for the item that was accompanied by a note from Marina that read: "At this time of my life I don't wish to have Lee's ring in my possession because, symbolically, I want to let go of my past that is connecting with Nov. 22, 1963."

In March 2017, I received another surprise phone call from Marina, who was as pleasant as before. She heard that I had attended a conference in Dallas sponsored by the research group JFK Lancer. The organization had honored me with the Mary Ferrell Award, named for the late woman who was legendary in collecting and archiving case material. Marina and I exchanged friendly small talk about how the years have aged us—I had just turned 86, and Marina was now 76—but left us no less committed to finding answers. She spoke of her husband, children, and seven grandchildren, and we made plans to get together the next time I was near her town for an extended stay.

But Marina had a mission with her call to me. She wondered if, given the advanced photographic analysis possible today, it might be possible to enhance the Ike Altgens photo that shows numerous people gathered at the entrance of the book depository. Most experts have agreed that the thin, dark-haired man on the left side is Billy Lovelady, an employee who testified to the Warren Commission that the photo is, indeed, him. Various color films also show the man in question, and they comport with the facial architecture of Lovelady. But some skeptics have always believed the man to be Oswald, which would mean he was outside while the motorcade passed by and not on the sixth floor, as authorities stated, or in the lunchroom, as Oswald claimed. Lovelady and Oswald do share a general resemblance. Recently, Ralph Cinque, a blogger who runs a website arguing for Oswald's innocence, raised the question that when Lovelady was asked during testimony to put a black ink "X" over his image in the photo, he may have instead marked the man to his immediate left— whose arms are covering his head, obscuring his face. Cinque asserts that the black X is on a black background and can't be detected with the naked eye. Lovelady can't be questioned because he died in 1979, yet all of the other employees who gave sworn testimony named him as among the employees on the steps, and not one of them stated Oswald was standing with them. I can see why the matter would be of great importance to Marina and her family. I couldn't give Marina any guidance except to say that the National Archives controls the Altgens original, so any permission for new testing would have to be approved by their curators.

Days after my 1992 meeting with Marina, I was coincidentally supplied with a copy of the KGB's 35-page secret official report on Oswald and the Kennedy assassination. At the time I had been writing the book *Cause of Death* with my two coauthors: my son Benjamin Wecht and Mark Curriden, who was then a reporter with the *Atlanta Journal-Constitution*. Since the Oswald report was in Russian, Curriden asked a Russian-speaking friend in the FBI to authenticate and interpret it. The report stated that the KGB believed that Oswald was a spy for the CIA or the U.S. military when he sought shelter in the Soviet Union in 1959. According to the translator, the more appropriate term was not "spy" but "snitch" or "informant."

The file said that Oswald was "under constant surveillance" during his stay in Russia. Among those it identified as KGB operatives informing the government on Oswald's activities were a neighbor in his apartment building, three co-workers at his factory, and two women with whom he had sexual relations. There was only a brief mention of Marina, who was only Oswald's friend at the time. According to the typed notes, Oswald worked alone, and the KGB was unable to ascertain any contacts he made with known American agents living and working in the Soviet Union. The notes described Oswald as "anxious," sometimes quick to anger, and with a weakness for liquor and women.

Many of the documents were nothing more than descriptions of Oswald and his typical workday and those he associated with after work. There was no background on his family and his brief stay in the military. One document stated that Oswald was taught Russian by the military intelligence division. However, it gave no date or specifics to support the statement. A completely separate document covered Oswald's decision to return to the United States. Although much of it detailed his and Marina's request to the U.S. government, there was one very interesting statement—that Oswald would assuredly be allowed to return if the American intelligence community believed he had fulfilled his purpose in Russia or if U.S. authorities had another task for him domestically.

One document in the Oswald file discussed the Kennedy assassination but gave very few details. It was more of a summary to close out Oswald's file. It stated that KGB agents and operatives did not believe the U.S. government's position that Oswald acted alone. In fact, the summary stated that, according to intelligence reports in a separate KGB file on the Kennedy assassination, there was evidence that factions within the American intelligence community—be it CIA, FBI, or military—played a role in the assassination. However, the report concluded that there was no indication that the murder was a government-orchestrated coup. To me, this meant that the agencies themselves were probably not involved in Kennedy's death but that various agents or officials within those branches supplied information or assisted in the cover-up. The report acknowledged the claims that the Castro government played a role but dismissed such a position as "capitalistic propaganda." The bottom line, according to the KGB summary: Oswald was not capable of plotting and carrying out the assassination of President Kennedy on his own. The KGB file listed friends with whom Oswald associated in Russia and upon his return to the United States. However, the file did not contain any names of Soviet agents who watched over or investigated Oswald. I found it quite ironic that the KGB was willing to open its files regarding the Kennedy assassination, but our own government refused to do the same.

The Journal of the American Medical Association

O nce again, the major American news media blew it when they threw national support behind two articles that ran in May 1992 edition of the *Journal of the American Medical Association* (*JAMA*). Written by national correspondent Dennis L. Breo, "JFK's Death, Part 1: The Plain Truth from the M.D.s Who Did the Autopsy," was an interview with two of the Bethesda doctors, U.S. Navy Commanders James J. Humes and J. Thornton Boswell. The pathologists announced they were standing by their autopsy report and that the president was shot twice from the rear, from a rifle fired above and behind him. One bullet went into his back and out his throat, and the other hit the back of his head. No shots came from the front, both doctors declared, and no one dictated what they wrote in their autopsy report. *JAMA*'s editor, a military pathologist named Dr. George D. Lundberg, endorsed the duo as telling the truth. Lundberg even held a press conference wherein he castigated dissenters as unintelligent and suggested they were motivated by profits or paranoia.

The usual suspects in the media reprinted the interviews and hailed the doctors' disclosure as "new evidence." Several newspapers, including the *New York Times* and the *Atlanta Journal-Constitution*, published articles about the interviews on their front pages. That same day, I was called by the producers of CNN's *Larry King Live* and asked to participate in a roundtable discussion that evening with Lundberg. I agreed. The first question I was asked was really the only one I needed to hear. "Does this new evidence or testimony change your mind about the way President Kennedy was assassinated?" the TV host inquired. "First, there is nothing new in this *JAMA* report," I boomed. "You can take these two guys [Humes and Boswell], freeze their bodies, unthaw them in a thousand years, listen to their story, and it will still be garbage. These are the very same two people who wrote this fairy tale and for them to now come out of hiding and repeat it does not make it nonfiction."

I scolded Lundberg for his one-sided article and for relying solely on the testimony of Humes and Boswell. And I mentioned again the angst of seeing the news media swallowing up this bitter medicine with a smile, while still tearing into Oliver Stone for any possible inaccuracies in his movie. I complained that Lundberg and his writer failed to point out that all the forensic pathologists on the House Select Committee panel, including Dr. Michael Baden, had been openly critical of the autopsy performed by Humes and Boswell. I also found it remarkable that Lundberg said he decided not to address the single-bullet theory in his article because it was "not relevant." I got a big chuckle from Larry King when I stated that saying that notion was not relevant to the Kennedy assassination was like saying the Nazis were not influential in World War II.

After *JAMA*'s "Part I" article, there were a number of excellent letters to the editor that *JAMA* was forced to print in a subsequent issue. Among them, two well-informed California experts—Drs. Gary L. Aguilar and David W. Mantik wrote scathing missives. It was especially encouraging to me to read these thoughts from physicians after the craven reactions from most of the other doctors who have piped in over the years, including those on the official commissions and committees. With few exceptions, I felt I was alone in carrying the water for responsible medical coverage of this case. Now it seemed I had company. Before long, Dr. Aguilar, an ophthalmologist, wrote me a letter of support. I called him and eventually visited him on a trip to the San Francisco area. Aguilar later introduced me to Dr. Mantik, who is a radiation oncologist with a Ph.D. in physics. Both men would later have the opportunity to inspect the autopsy materials at the National Archives, as I had. Each of these experts has written incredibly detailed papers on the Kennedy case, and I've had the privilege of appearing on numerous assassination study panels with them.

In that same *JAMA* issue, Dennis Breo wrote another article, "JFK's Death, Part II: Dallas M.D.s Recall Their Memories." This piece attacked Dr. Charles A. Crenshaw, whose book, *JFK: Conspiracy of Silence*, about his experience in the emergency room at Parkland Hospital, had just been released. Crenshaw had written that the huge defect in the occipital area at the back of Kennedy's head was clear proof of an exit wound. The *JAMA* article quoted other Parkland doctors who denied Crenshaw's claim. As a unit, these doctors claimed their findings lined up perfectly with what the Bethesda autopsists said—yet, their comments were at variance with their sworn testimony to the Warren Commission, the House Select Committee on Assassinations, and other official interrogators.

The Parkland crew even tried to diminish Crenshaw's credibility by telling the *JAMA* author a whopper about when Lee Harvey Oswald was in the emergency room two days after Kennedy's death. As Crenshaw wrote in his book, a Parkland telephone operator received a call from a man with a loud voice, sounding like President Johnson and demanding to speak to a doctor in the E.R. She rang the room, Crenshaw happened to pick up the phone, and LBJ identified himself and told him the doctors needed to get a deathbed confession from Oswald. Of course, Oswald died without saying a thing to the doctors. The *JAMA* article quoted Dr. Charles Baxter, another Parkland surgeon, who scoffed that LBJ never had a phone conversation with Crenshaw, hinting that the grandiose story was intended to increase book sales. But Crenshaw had never tried to embellish the call as anything made to him personally, and reporters who looked into the claim found ample proof of the call. Phyllis

Bartlett, the nurse who patched in the call to Crenshaw, also verified his account. Dr. Crenshaw repeatedly asked *JAMA* for a retraction, which was denied. So he and one of his coauthors J. Gary Shaw, filed a "slander with malice" lawsuit on November 29, 1992, 29 years after JFK's death. Almost two years later, after a court-ordered mediation, the matter was settled, and *JAMA* ended up writing a check for its colossal error.

Many JFK researchers raised questions about why the third autopsy doctor, U.S. Army Lieutenant Colonel Pierre A. Finck, wasn't included in the May 1992 interview. Was he being purposefully evasive? Was this a sign that he disagreed with his cohorts' stand? To settle the matter, *JAMA* flew author Breo to Geneva, Switzerland, where Finck had moved. A rather snarky Finck went on the record for *JAMA*'s October 1992 issue, in an article titled "JFK's Death, Part III: Dr. Finck Speaks Out, 'Two Bullets, From the Rear.'" Although the first article quoting Drs. Humes and Boswell annoyed me, and the second one left me shaking my head, this third one really got under my skin. Finck, who claimed not to have seen Oliver Stone's movie, nonetheless had the audacity to tell Breo, "I understand that the film *JFK* got only two things right: the date and the victim! All these fantasies and add-ons create fiction, not history. The danger is that the fiction will be mistaken for history."

Alas, it seems Finck was the one spreading fantasies. "I have nothing to hide," he was quoted as saying. "I am not part of a conspiracy. There was no military interference. The direction of the fatal wound traveled from back to front." This statement floored me. The morning after I had given my critique of the Warren Commission report at the 1966 annual meeting at the American Academy of Forensic Sciences, Finck seemed perplexed, unhappy, and uncomfortable, and told me wished he could talk about it but wasn't permitted to. Then there was his sworn testimony in 1969 in the Clay Shaw case that appeared to completely contradict what he was now saying.

To vent my frustration, I immediately fired off a letter to *JAMA* that was published in a later issue:

Dr. Finck now states in his interview with you that there was no interference with the autopsy by an army general. In 1969, testifying under oath in the Clay Shaw trial in New Orleans, Dr. Finck stated that he and his colleagues were ordered by a general (whose name he was unable to remember) not to dissect out the bullet wounds of JFK's back and neck. Which statement do you think is more likely to be true—the one made six years after the autopsy under oath, or one made 29 years later in an unsworn, self-serving interview? Dr. Finck now states in his interview that the postmortem examination on JFK was a "complete autopsy." However, in his written report to the commanding officer at the Armed Forces Institute of Pathology in 1963, just days after the autopsy was completed, Dr. Finck stated that the autopsy was "incomplete." —Cyril Wecht, M.D., J.D.

The Assassination Records
Review Board

O n July 24, 1963—four months before he died—President Kennedy met with a delegation of high school juniors from each state on the lawn of the Rose Garden. There is news footage of the commander-in-chief interacting with the youths, including one tall, curly-haired student from Arkansas. It was the 16-year-old's first trip to our nation's capital, but that day would give his life direction and turn the would-be professional saxophone player to a career in public service.

The young man muscled his way forward as Kennedy went down the line, looking at each student and shaking his hand. When it was his turn, the teen offered his hand, shared solid eye contact with the president, and nodded to whatever encouraging word JFK gave him. Then, as Kennedy moved to the next boy, the lad looked at his hand as if he would never wash it again.

"It had a very profound impact on me," remembered that boy, William Jefferson Clinton, who would go on to become our 42nd U.S. president. "It was something that I carried with me, always." Clinton told his pals that one day he would have JFK's job as president of the United States, and he did for two four-year terms beginning in 1993.

Clinton's shared values with Kennedy were noticed by JFK researchers who believed the younger president might be open-minded to learning why his hero was assassinated. As expected, when Clinton took over from President George H.W. Bush, he inherited the JFK Assassination Records Collection Act, which sought to evaluate and release case documents to the public, unless there was a good reason for them to remain secret. The act provided for the release of materials 25 years old or older, but Clinton also mandated that new documents could only be classified for 10 years unless a review deemed that classification was warranted.

The five members of the now-titled Assassination Records Review Board (ARRB) were appointed by Clinton and sworn in on April 11, 1994. Its chairman was John R. Tunheim, an adjunct professor at the University of Minnesota Law School, who was recommended by the president of the American Bar Association. In 1995, Tunheim was nominated by Clinton to a vacancy on the U.S. District Court in Minnesota and was elevated to the chief judge position in 2015.

Tunheim's panel members were Henry Franklin Graff, a historian on the presidency and professor emeritus of history from Columbia University; Kermit L. Hall, a legal scholar and dean of the College of Humanities at Ohio State University; William L. Joyce, an associate university librarian for Rare Books and Special Collections at Princeton University; and Anna K. Nelson, an adjunct professor of history at the American University and key staff member who helped write the Presidential Records Act that declassified documents after President Nixon left office. Their written report, signed unanimously by all five panelists, was dated September 30, 1998, and sent to Clinton.

The board's executive director was David G. Marwell, who had previously directed the Berlin Document Center where he traced Nazi war crimes. He left the ARRB in 1997, the original date the board's work was due to be completed, but when it was extended by a year, his replacement was T. Jeremy Gunn, the board's associate director for research and analysis, and its general counsel. In the final months of the board's work, as its report was being written, the executive director was Laura A. Denk, who had served as the chief analyst for its FBI files.

The board's senior staff included Thomas E. Samoluk, Tracy J. Shycoff, Ronald G. Haron, and K. Michelle Combs. Eileen A. Sullivan handled the press requests, and Charles C. Rhodes was its computer specialist. A number of crucial experts were consulted for their expertise in various areas. Douglas P. Horne had been a general senior analyst but was promoted to chief analyst for military records, a post previously held by Major Timothy A. Wray. Robert J. Skwirot performed that same task for CIA records, as Kevin G. Tiernan did for FBI records. Other senior analysts were Joseph P. Freeman and Irene F. Marr, and general analysts were Sarah Ahmed, Marie B. Fagnant, James C. Goslee II, and Peter H. Voth. Sitting in on some of the sessions were Mark Heilbrun, a Senate Intelligence Committee staffer, and Dennis J. Quinn, who was familiar with the medical and autopsy evidence. Jerrie Olson served as the executive secretary, Catherine M. Rodriguez was the technical assistant for research and analysis, and Janice Spells was the administrative assistant.

Meetings consisted of both open and closed-door sessions in Washington, D.C., Dallas, Boston, New Orleans, and Los Angeles. The goal was to review documents that the Warren Commission and other investigative committees had held secret, and sworn testimony was taken from many of the same individuals who had spoken to previous governmental sessions, such as the Parkland physicians and the Bethesda autopsy doctors.

This time, authors, researchers, and scientific experts who had new takes on photographic and other evidence were called and even asked about documents they'd like to see. They were also allowed to name witnesses whom they felt should be compelled to answer questions for the board. Early in its proceedings I flew to Washington, D.C., for a meeting with Tunheim and his top staffers. They had a transcript of my lengthy testimony before the House Select Committee on Assassinations, and I was able to emphasize the areas I felt they should pursue. You can be sure I mentioned the president's missing brain.

The ARRB's spirit of openness was a striking difference from previous panels, and that road traveled both ways. *Best Evidence* author David Lifton donated a high-resolution copy of the Zapruder film, as well as compact discs, video and audio tapes, and transcripts of the many people he had interviewed over the years. Then he thanked the panel for releasing the House Select Committee on Assassinations testimony from a man named Gerald J. Bruno, who was the Democratic National Committee advance man for the president's trip to Dallas and had written a 1971 book about it. Bruno chose the route for the motorcade and worked the media ahead of the visit, so his testimony should have been critical. But as Lifton pointed out, the Warren Commission not only failed to interview Bruno but didn't even seem to know who he was. At Lifton's urging, Bruno was deposed by the HSCA, but when its report was released, the political operative's testimony was mysteriously sealed for 50 years. Thanks to the ARRB, that testimony was finally made available to the public. More important than the actual testimony is the question of why it was sealed for so long. There is no answer for that. I will add that Bruno was not only JFK's advance man for his fatal trip but also performed the same task for Senator Robert F. Kennedy when he made his deadly trip to Los Angeles in 1968.

Homicide prosecutor-turned-author Robert K. Tanenbaum was the former deputy counsel for the HSCA and wrote a fictionalized account of his experience titled *Corruption of Blood* (published in hardcover by Dutton Adult in 1995 and as an e-book by Open Road Media in 2010). He explained to the board why he and chief counsel Richard Sprague left the HSCA after being stonewalled whenever they sought information about Lee Harvey Oswald's anti–Castro activities and his links to the CIA and FBI. Tanenbaum and his team had discovered a transcript from the Warren Commission in which member and ex–CIA Director Allen Dulles personally put the kibosh on exploring these avenues. Tanenbaum also complained that CIA agent David Atlee Phillips was caught lying about a photograph from Mexico City that purportedly showed Oswald at the Russian Embassy where he phoned the Cuban Embassy—a call that was recorded, and then lost, according to Phillips. Numerous witnesses denied that the photo showed Oswald and stated that it was not his voice on the recording—but the ball was dropped when it came to investigating this evidence. A source had provided photos of Oswald, Clay Shaw, and David Ferrie, and there was credible information putting Oswald together with CIA mercenaries in Louisiana. But the HSCA shut down that part of the probe, even disallowing the group from making long-distance phone calls or using postage stamps. Tanenbaum urged the panel to seek evidence about the Alpha 66 anti–Castro activists who were central to this part of the story.

James DiEugenio, author of *Destiny Betrayed: JFK, Cuba, and the Garrison Case* (published in hardcover by Sheridan Square in 1992 and as a paperback by Skyhorse Publishing, 2012), suggested that the board investigate CIA spooks Richard Helms, James Jesus Angleton, and Robert Maheu—the last of whom also worked for the FBI and with the Mafia. He specified communications that needed to be declassified, and that in the years since the Jim Garrison prosecution of Shaw failed, new information proved that Shaw was, indeed, involved in CIA projects. And he wanted the full files on Ruth and Michael Paine released, stating that Ruth had been asked more questions than anyone else by the Warren Commission, but the HSCA never called her to testify. He was convinced there was much there to yet be unveiled.

Researcher Debra Conway spoke of the work she does as administrator of JFK Lancer, a website that collects and posts valuable documents. She asked the board to gain control of the Zapruder film, making the best possible version available for researchers to view, and to use the JFK Assassination Records Act to preserve and protect all the photographic and video evidence in the case. She praised the board for its recently disclosed files on the Mexico City angle.

John Patrick Judge co-founded the Committee for an Open Archives in 1990 to push for full public disclosure on the John F. Kennedy case. Prior to the JFK Records Act, Judge and his group had already been instrumental in getting many files declassified. Judge was also the executive secretary for the Coalition on Political Assassinations (COPA), a group for which I served as first elected chairman. COPA broadened the scope of its predecessor to include the deaths of Senator Robert Kennedy, the Rev. Martin Luther King, Jr., and other politically-motivated murders. Judge hosted the annual COPA conferences where I got to know him well. In general terms, Judge explained to the board how both nonprofit groups had wide grass-roots support and monitored the schedules for declassifying documents. Judge believed that JFK's demise was a coup d'etat engineered by the U.S. Joint Chiefs of Staff and took particular pride in seeing that military files were released. He also impressed upon the panelists that they should not accept as fact if a federal agency tells them something is unavailable. Judge died in 2014 after a stroke and is fondly remembered as the people's watchdog.

William Kelly, the other co-founder of the Committee for an Open Archives, was a journalist who wanted materials released involving John Martino, who was affiliated with commandos in Cuba and connected with notable organized-crime figures like Santo Trafficante and John Roselli. Kelly also referenced legendary Los Angeles television news producer Peter Noyes, whose early book *Legacy of Doubt: Did the Mafia Kill JFK?* (published by Pinnacle Books in 1973, and republished as an ebook in 2010) tied Mafia chieftain Carlos Marcello into the case. Noyes' research zeroed in on a criminal named Jim Braden, whose original name was Eugene Hale Brading. Braden had been busted as an unauthorized person on the third floor of the Dal-Tex building, across from the book depository, right after the assassination. Brought to the sheriff's office and unable to show identification other than a credit card, he said he was in town on oil industry business, had popped into the office building to look for a phone, and had no knowledge of anything to do with the assassination. Noyes' book suggests that cops should have taken a closer look at this man who had ties to the Hunt Oil company, organized crime, and right-wing mercenaries, and rumored connections to David Ferrie and Jack Ruby. Instead, Braden was released.

Later, researchers began questioning whether Braden might have been part of a shooter team in a window of the Dal-Tex building, which would have given him an excellent firing line for a bullet coming from behind Kennedy. Assassination scholar Robert Harris has made a number of interesting videos on You Tube, including one on the single-bullet theory and a possible trajectory from the Dal-Tex building's third floor.

After Judge's death, COPA disbanded, and Bill Kelly helped to form Citizens Against Political Assassinations (CAPA), of which I serve as chairman of its Executive Committee. You can see CAPA's efforts to "demand transparency, action, and accountability" at its website.

Gary Aguilar, a practicing ophthalmologist from San Francisco whose knowledge about the medical evidence was riveting, told the board about a six-page document that had been restricted by the CIA. It was an interview with Pierre Finck, the Bethesda doctor who was the only forensically trained autopsy pathologist who had worked on the president. According to the autopsy report that Drs. Finck, Boswell, and Humes signed off on, the fatal head blow entered JFK's skull to the right and just above the external occipital protuberance. Aguilar even brought a skull to demonstrate the wound track to the panelists. However, photos and X-rays proved that the wound was on the parietal bone, 10 centimeters higher than what the doctors had put in writing. Aguilar believed Finck's classified interview must have been about that inconsistency and also mentioned a statement Finck had made about a photograph of the disputed wound that Aguilar discovered was missing from the file. Additionally, Aguilar offered proof of the Bethesda doctors making conflicting statements to a reporter, and Aguilar wanted the board to speak with that person to settle the dispute.

James H. Lesar explained to the board that its work had the chance to restore the trust of the American people in their government. The documents that were sealed at the request of the CIA and FBI have done more damage to the psyche of most citizens than whatever revelations might be in those documents. The FBI had sealed information about Mafia activities under the claim that it did not involve the assassination, and such a Catch-22 was unacceptable. Lesar also made an unbelievable announcement, that "the JFK Act excluded from its definition the Kennedy X-rays and autopsy photographs." Calling that a stunning irony, he said that these items were the "most probative evidence" on the question of whether there was a conspiracy. He urged the panel to amend the scope of the act and let the People have what belongs to them. It would have been a perfect time for him to mention that President Kennedy's brain had gone missing but, alas, that didn't happen.

In all, 61 witnesses were called and plenty of documents cited that the ARRB was asked to obtain. However, it didn't always get the cooperation they hoped for. A case in point involves George G. Burkley, JFK's personal physician who had been a rear admiral at the time of the assassination but had been later promoted to vice admiral. Dr. Burkley died in 1991 and wasn't available to give testimony to the panel, but in 1976, his attorney, William Illig, had contacted the chief counsel of the HSCA, Richard Sprague, with news that Burkley believed there had been a conspiracy. Sprague left the committee a couple of days after his conversation with Illig, who was not called to give testimony.

The comment about Burkley was much different than a brief affidavit that the admiral would submit to the HSCA in 1978, in which he stated that he had accompanied the president on Air Force One for the trip to Texas, rode in the motorcade, saw JFK's wounds at Parkland, sat near the casket on the flight back to Washington and in the ambulance to Bethesda, and attended the autopsy. Burkley, who signed the death certificate, also wrote in his legal document that he supervised the transfer of the president's brain and other autopsy materials to the National Archives where—as we know—they vanished.

Burkley was not questioned by the Warren Commission, the Ramsey Clark Panel, the Rockefeller Commission, or the HSCA. In 1967, he gave an oral history interview for the JFK Library, but the person who conducted the session had no medical background, and there was scant mention of the assassination. Burkley was not asked about inconsistencies between the Dallas and Bethesda doctors, or the missing brain and autopsy items. The interviewer did ask one solid question: "Do you agree with the Warren Report on the number of bullets that entered the president's body?" Burkley's response was: "I would not care to be quoted on that." During the ARRB investigation, a staff member asked Burkley's daughter, the executor of his estate, if the panel could obtain the pertinent files from Illig's law firm. She refused to grant permission.

And when the ARRB contacted Marion Ebersole, the widow of Dr. John H. Ebersole, the acting chief of radiology at Bethesda who took X-rays before JFK's autopsy, she told them she didn't have her husband's personal papers or any assassination records. In his testimony before the HSCA—to which I was a witness—Ebersole mentioned Russell H. Morgan, the Johns Hopkins radiologist who was on the Clark panel and had said at a professional conference that no radiologist was present at JFK's autopsy. Ebersole fired off a blistering correction but did not receive an acknowledgment from Morgan. Ebersole also testified about an article he had in his files that included Morgan's quote. It's unknown what happened to that letter, the article, or Ebersole's other files. It's certainly possible the doctor got rid of them, but when I think back on his testimony before the Ramsey medical panel, he was very clear about what he said and thought.

Naturally, there were authors, researchers, and sundry interested parties who opposed the premise of a conspiracy who gave testimony and materials to the ARRB. The board felt it was only fair that their inclusions be on the record. If someone didn't care to comply with a request for documents, they could just say no. The ARRB had no power to hire a SWAT team and storm a residence or office to procure what it needed. Unfortunately.

When the ARRB issued its written report, it had declassified documents from every alphabet agency in the U.S. government, as well as presidential libraries, and the National Archives. Between 1994 and 1998 alone, two million documents about the murder of President Kennedy were declassified, a hailstorm of unprecedented access for the public and, especially, for the case scholars who were best able to analyze each piece of paper. Five million pages of JFK assassination records are now available for viewing at the National Archives in College Park, Maryland, or searchable online.

Did the ARRB's efforts lead to any indictments or arrests in the president's murder? Of course not. And it also didn't open everything, since there are volumes of information still off-limits to the public. But every so often there's an enormous "document dump" that tantalizes the buffs and helps lead to everyone's better understanding. For that, we can be grateful.

The ARRB's report recommended that future declassification boards be independent in structure and qualification of the appointments, that congressional legislation be implemented for an enforceable review and appeals process, and that there be a serious look at the amount of time that documents are allowed to remain classified. Citing concern that critical records were withheld from the board, it advocated a "compliance program," although there were no specifics listed for what that would entail. But without the addition of a "battering ram" provision, I'm afraid we may get more of the same stalling tactics and failure to comply.

In early June 1993, the JFK community began hearing that ex-governor John Connally was having serious medical woes from pulmonary fibrosis and wasn't expected to live much longer. I teamed up with the ARRB to draft a letter to then–U.S. Attorney General Janet Reno to explain that the governor had metallic fragments or shavings in his body that might have evidentiary value in the assassination investigation. The letter stated: "Subjected to neutron activation analysis and other scientific procedures, these fragments may be able to resolve the controversy as to whether President Kennedy was assassinated as the result of a conspiracy."

We recommended that the Justice Department issue an order to allow a qualified forensic pathologist to remove any metallic pieces that could then be sent to a metallurgy lab to see if there was a match to the magic bullet CE-399 that was supposedly found on the Parkland stretcher. Without spelling it out, we knew that if there was no link, we could prove without a doubt that 399 was phony, and, on that basis, the case should be reopened.

We did not want to be insensitive to the Connally family, so we held off on sending the letter until news hit on June 15 that the former governor had died. We then had someone in Washington, D.C., hand-deliver the letter to the attorney general's office. The point was made that there was a need for quick action because the family would soon bury Connally. The Justice Department could choose a qualified forensic pathologist and radiologist to procure the fragments, and we asked that a board-certified, independent representative be allowed to observe and consult. I explained that the removal of fragments could be performed without leaving detectable damage if the family wanted an open-casket funeral.

The attorney general reacted with lightning speed and told us she would send an FBI agent to speak with Nellie Connally, because it would be necessary to obtain her permission before any further action could be taken. However, Mrs. Connally turned down the request, and her husband was buried with his metal shavings intact.

When Mrs. Connally died in 2006, I didn't bother asking the children for permission to exhume their father and do the testing. I'm confident they would have heard about my earlier request and, if interested, could have pursued it with me. For the record, it's still an option, if they decide to change their minds. It remains a matter of legitimate national public interest.

President Nixon seemed star-struck by Connally, the handsome Texan with the bigger-than-life personality. Despite the latter's decades-long obeisance to the Democratic party, Nixon offered to appoint Connally as U.S. secretary of the treasury. But Connally would only take the job if Nixon could find a nice gig for George H.W. Bush, the Republican stalwart who had supported Nixon in the 1968 race while Connally had backed Senator Hubert Humphrey. Bush had served a term in Congress but had lost two elections for the Senate, and Connally felt he'd earned some good fortune. Nixon appointed Bush as ambassador to the United Nations, thus kicking his political profile into high gear. In the run-up to the president's 1972 re-election, Connally led "Democrats for Nixon" and, in 1973, switched over to the Republican team where he remained until his death. When Vice President Spiro Agnew left office in a financial scandal, Nixon replaced him with Gerald Ford, rather than Connally, realizing that the party jumping had made enemies in the House and Senate. A month before Nixon would himself resign in 1974, Connally was indicted for allegedly pocketing $10,000 from a lobbyist. On trial the next year, he called a number of big-name character witnesses, including Jacqueline Kennedy, Lady Bird Johnson, and the Rev. Billy Graham. He was acquitted. Both Connally and Bush were early candidates in the presidential race of 1979 but were crushed by Ronald Reagan's momentum.

I never saw the governor's medical reports beyond those in the Warren Commission Report that discussed his treatment at Parkland Hospital when he was shot. But there is the distinct possibility that the bullet damage he sustained to his lung led to the disease that caused his death. Pulmonary fibrosis stems from scar tissue that gets thicker and more painful over time. He would have suffered greatly.

Media Matters

In the years after the filing of reports by the various commissions, the president's assassination was put on the public's back burner, although each November would bring press coverage, with me doing my part to remind people of the mishandling of the investigation. But the weeks leading up to November 22, 2013, marking the 50th anniversary of JFK's murder, brought a profusion of television and radio documentaries. Most of them took an "Oswald acted alone" stance, and a common theme was to ostensibly use "new technology" to solve the crime—although, against all scientific certainty, the results were predetermined before anything was begun, and the editing reflected that. There's no way I can relate all the appearances I made during this time, but two stand out for what I was able to communicate and how I learned new info.

Fox News' *The Kennedy Assassination: Conspiracy or Murder?* was a special hosted by my old friend, Geraldo Rivera. Geraldo, after all, was the first national broadcaster to reveal the Zapruder film to the public in 1975, and his knowledge of the case was vast.

We first met around 1971 when Geraldo was a young attorney and reporter for New York's WABC-TV *Eyewitness News.* He interviewed me for his investigation into the inhumane and abusive conditions of mentally-ill patients at the Willowbrook State School in Staten Island. His solid work merited him a Peabody Award for Excellence in Broadcasting, and he was quickly promoted to doing reports for the ABC network and others. Over the years I made countless appearances on his various TV and radio projects, wherever he happened to have a show at the time. When he needed a talking head to discuss a contentious death in the news, from terrorism to police shootings, or celebrity demise, from Anna Nicole Smith to Elvis Presley and beyond, I was the medical examiner he usually called first. In 2011, when Dawna Kaufmann and I co-authored *From Crime Scene to Courtroom*, with its chapters on Michael Jackson, Casey Anthony, and others, Geraldo graciously penned the foreword.

Geraldo's JFK TV show certainly covered a lot of ground. He began by stating that an unattributed 59 percent of Americans felt they had been lied to about the assassination. Then he ran a 40-year-old interview he conducted with Marguerite Oswald who said that her son had been an intelligence agent and was framed in the president's murder. She bragged to Rivera about her collection of books that were sympathetic to Oswald and recounted the story of how an FBI agent had shown her Jack Ruby's photo before the nightclub owner killed Oswald.

Geraldo conducted fresh interviews with Vincent Bugliosi who promoted his book and called conspiracy talk "moonshine"; another author who claimed a Secret Service agent accidentally shot the president; a former CIA covert operative who said Oswald might have fired the shots; and Mark Lane who said the CIA did it, and Oswald wasn't involved at all. Journalist Jefferson Morley spoke about Oswald's connections in Mexico City and how the CIA anti–Castro agents tracked him in New Orleans, showing a declassified cable signed by five senior counter-intelligence officers 42 days before the assassination with Oswald's CIA case number and a notation that he "is maturing"—suggesting that he was being groomed for an intelligence assignment.

I was the final guest via a satellite remote from my Pittsburgh Fox-TV affiliate, and Geraldo described me as "knowing more about what happened that day in Dallas than any man alive." I expected that he would then have me describe the medical issues, but instead he simply asked: "Who killed JFK?" Taken aback at this unexpected question and mindful of how little time we had left in the program, I rattled off that a small group of CIA and military instigators gave the orders, angry that Kennedy was removing ground troops from Vietnam and dismantling the CIA after disastrous missions in Cuba, Iran, Guatemala, Chile, and Asia. I accused the CIA of operating as a separate, out-of-control government and quoted the comic strip character Pogo that once stated: "We have met the enemy and he is us." I spoke of Robert McClelland, the senior surgeon at Parkland Hospital, who had seen hundreds of gunshot wounds in Dallas and had no doubt as he observed Kennedy's wounds that the fatal head shot was fired from the president's right front, and my view that JFK had actually been struck twice in the head and once in the back—which led me to this gust of verbiage: "The sine qua non of the Warren Commission Report is the single-bullet theory, one bullet producing seven wounds on two men. The trajectory is absurd. The bullet only lost 1½% of its total weight, although it left fragments of itself in four anatomic locations in Kennedy and Connally, and the bullet emerged near pristine. The government itself conducted an experiment shooting into goat carcasses to simulate Connally's rib fracture and into human cadavers to simulate Connally's radial fracture. They could not produce a bullet that came anywhere near the pristine condition of CE-399, the hero of the single-bullet theory that allegedly had to have broken both a rib and a radius of this 6'4", big-boned man. This is hard forensic scientific evidence. The missing brain, the burned notes in the fireplace by Humes on Sunday night, the missing of the bullet hole by the autopsy pathologists on Friday night—the whole thing is a total fiasco. It's a debacle!" Geraldo laughed, "OK! On that note, take a breath, Dr. Wecht. You're wonderful. I really appreciate it."

Fox News also presented a program titled *50 Years of Questions: The JFK Assassination*, hosted by Bill Hemmer. Archival footage and recent interviews were shown, with Ruth Paine, Clint Hill, presidential historian Robert Dallek, Bill O'Reilly,

Mark Lane, and a ballistics expert who re-created how Oswald could have fired the shots, and others.

I was brought to their New York video editing facility to observe a computer animation of the Zapruder film with another expert, John T. Orr, an ex–Justice Department attorney who had also studied the Kennedy materials in the National Archives. Like me, when I had earlier written to then–Attorney General Janet Reno requesting that she ask the Connally family for metal fragments from the ex–Texas governor's cadaver after his death—the request Nellie Connally declined—Orr had independently written a lengthy report for Reno, asking about other evidence.

As the video editor showed us the various frames, and I described the folly of the single-bullet principle, I was happy to see that the animation was accurate. Many of the ones I had seen elsewhere consisted of moving John Connally's seated position to the left to better justify their magic-bullet scenario. I explained how the bullet that hit Kennedy and missed Connally likely continued onward to crack the limo's windshield, leaving a dent on the chrome. But that shot could not have come from the Texas School Book Depository, I asserted. The computer editor traced a reverse angle for a fatal head shot from behind and the trajectory lined up with the roof of the County Records building. Orr opined that there were four shots, with Oswald firing the fourth shot that missed JFK. We discussed how the snow-flaking pattern seen in the X-rays of Kennedy's skull suggests an expanding soft- or hollow-point bullet that pulverizes its target, rather than a military bullet that is what Oswald was said to have used.

Orr also said more proof of a second shooter was a bone fracture in JFK's back at the level of the first thoracic vertebra, indicating a bullet entering Kennedy's back, traveling downward, hitting bone and ricocheting upward. The Warren Commission said that bullet traveled downward but never hit bone, and the HSCA's dimensions placed the wound four inches lower. I added that the only way for a bullet to deflect is if it hits something firm, like bone.

Orr believed that his courthouse-roof shooter fired into JFK's head with a tumbling bullet that went on to strike Connally's wrist. His report to Reno mentioned the need to test five bullet fragments from inside the limo. To accomplish this, the FBI brought in another expert, Dr. Michael Zimmerman, a pathologist whose specialty was studying ancient mummies. He rehydrated the fragments and discovered traces of mummified human skin and muscle tissue but no hair. Yet, suddenly and without comment, the Bureau halted the lab work. Orr had also requested tests be done on a fragment with white fibers and a black speck that could be ammunition residue— and Hemming reported that a much earlier bullet worksheet had requested the same items be tested—but not only was that testing ignored, its mention was omitted from the HSCA's final report. Given the evidence we have to work with, there's no way of knowing whether Orr's theory of where the shots came from is accurate, but we're in solid agreement that the need for more testing is crucial.

Hemmer ended his program by reminding the audience that, in 1992, Congress passed the JFK Assassination Records Act to give the public access to some five million pages of governmental files, and that by 2017, all assassination records will be made available unless they jeopardize national security. We would all come to discover that "cone of silence" would be extended again.

My show-business connections served me well during the 50th anniversary projects but before and after that date as well. Those with television programs often seek me out as a guest when there's a puzzling celebrity death or cataclysmic event in the news where I can explain medico-legal procedures. The intelligence and capacity for details on the part of these news anchors and hosts make sitting with them a pleasure—and sometimes after a program ends, I will continue talking with the individuals off-camera, because their curiosity is so pronounced. I made countless appearances on CNN's *Larry King Live* when that was a nightly prime-time series and relished time speaking with CNN's Dr. Sanjay Gupta; Fox News' Judge Jeanine Pirro; and news pros Ashleigh Banfield, Katie Couric, Greta Van Susteren, and Catherine Crier, plus syndicated daytime talker Dr. Phil, among so many others. And it's always a welcome call when a producer from ABC News' *20/20* and *PrimeTime Live*, NBC's *Dateline*, and CBS' *60 Minutes* and *48 Hours* extend an invitation to comment on one of their projects.

In 2015, I appeared in a documentary about the shooting death of rock star Kurt Cobain of the band Nirvana. Titled *Soaked in Bleach* after the lyrics in one of Cobain's songs, it addresses the mystery of whether the drug-addicted musician committed suicide or died at the hands of someone else. Directed by Benjamin Statler, and produced and written by Statler, Donnie Eichar, and Richard Middleton, the film includes re-creations and archival footage, and is now available for viewing on streaming services. The next year, Eichar executive-produced and wrote a Lifetime Movie Network documentary titled *The Body Detective*, in which I was asked to reopen a West Virginia case from 1997. Authorities had determined that 54-year-old Teresa Rollins died in a freak accident, but I proved that she had been murdered. Her family members were very grateful for my help, and I was pleased that they finally found justice and we were able to chronicle it in movie form.

This year, I appeared in a film titled *Cyril*, by Mark Clayton Southers, one of Pittsburgh's leading playwrights who is making his documentary debut. I engaged in some evocative dialogue on racial relations and crime, and discussed three of my prominent cases: the homicide trial of former football legend O.J. Simpson; the sexual assault and violent murder of six-year-old Boulder, Colorado, girl, JonBenét Ramsey; and the assassination of President Kennedy. The film should be released in the near future, so keep your antennae up for it.

And in another medium, 2020 marked the release of my autobiography, *The Life and Deaths of Cyril Wecht: Memoirs of America's Most Controversial Forensic Pathologist* (via Exposit, an imprint of McFarland & Company, Inc., Publishers). Written with Jeff W. Sewald, a Pittsburgh-based award-winning journalist and filmmaker, the book covers my personal and political intrigues, as well as my most noteworthy cases. The book has been well-received, and at countless interviews and signings, I enjoy engaging with readers, some of whom are old acquaintances and many who are younger and inspired by my work. It seems as if everyone asks my views on the Kennedy assassination, and I never fall short of avenues to examine.

JFK's death is also a powerful subject to many celebrities I'm pleased to consider my friends, including Oliver Stone, Alec Baldwin, Rob Reiner, and others. They're in the right age-range where their lives were profoundly affected by our nation's political murders, and while they have careers that have taken them around the world with movies and TV series, in all genres, they like discussing the topic with me, and the feeling is mutual.

Moving Forward

In the fall of 2000, I founded the Cyril H. Wecht Institute of Forensic Science and Law at the Duquesne University School of Law in Pittsburgh. With the popularity of true-crime cases and trials in the news, there was a burgeoning interest for students seeking graduate degrees and professional certificates from a prestigious outlet. Courses in law, nursing, law enforcement, pharmacy, the health sciences, business, the environmental sciences, and psychology appealed to our diverse group of enrollees who realized this knowledge would lead to intellectual stimulation and satisfying careers. The Wecht Institute also hosts seminars all year long, as well as an annual conference that convenes local and national experts from a wide array of disciplines to shed light upon particular issues. As the first and only set of forensic science programs housed at a law school, the Wecht Institute is nationally unique. It hit the ground running and hasn't looked back, thanks to its administrator, my son Benjamin Wecht. I continue to serve as chairman of the Advisory Board.

Because so many students recognized me from media appearances, there was constant inquisitiveness about my views on the Kennedy case and other political assassinations. I was gratified to see so many bright students asking the right questions and wondering how they could move the JFK investigation into new horizons. It was a natural progression for us to use the institute for creating a series of ongoing symposiums. The first one was held in 2003 to mark the tragedy's 40th anniversary.

"Into Evidence: Truth, Lies, and Unresolved Mysteries in the Murder of JFK" was a three-day event and a resounding achievement. Presenters included many individuals you've read about in this book and others new to you, among them Dr. Michael M. Baden, who chaired the House Select Committee on Assassinations' Forensic Pathology Panel and for 25 years worked in New York City's Office of the Chief Medical Examiner; Dr. Walt Brown, who is a historian, an author, and a former special agent for the U.S. Department of Justice; Gary T. Cornwell, who served as legal counsel for the HSCA; James DiEugenio, author of two books on the JFK assassination and consultant for the film *JFK*; Roger Bruce Feinman, who lectures and previously worked with the late Sylvia Meagher on Warren Commission research; Robert J. Groden, who was a photographic consultant to the HSCA and the film *JFK*; Mark Lane, author of *Rush to Judgment*; Dr. Henry C. Lee, who is a world-renowned criminalist and chief emeritus of the Connecticut State Crime Lab; James H. Lesar, who is a specialist in Freedom of Information Act litigation; Dr. David W. Mantik, whose expertise as a physicist and radiologist brought new understanding of the president's X-rays; Dr. Joan Mellen, who is an English professor and wrote a biography of Jim Garrison; Jefferson Morley, who as a veteran Washington journalist uncovered secrets of the CIA; Dr. John Newman, who served as a military intelligence officer and has written two books on the assassination; Dr. Thomas T. Noguchi, who was the chief medical examiner for Los Angeles County and performed the autopsy on Senator Robert F. Kennedy; Dr. Randolph Robertson, who is a diagnostic radiologist and assisted the Assassinations Records Review Board; Zachary Sklar, who wrote the screenplay for *JFK*; Arlen Specter, who was the senior U.S. senator from Pennsylvania and an assistant counsel to the Warren Commission; Robert K. Tanenbaum, who served as deputy chief counsel for the HSCA and worked as a homicide prosecutor in New York; Dr. Josiah Thompson, who is a private investigator and is author of Six Seconds in Dallas; and John R. Tunheim, who is federal judge and chairman of the ARRB. And I delivered my lecture on the single-bullet myth, which got a boisterous reaction from the crowd. An eight-volume set of DVDs was released for this event.

In 2013, for the 50th anniversary, the Wecht Institute held another monumental international symposium, this one titled "Passing the Torch." Many of the previous experts also appeared for this conference, with additions that included Oliver Stone, who directed *JFK*; David Talbot, who is a journalist and author of a book about Allen Dulles and the CIA's role in the JFK case; Lisa Pease, who is coeditor of *Probe* magazine and an author; Dr. Robert N. McClelland, who worked on JFK as a Parkland Hospital surgeon; Patrick J. Speer, who is an assassination researcher; and John Judge, who was a historian lecturing on "A Call to Action: Why the JFK Assassination Still Matters and What Needs to Be Done." A 13-volume set of DVDs was made of that three-day event. Both boxed sets were released by the Forensic Sciences and Law Education Group, LLC. I presented lectures at both events and participated in several panels throughout. It was a delight to see such elevated discussions on a topic that clearly still inspires and incites people.

In 2017, Citizens Against Political Assassinations, of which I am chairman/ president, began holding annual symposiums on President Kennedy's demise. These generally occur over two or three days each November in Dallas. The people who are brought together for these most interesting events partake in cutting-edge discussions by individuals with unique qualifications on the subject. It's said that CAPA is "where the eagles soar," and I heartily concur.

The CAPA Board of Advisors include Bill Kelly, Jr., who is a journalist, historian, and member of CAPA's Executive Committee and was instrumental in getting the JFK Assassination Records Act passed by Congress; Glenda De Vaney, who is a retired civilian paralegal from the Department of the Navy serving as CAPA's secretary and program director; researcher Michael Nurko, who is a researcher serving

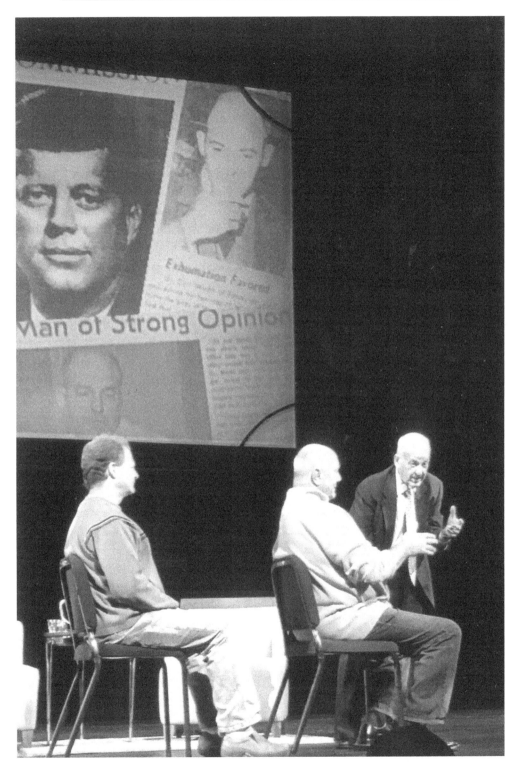

Demonstrating the single-bullet hoax at a JFK conference at the Wecht Institute (Wecht Collection).

as treasurer, and who is a former member of the Democratic National Committee; Dr. Gerald McKnight, who is a retired professor of history and author of two books on political assassinations; Newman (mentioned above); Dr. Peter Dale Scott, who is a former Canadian diplomat, English professor, and author of books that detail America's "Deep State" connections to Kennedy's murder; Bill Simpich, who is a civil rights attorney and author of a book that asserts that Lee Harvey Oswald was a framed double agent; Gary Aguilar, who is an ophthalmologist, a lecturer on JFK's medical evidence, and one of the few civilian physicians to have viewed the restricted autopsy evidence at the National Archives; Abraham Bolden, Sr., who is a former Secret Service agent recruited by President Kennedy and wrote a book about how the government tried to end his career; Alan Dale, who is a JFK webmaster, editor, and contributor to the Assassination Archives and Research Center; Dr. Marie Fonzi, who is the widow of HSCA investigator Gaeton Fonzi and has uncovered crucial connections between Cuban exiles and CIA black operations; Wayne S. Smith, who was appointed by JFK to the Latin American Task Force and has written several books about Cuba and Fidel Castro; David Talbot, who is a journalist, founder of Salon. com, and author of books about the Kennedys and the CIA; Robert Tanenbaum, who was a homicide prosecutor before he served as the HSCA deputy chief counsel and has authored best-sellers; Benjamin Wecht (mentioned above); and Douglas Caddy, who is a Houston attorney with expertise extending from the JFK case to the Watergate scandal.

The CAPA brain trust invites guest lecturers who don't just sit on past laurels to sell books or repeat stories. These orators expand their own knowledge base, writing fresh materials, using multimedia demonstrations, and seeking out new forensic techniques that can lead off into directions never before considered. That's the beauty of science—it's living and breathing and mutable.

Due to the COVID-19 pandemic, the 2020 CAPA conference was a remote event that allowed for an even greater lineup of speakers. Among them were Russell Kent, who is a British-based physiologist and author of the upcoming book *JFK Medical Betrayal: How Successive Panels Failed the President*, which reveals why my medical evidence testimony to the HSCA threw the forensic pathologist panel into an absolute panic and—unbeknownst to me at the time—how drafts were secretly rewritten to cover up their shortcomings in supporting the single-bullet theory; John Barbour, who screened his documentary *The American Media and the Second Assassination of John F. Kennedy* about the cover-ups in the case and discussed his previous film about Garrison, the New Orleans district attorney who failed to get a conviction in the only case ever filed for JFK's murder and was the character played by Kevin Costner in the film *JFK*; Aguilar, who discussed what the science tells us happened in Dealey Plaza and how the Warren Commission Report was woefully inadequate; David Denton, who studied the declassified JFK files and its revelations about the CIA and Cuban exiles, related what to look forward to in future disclosures and why citizens should not group this case with today's fake-news conspiracies;

James Wagenwoord, who described how he worked at *Life* magazine in the 1960s and how JFK's decision to withdraw forces from Vietnam led to his murder; Dick Russell, who authored *The Man Who Knew Too Much: Hired to Kill Oswald and Prevent the Assassination of JFK* about Richard Nagell Case, a U.S./Russian double agent; Alan Dale, who is a journalist and host of *JFK Conversations*, an online discussion group for all facets of the president's assassination; Dr. Mantik, who discussed new analysis of JFK's head wounds and whether the president's autopsy X-rays were altered; Brandon Birmingham, who discussed what the jury heard and what it was denied in the Jack Ruby trial from his perspectives as a judge and former cold-case prosecutor; Russ Baker, who describes himself as a "muckraker journalist" and discussed linkages of the life of Kennedy with George H.W. Bush, George de Mohrenschildt, and Texas oilmen; and Robert Groden, who produced the documentary *JFK: The Case for Conspiracy*, which explained what the Parkland Hospital doctors observed when they tried to save the president's life. In addition, there was a pre-recorded interview with two Parkland doctors, Robert McClelland and Ron Jones.

Many of the speakers and I participated in a special half-day discussion on "JFK and the Media," which was moderated by Washington, D.C., author and lawyer Andrew Kreig, who is a co-founder and executive director of the Justice and Integrity Project, which confronts government malfeasance and deception. It was a lively session with plenty of expressed indignation.

Because the conference was virtual, readers of this book can go to the website https://vimeo.com/showcase/7840555—using the password 2020capajfk—to see all of the content. Readers can visit CAPA's website at https://capa-us.org.

A critical component of CAPA's symposiums is the outreach to high school and college students, who are at the beginning of their tantalizing trip into this great historic mystery. A portion of each event is dedicated to these youthful attendees who need to find out who JFK was so they can then learn why he was killed and who benefited from his death. Filmmaker Andrew Kiel created a wonderful collage of entertaining and educational footage of Kennedy's election, inauguration, press conferences, and the Cuban missile crisis. At this writing, booking speakers is in process for the 2021 conference. Check the CAPA website for details.

One never knows when a valuable piece of information might come into play, so we keep a collective open mind. It's a bit like PBS' series *Antiques Roadshow* where viewers bring in a piece of art or jewelry from their attic and have it appraised by the show's experts. Maybe it's junk, maybe it's worth millions, but until you ask, you won't know. For the Kennedy case, young people whose grandparents might have left letters, photos, or arcane family lore come to us for assessment of their discovery. Will it be a crucial piece of the puzzle that will help solve the case? This is unknown until it is shared with a key person on CAPA's extensive team who will evaluate its worth.

CAPA's outreach is global. There is a 30-something married mom of two in

Dunedin, New Zealand, who has helped CAPA with social media and closely follows JFK news via various podcasts. Frankie Vegas also works with Greg Parker's group, Reopen Kennedy Case, and helped him organize a conference in Melbourne, Australia. I've never met Frankie, but I feel close to her—mostly because she has my face tattooed on her right thigh, a masterpiece by ink artist Aja Ann. Frankie also has a tattoo of President and Mrs. Kennedy on her upper left arm by another artist. In the tattoo that features me, the eye in the triangle is President Kennedy's as depicted in *Life* magazine, and the word "Darling" appears not because Frankie has a crush on me—but as a jape at Vincent Bugliosi who once called me "the darling of conspiracy theorists."

The CAPA lawyers in our midst file FOIA requests and push for having documents declassified. When President Donald Trump took office in 2017, he promised that as an outsider, he would not be afraid of opening long-dormant JFK files. Some 35,000 documents were made available but with redactions and protests from the FBI and CIA. The next year, another 19,045 documents were released, but 15,584 were held back for purported national security reasons. The National Archives has another 520 files locked away that can only be unsealed under a judge's order. Full declassification of the remaining documents was supposed to occur on October 26, 2021, under our current leader, President Joe Biden. But three days before the deadline, he announced there would be a delay, citing the COVID-19 outbreak which has slowed down the process of digitizing the material. Papers deemed "appropriate for release to the public" are now scheduled for release on December 15 of this year, with the balance available in December 2022. Either way, Biden will get to take the credit for getting the job done, or the blame for continuing to stonewall. Of course, just releasing information is meaningless without the observations of people equipped with the wisdom to decipher the material. We remain ready and hopeful.

At CAPA, our mission is to demand transparency, action, and accountability, and regardless of one's age, political persuasion, or professional background, the murder of John F. Kennedy is a blow to the heart of our nation's freedom and cannot go unchecked. As President Abraham Lincoln once reminded us, ours is a government "of the people, by the people, and for the people." And we the people must demand answers and expose the lies we have heard for 58 years. I hope this book encourages each reader to find ways to get involved and never give up. After all, in the words of Kevin Costner's character in a great Oliver Stone film: "It's up to you."

Acknowledgments

A book like this doesn't get written without a team of associates, friends, and family—and I'm grateful to every one of them.

I wish to credit my stalwart coauthor, Dawna Kaufmann, for taking the random stories about my JFK adventures over the years and weaving them into a smooth narrative. An accomplished true crime journalist, Dawna was the only reporter to ask the right questions and attain a full confession from former FBI Associate Director W. Mark Felt, Sr., that he was "Deep Throat"—the *Washington Post's* secret source during the Watergate scandal—solving the biggest media mystery of the 20th century. She has written hundreds of celebrity death and crime stories for a variety of publications, all with an emphasis on probing interviews and forensic science, which is how we met and became friends. She is also an award-winning creator of theatrical and televised entertainment, producing prime-time network TV, and writing for *Saturday Night Live* and many other series. Full of knowledge and personality, Dawna is a popular guest on news and documentary projects, and radio and podcasts. A schoolgirl when President Kennedy was assassinated in 1963, she was deeply shaken by his death—and that of his brother, Senator Robert Kennedy, five years later—and vowed to never rest until she could learn the facts behind these historic disasters. I'm pleased that this book has given Dawna answers as she's helped me communicate them to readers.

This is the fourth book Dawna and I have written together. Each of our previous works feature multiple cases and trials: *A Question of Murder: Compelling Cases from a Famed Forensic Pathologist* covers the drug overdoses of Anna Nicole Smith and her son, the homicides of two San Diego children, and mass "involuntary euthanasia" at a New Orleans hospital in the wake of Hurricane Katrina (Prometheus Books, 2009); *From Crime Scene to Courtroom: Examining the Mysteries Behind Famous Cases* examined the deaths of Michael Jackson, Casey Anthony, Drew Peterson, Brian Jones, and others (Prometheus Books, 2011); and *Final Exams: True Crime Cases from Forensic Pathologist Cyril Wecht*, which covers lesser known horrific and puzzling cases from across America (Planet Ann Rule, 2014; with an updated version released in 2021 by McFarland/Exposit Books, Inc.).

I would also like to thank my accomplished and kind secretary Florence Johnson; our eagle-eyed editor, Brett Bush; friends Randy Kasper, Chris Loos,

Anne-Marie Nash Valdivia, and Debra Storch; the magic elves at our publisher, Exposit, and its parent company McFarland; coauthor of my autobiography, Jeff M. Sewald; author and lecturer Russell Kent; and the individuals who supplied photos that illustrate points in our book: AP Images' Kevin O'Sullivan; Randy O. Sacia; Robert J. Groden and the Groden Collection; April Foran and David Lopez of Parkland Health & Hospital Systems; Ben Wecht; Frankie Vegas; and Andrew Krieg. A sincere shout-out goes to Oliver Stone for his fellowship and for writing the foreword.

I've lived 90 years of good health and intellectual stimulation but have never lost sight that the most important thing in my life is my family—my wife and my children and, later on, my grandchildren. We get together for dinner most Sundays and have enjoyed group vacations around the world. The assassination of President Kennedy has been a factor in all of my children's and grandchildren's lives and they've watched my frustrations and victories since they were in diapers. Now that the kids are adults with families of their own, I salute them for their support, in birth order: David N. Wecht, Pennsylvania State Supreme Court justice, his wife, Valerie, and their children Nathan, Jacob, Alexander, and Emma Jane; Daniel A. Wecht, clinical professor of neurosurgery at the University of Pittsburgh School of Medicine, his wife, Anna, and their children Sophie, Gabriel, and Sarah; Benjamin E. Wecht, Program director of the Cyril H. Wecht

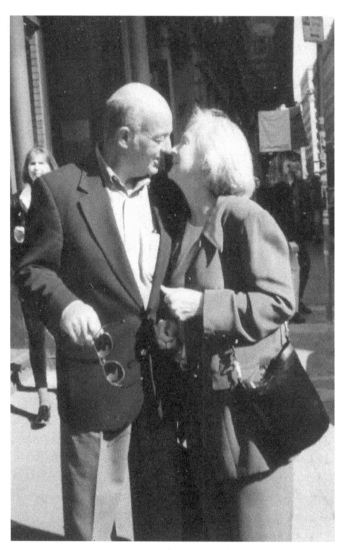

October 21, 2021, Sigrid and I celebrated our 60th wedding anniversary. She's been with me for every step of my work on the JFK case and I couldn't have asked for a better life partner (Wecht collection).

Institute of Forensic Science and Law at Duquesne University, his wife, Flynne, and their children Dylan and Zoe; and Ingrid A. Wecht, obstetrician-gynecologist and a senior staff member at West Penn Hospital, her husband, Harold, and their children Macey and Jessica.

But my greatest appreciation goes to my wife, Sigrid Wecht, a family law attorney and office manager of Cyril H. Wecht and Pathology Associates—and, always, my inspiration.

Index

CPSIA information can be obtained
at www.ICGtesting.com
Printed in the USA
BVHW051007060222
628232BV00013B/1319